THE NEW

DR. NOWZARADAN

DIET PLAN AND COOKBOOK
BIBLE | 5 BOOKS IN 1

A Healthy Collection of
1200-Calorie Recipes and Meal Plans
on a Budget Suitable for Every Age,
with 7 Unspoken Secrets

Juan Smith

©Copyright 2022 - All rights reserved

The content contained within this book may not be reproduced, duplicated, or transmitted without direct written permission from the author or the publisher.

Under no circumstances will any blame or legal responsibility be held against the publisher, or author, for any damages, reparation, or monetary loss due to the information contained within this book, either directly or indirectly.

Legal Notice

This book is copyright protected. This book is only for personal use. You cannot amend, distribute, sell, use, quote or paraphrase any part, or the content within this book, without the consent of the author-publisher.

Disclaimer Notice

Please note that the information in this document is for educational and entertainment purposes only. Every effort has been made to provide accurate, up-to-date, complete and reliable information. There are no warranties of any kind, expressed or implied. Readers acknowledge that the author is not engaged in providing legal and financial, medical, or professional advice. The contents of this book have been derived from various sources. It is recommended that you consult a licensed professional before trying the techniques described in this book.

YOUR FREE GIFT

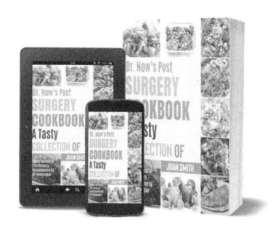

As a way of saying thanks for your purchase, I'm offering the book "Dr. Now Post Surgery Cookbook" for FREE to my readers!

To get instant access just scan this QR code:

Inside the book you will discover:

- Key Notes on the Diets
- The benefit of Dr. Now Diet Plan
- Lots of Recipes to Taste
- Science Behind the Dr. Now Diet
- And much more...

If you are ready to change your life forever, get in shape and forget the idea of classic diets, make sure to grab your FREE gift!

Table of Contents

ABOUT THE AUTHOR 5

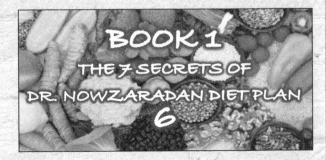
BOOK 1
THE 7 SECRETS OF DR. NOWZARADAN DIET PLAN 6

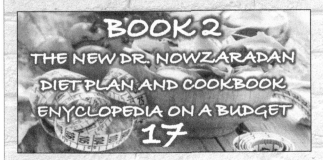
BOOK 2
THE NEW DR. NOWZARADAN DIET PLAN AND COOKBOOK ENYCLOPEDIA ON A BUDGET 17

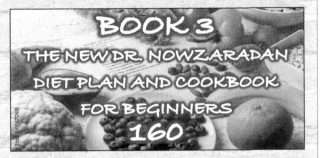
BOOK 3
THE NEW DR. NOWZARADAN DIET PLAN AND COOKBOOK FOR BEGINNERS 160

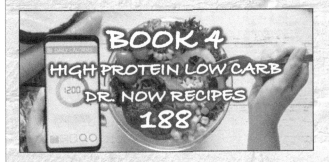
BOOK 4
HIGH PROTEIN LOW CARB DR. NOW RECIPES 188

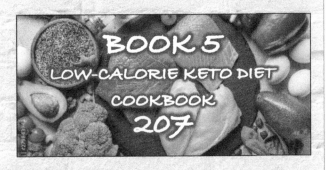
BOOK 5
LOW-CALORIE KETO DIET COOKBOOK 207

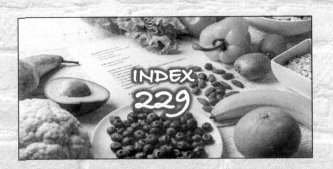
INDEX 229

ABOUT THE AUTHOR

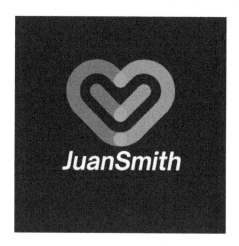

Juan Smith is the pseudonym of a patient of Dr. Nowzaradan. After reaching over 600-lb at the age of 33, Juan made the decision that saved his life. Juan underwent surgery years ago, and he followed the Dr. Now diet closely both before and after the operation.

So, within a few weeks, he reached a weight of 175-lb, which he has since maintained to this day.

"Our house has become my prison, and soon it will also be my coffin," he often repeated to his mother and father, who stood by him and supported him.

To pay tribute to Dr. Nowzaradan, Juan decided to write a series of books on the "Now Diet" to make other people in the situation he was in feel motivated to take the path that led him to a new life.

THE 7 SECRETS OF
DR. NOWZARADAN
DIET PLAN

The Unspoken Truths
about the Nowzaradan Diet

Juan Smith

INTRODUCTION

If you are interested in losing weight, Dr. Nowzaradan's diet plan is one of the best options. It focuses on eating the right kinds of food in the right quantities and staying active. It also recommends that you avoid carbohydrates, alcohol, and stress.

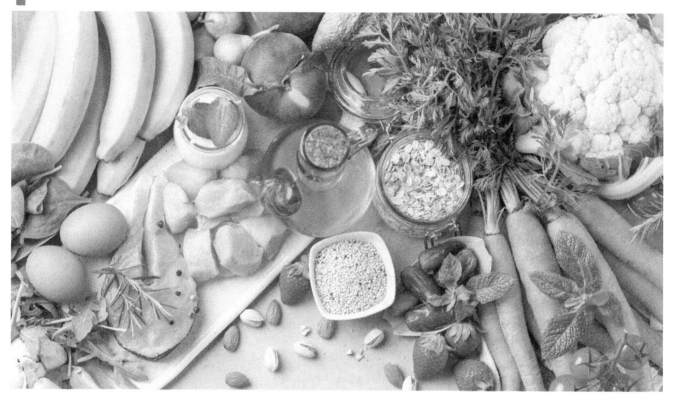

Benefits of Dr. Nowzaradan's 1,200-calorie diet plan

The 1,200-calorie diet plan was developed by Dr. Nowzaradan to help obese and overweight individuals lose weight. It emphasizes eating smaller portions and eating two to three times per day. The diet requires strict tracking of calorie intake. Besides reducing obesity, this diet plan can lower the risk of surgery. Patients undergoing bariatric surgery should consider a diet plan that reduces their intake of carbohydrates, fats, and sugar. By restricting calories to less than 1,200 per day, patients can avoid the risks associated with surgery and regain their health.

This diet plan allows patients to lose weight fast and with fewer side effects. People on this diet plan can reduce their stress level as it teaches them proper eating habits. It also helps them reduce their postoperative pain. While it has many advantages, the 1,200-calorie diet plan is not sustainable long-term. It is important to note that Dr. Nowzaradan's diet plan is designed for people who have to lose significant amounts of weight or need surgical procedures to reduce their size.

A study by the Department of Pathology at the University of California found that people following the diet reduced their blood sugar and insulin levels. Additionally, the diet reduced inflammation and the level of cholesterol.

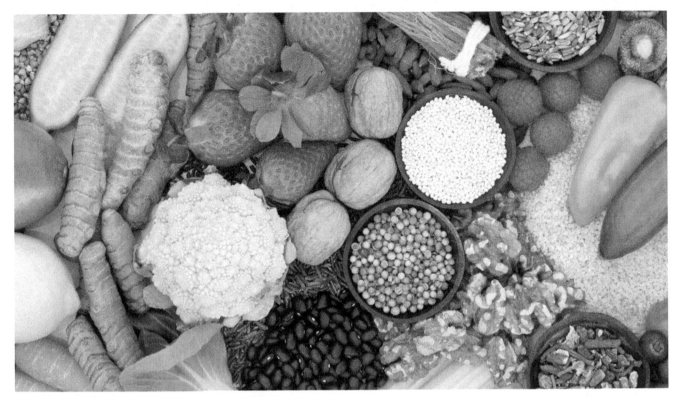

Exercise plans allowed under Dr. Nowzaradan's diet plan

The diet plan includes a range of nutritious foods, including foods high in protein and fiber. In addition to healthy foods, the plan allows for low-calorie meat, fruits, vegetables, and nuts. However, it is recommended that you avoid processed meats.

Requirements for following Dr. Nowzaradan's diet plan

These restrictions are reasonable and are aimed at ensuring that you're eating a healthy diet.

Dr. Nowzaradan is an Iranian-American surgeon. He is a well-known doctor and has been featured on the popular television show My 600-lb Life. The show chronicles the lives of his patients as they lose weight and get into better physical shape. In addition to his diet, Dr. Nowzaradan also offers individualized exercise and nutrition plans.

The diet calls for the consumption of unprocessed foods with low fat content. Sugary condiments and fried meats are also excluded. The diet also promotes small portions and emphasizes fruits and vegetables.

The diet requires the dieter to consume around 1200 calories a day and to increase fiber in the diet. The diet is designed to help the patient lose up to 30 pounds in four weeks. This is done by reducing fat, restricting carbohydrates, and increasing fiber. It encourages healthy eating habits and helps the dieter become more aware of smaller portions.

Low-calorie diets may also lower the chance of developing certain diseases and assist a person in weight reduction, encouraging them to continue with the diet. However, weight is neither the only nor the most accurate indicator of health. A person's health will not constantly improve just because they lose weight

CHAPTER 1. HOW TO GET STARTED

The Nowzaradan diet is a unique plan that helps people lose weight safely and sustainably. This diet follows a 1,200-calorie daily plan, endorsed by Dr. Younan Nowzaradan, an award-winning TV doctor famous for his work with morbid obesity.

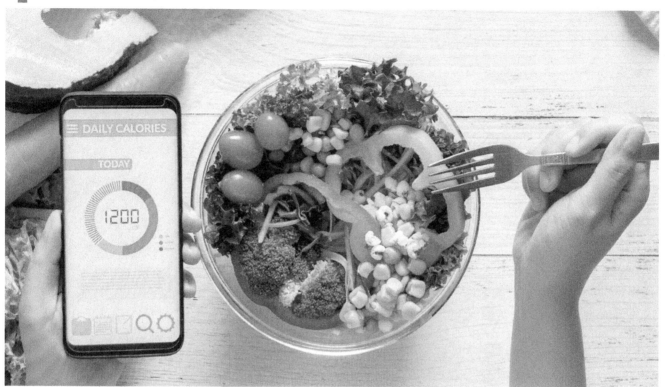

Dr. Nowzaradan's 1,200-calorie diet plan

The 1,200-calorie diet plan is an effective weight loss, requiring only 1,200 calories daily. The low-calorie diet promotes a healthy lifestyle and helps patients lose weight and improve appetite control. The plan requires patients to learn proper nutrition and reduce their intake of high-calorie food. It is not intended for regular people but for people who are morbidly obese and are preparing for surgical procedures.

While the diet plan is a good option for morbidly obese people, it is not a good option for non-morbidly obese people looking to lose weight quickly. It requires strict adherence to the plan and the following of a medical professional.

While the 1200-calorie diet may seem like a strict diet, it has been proven safe and effective for weight loss. The plan includes a seven-day meal plan and recommended foods. If you follow the diet plan correctly, there is no reason to skip meals or eat unhealthy food.

Dr. Younan Nowzaradan's approach to weight loss

The Iranian-American surgeon, Dr. Younan Nowzaradan, has built his empire by helping morbidly obese people lose weight and turn around their lives. He is 75 years old and weighs 82 kg. In addition to his practice, he's affiliated with several local hospitals. His approach to weight loss is highly effective, and his patients have lost incredible amounts of weight using his diet plan.

The diet is made up of a combination of low-calorie, high-protein products. He restricts calories to around 1200 per day. While it may seem like a drastic and unrealistic plan to lose weight, Dr. Nowzaradan claims that it's an effective way to lose weight without depriving the body of essential nutrients.

The first step in Dr. Nowzaradan's plan is an intensive consultation. Then, after determining the cause of the weight problem, he'll recommend a diet to help you lose excess fat.

While bariatric surgery alters the body's metabolism by manipulating a hormone in the gastrointestinal tract, it's not a permanent solution. Over time, the body's metabolism reverts to pre-surgery levels. A healthy lifestyle is essential for lasting results.

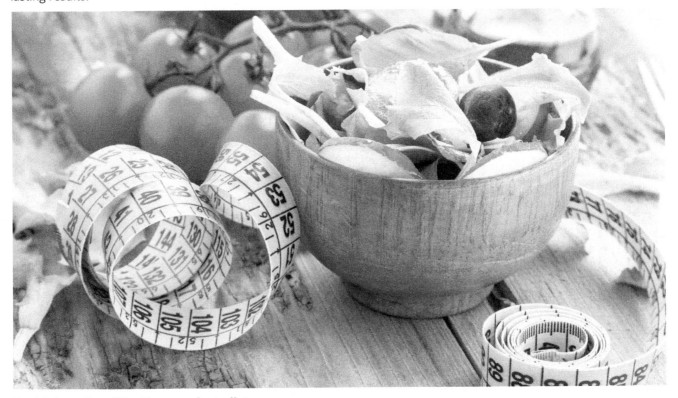

Health benefits of Dr. Nowzaradan's diet

Unlike many other diet plans, Dr. Nowzaradan's diet does not call for any specific foods to be consumed in large quantities. Instead, the diet calls for a diet consisting of lean proteins, vegetables, and non-starchy carbohydrates. In addition, however, you must avoid processed meats and other foods high in fat and sugar.

If you follow the diet, you should only consume about 1200 calories daily. This amount is low enough for people who are not severely obese. The best types of food to include in your diet are those rich in fiber, protein, and low in fat.

The diet plan designed by Dr. Nowzaradan is a great way to lose weight effectively. It provides the essential nutrients for weight loss and encourages a healthy lifestyle after weight loss surgery. However, the diet should not be followed for a long period of time.

The diet has moderate food restrictions. Fruits with low glycemic index and low sugar content are recommended, while processed meats and fats are discouraged. However, the plan includes plenty of lean protein and vegetables.

CHAPTER 2. THE SECRET PRINCIPLES

Meal planning is beneficial as it keeps you on track. The diet plan is a lifestyle change, not a quick fix.

High-protein, low-carb, calorie-restricted diet

A high-protein, low-carb diet has several health benefits. In particular, it promotes bone health by lowering the risk of osteoporosis. Additionally, protein-rich foods are good for the body's absorption of calcium, which increases bone strength and reduces the risk of osteoporosis.

A high-protein diet should be based on lean meats, whole grains, berries, and vegetables. You should not eliminate any foods from your diet but eat more lean meats and fewer refined carbohydrates and sugars.

A high-protein, low-carb diet can help manage your blood sugar levels. By reducing your carbohydrate intake, you'll be able to maintain your muscle mass while burning more fat. While high-protein, low-carb diets are generally safe, you should talk with a dietitian or doctor before starting one. Some examples of vegetables are leafy greens, cucumber, cabbage, and mushrooms. Additionally, you can include some soy and pea protein powders in your diet.

Elimination of toxins

This diet plan focuses on natural foods to remove toxins from the body. It contains several fruits and vegetables that aid the body in detoxification. It also includes lots of water to get the digestive juices flowing. It can be followed for three or ten days.

However, you must be aware that the Nowzaradan diet plan is not intended for people with specific weight loss goals. It is a general diet plan and not designed to help you lose weight quickly.

Limitation on food intake

Limitation on food intake is an essential aspect of the Nowzaradan Diet Plan. Although the plan does not require a complete diet ban, certain foods are banned, including fatty foods, popcorn, oatmeal, protein shakes, and processed meats. Additionally, avoiding refined sugars, olive oil, and butter is essential.

The Nowzaradan Diet Plan recommends a calorie-controlled diet before and after bariatric surgery. The procedure is still relatively new, but thousands of people have undergone it. People who have had the procedure must follow a strict diet to reduce the size of their liver and decrease the risk of complications.

Consultation with a doctor

Before beginning a diet plan, you should consult with a doctor. The diet should be based on the dietary recommendations of a health care provider, not on a calorie restriction. In addition to discussing your goals and health history, you will also need to discuss your present weight and family history. Your doctor will also discuss any pre-existing health problems you may have.

It is important to avoid high-fat foods and sugar, while still consuming plenty of water. In addition, you will want to limit your bread intake, using low-calorie flour instead. This will help reduce your risk for complications of surgery.

Dr. Nowzaradan is an Iranian-American physician who has treated many obese patients. His diet plan is based on a low-calorie, well-balanced diet and a focus on high-protein foods and vitamins.

Although the Nowzaradan Diet Plan is a safe and effective diet, it is important to talk to your doctor before beginning this diet plan. It is essential to have a healthy body and a happy, healthy life. If you are considering surgery, this plan may help you lose significant weight without surgical complications.

CHAPTER 3. THE 7 SECRETS OF DR NOWZARADAN'S DIET PLAN

Dr. Nowzaradan lives in Houston, Texas. His diet plan has helped many patients lose hundreds of pounds. His diet plan also requires patients to lose at least 30 pounds within 30 days before undergoing weight loss surgery. The diet plan follows a strict nutritional regimen designed by Dr. Nowzaradan. He recommends a low-fat, high-protein diet for patients. The diet plan also includes a list of high-calorie foods. However, the plan isn't appropriate for everyone.

While the diet plan is low in calories, it is essential to understand that the calorie intake is deficient. It should be noted that a person of 600 pounds should consume at least one square meal per day. In addition, the plan recommends consuming lean protein sources and non-starchy vegetables.

1. It puts your body into ketosis

The diet plan follows the principle of restricting caloric intake while increasing the number of macronutrients consumed. This helps patients lose weight and curb their appetite. It also involves education for patients, who must relearn proper nutrition.

Unlike most other diet plans, Dr. Nowzaradan's diet plan puts your body into a state of ketosis. This process is very effective in losing weight and improving health.

2. It reverses detrimental habits

If you want to lose weight and reverse damaging habits, Dr. Nowzaradan's Diet Plan can help. This medically supervised diet program considers factors such as your current weight, family history, and preexisting health conditions. It advises patients to limit high-fat, sugary foods, and drink plenty of water. The best bread options are made from low-calorie flour.

3. It helps dieters commit to a healthy lifestyle after surgery

After undergoing a weight loss surgery, you will need to eat a diet that supports your body's ability to reduce excess fat. This plan focuses on small meals containing about 600 calories twice a day.

While most dieters find it difficult to stick to a diet after surgery, the Dr. Nowzaradan Diet Plan is designed to make the process easier and more rewarding. The plan includes a comprehensive list of foods to avoid. Typical breakfasts include low-fat cottage cheese, plain Greek yogurt, and oatmeal. Lunches include lean protein and starchy vegetables.

In addition to reducing calories to a daily limit of 1200, the diet focuses on eating healthy foods with high amounts of fiber.

The diet plan is a vital part of a successful weight loss journey. Ultimately, it will help you commit to a healthy lifestyle after your surgery and achieve your goal. Whether you have a gastric bypass, gastric sleeve, or lap band, Dr. Nowzaradan's diet plan will help you maintain the weight-loss results you desire.

4. It provides gentle motivation and encouragement

Since each patient is unique, the plan involves significant customization and behavioral changes. There is a customized meal plan and a list of foods to avoid. It also involves regular checkups and follow-up sessions. This type of program provides gentle motivation and encouragement.

5. It is effective for people with a wide range of health conditions

Dr. Nowzaradan has helped people with a wide range of health conditions. He has seen children, as well as adults, lose weight. He has also treated patients with metabolic and inherited disorders. The diet plan's effectiveness can be attributed to its evidence-based principles. It recommends high-fiber foods and low-fat foods instead of protein bars and shakes.

6. The diet plan is adaptable and scalable

The diet plan is adaptable and scalable. It is best used by people who are committed to losing weight and adopting a healthy lifestyle. The program is suitable for people who need to lose significant weight. However, it can effectively be used with other treatment measures, such as weight loss surgery, medication, and additional counseling.

Dr. Nowzaradan's diet plan was originally designed to help people lose weight before undergoing weight loss surgery. It is also effective for patients who require help losing weight after a weight loss surgery.

7. It includes a customized meal plan

The customized meal plan involves limiting high-fat, high-calorie foods. It also recommends increasing protein intake. The meal plan provides the maximum caloric value while eliminating processed foods.

Given that it involves reduced portions and calorie intake, this diet plan is an easy-to-follow diet. Its excellent science-based approach makes it a valuable medical program for patients with metabolic and nutritional disorders. It works by reducing caloric intake and increasing the number of macronutrients consumed.

CHAPTER 4: THE DISEASES THAT ONLY THE NOWZARADAN DIET CAN CURE

Before beginning the Nowzaradan Diet, you should assess your current eating habits. You can use the assessment tools provided by the book. Then, implement the Nowzaradan Diet. The diseases that only the Nowzaradan Diet can cure include:

1) Cardiovascular disease (heart attack and stroke)

2) Diabetes mellitus type 1 and 2

3) High blood pressure

4) Breast cancer

5) Lupus

6) Non-Hodgkin's lymphoma

Proper diet follow-up will prevent the return of the diseases once your diet is completed.

When you complete the Nowzaradan Diet, you will have successfully restored your health to that of a "Nowzaradan" and followed the instructions regarding proper follow-up with your physician.

The Nowzaradan Diet remedied illnesses that no drug could have.

The Nowzaradan Diet helped several people to live normal life expectancies.

The Nowzaradan Diet helped to rebuild the immune systems of cancer patients.

Since the diet is a modification of the Paleolithic Diet, other diet supplements can be used along with the Nowzaradan Diet.

The only required supplement is flaxseed oil. Not only does flaxseed oil provide vitamins A, B, and E, it also helps the body eliminate cancers.

The use of flaxseed oil is popular in the Paleo Diet. The Nowzaradan diet also uses flaxseed oil, probably because the diet also reverses diseases that Paleo Diets do not like Type II diabetes, high blood pressure, and high cholesterol.

Flaxseed oil helps prevent insulin resistance and is a major diet supplement.

A diet would probably be boring if one only ate fruit, fish, and meat, but the Nowzaradan Diet allows more varieties than the Paleo Diet.

The idea of adding spices and herbs is a good variety to make the diet more interesting.

A good example is adding vanilla and cinnamon for sweet dishes, cumin for chicken, and coriander or garlic. The Nowzaradan Diet also allows salt. It is supposed to be healthier than artificial preservatives and is a major ingredient in most food we eat.

CHAPTER 5: THE TRICKS AND TIPS TO STAY ON THE NOWZARADAN DIET PLAN

A diet plan like the one developed by Dr. Nowzaradan can be helpful to those who are struggling with their weight. The diet plan is not only about reducing calories, but also focusing on a balanced diet. In some cases, the diet plan may be insufficient for a person to lose a significant amount of weight. This is because everyone burns more calories than that and needs more energy than 1,200 calories per day. Therefore diets that provide a smaller number of calories force people to burn more fat to compensate for the lack of energy.

The diet plan can help people lose weight, but it is not an easy journey. It takes tenacity and consistency. Even weight-loss surgery will not help if a person isn't able to maintain the lifestyle. Fortunately, there are several diet plans out there to help people reach their ideal weight.

The plan allows for a maximum of 1,200 calories each day and discourages snacking, as snacking can lead to binge eating. However, it doesn't mean that dieters should cut out all snacking. Eating small snacks in between meals will help a dieter stay on track.

Unlike other diet plans, the Dr. Nowzaradan plan demands a stricter calorie restriction than most diets. The program also requires a person to be habitual in the diet, particularly for people who are seriously obese.

Dr. Nowzaradan has a weight-loss clinic in Michigan. There are three diet plans from Dr. Nowzaradan, but which will work best for you? The plans are based on the newest research and are based on actual success stories. This diet plan is also designed to help patients recover quickly after bariatric surgery.

It is calorie-restrictive

The Nowzaradan Diet Plan is a calorie-restrictive plan designed to help morbidly obese patients lose weight quickly. This plan emphasizes low-calorie, healthy foods while avoiding high-fat, high-calorie foods. Furthermore, restricting calories to 1200 or less has several negative side effects, including slowing your metabolic rate and altering your hunger hormones.

The Nowzaradan Diet Plan calls for eating small, frequent meals two to three times per day. The recommended daily calorie intake is about 1200 calories. Another important factor to consider when following a low-calorie plan is the types of food you eat. The plan emphasizes low-calorie, protein and fiber-rich foods.

As with any diet, the Nowzaradan Diet Plan requires planning and preparation. In order to be successful, it's best to consult a dietitian or doctor before starting the diet. Moreover, the Nowzaradan Diet Plan should be used only as a last resort for extremely obese people. There are many other, more effective solutions available for weight loss.

The Nowzaradan Diet Plan is a calorie-restrictive plan for bariatric surgery patients. The plan's main goal is to help patients lose weight before their bariatric surgery. Surgery is a risky procedure, and it's essential for obese patients to lose weight before the operation.

It is Low-Carb

Despite the name, The Nowzaradan Diet Plan is not a low-carb diet. Instead, it is a diet that encourages healthy eating. It includes a few rules and guidelines to follow, such as eating only small portions. The plan also encourages a healthy lifestyle by avoiding foods high in calories such as processed snacks, sugar, and starchy vegetables. Additionally, it encourages people to avoid alcohol and calorie-dense drinks.

This diet is recommended for patients who are very obese, under the medical supervision of a physician. The plan emphasizes whole and natural foods as well as a commitment to change eating habits before surgery. It's also important to note that the diet requires a significant change in lifestyle, including a commitment to change eating habits before surgery and to maintain a healthy lifestyle afterward.

It is High-Protein

The Nowzaradan Diet Plan is a high-protein diet that allows you to eat many healthy, high-protein foods. The plan also allows for a large variety of carbohydrates and low-calorie fat-based foods. Some foods included in the diet are low-fat cottage cheese, low-fat egg whites, oatmeal, and turkey sausage.

The Nowzaradan Diet Plan has gained widespread attention since it was featured on a popular reality show on TLC. It is a high-protein, low-carb diet that morbidly obese individuals follow to prepare for surgical procedures to reduce their body weight. The plan features a 1200-calorie menu, as well as tips for determining whether the diet plan is right for you.

THE NEW

DR. NOWZARADAN

DIET PLAN AND COOKBOOK ENYCLOPEDIA ON A BUDGET

The Ultimate Collection
of 365 Tasty 1200-Calorie Recipes
for Every Age
and 93+1 Healthy Meal Plans

Juan Smith

INTRODUCTION

Incorporating many foods rich in nutrients is not incompatible with adhering to a low-calorie diet plan. Because there is only room for 1,200 calories, there is no room for foods that aren't completely nutritious. Therefore, doing so is a need.

The most important thing is to eat a diet rich in low-calorie, high-fiber fruits and vegetables, low-fat, whole grains, and lean proteins.

So, for example, you would need to trade one teeny little rule for three-quarters of a cup of blueberries to get one fruit serving. Also, due to rounding off, different scales, or different calculation methodologies, the same numerical values may vary somewhat from one list to the next.

If you eat the recommended number of servings from each food category, however, you can be certain that you will have a diet that is high in nutrients while being low in fat and calories.

Additionally, it may be difficult to accurately measure or estimate the appropriate serving size when it comes to some dishes. An upcoming clearance sale will become available. Some in handy.

CHAPTER 1. ALL ABOUT THE NOWZARADAN DIET PLAN

Dr. Younan Nowzaradan, who is renowned for performing surgery on patients who are obese on the TLC reality program "My 600-Lb. Life," is the brains behind the Dr. Now Diet, which is a very stringent low-calorie and low-carbohydrate eating plan. The Dr. Now Diet was designed by Nowzaradan. Patients who weigh more than 600 pounds before weight-loss surgery are followed by the program both before and after the procedure.

In order to better prepare patients for bariatric surgery, Nowzaradan recommends that patients follow the diet prescribed by Dr. Now. Nowzaradan is the author of the book "The Scale Does Not Lie, People Do," which was published in 2013.

Bariatric Surgery

- **Gastric bypass.** The Roux-en-Y gastric bypass, which is more often referred to as just gastric bypass, will make your stomach smaller. Surgeons will use the upper portion of your stomach to construct a tiny pouch in your abdomen. As part of the bypass procedure, a little section of your small intestine, known as the jejunum, will be connected to a hole in this new pouch. Because of this, the quantity of food that you are able to ingest is decreased, and you are able to take in less calories as a result.
- **Sleeve gastrectomy.** When you have this particular operation, about three quarters of your stomach will be removed. What is left is a segment that is either in the form of a tube or a sleeve, and it can only hold a small portion of the food it once did. According to Dr. Xiaoxi Feng, a bariatric surgeon at the Cleveland Clinic in Ohio, the effects of this treatment are irreversible.
- **Duodenal switch.** This method, which is more formally called as biliopancreatic diversion with duodenal switch, is a hybrid procedure that combines aspects of sleeve gastrectomy and bypass. According to Feng, bariatric surgeons perform a more comprehensive version of gastric bypass surgery during the duodenal switch operation.
- **Lap-band.** Laparoscopic gastric banding, also known as an adjustable gastric band, is a treatment that involves the implantation of a soft implant that incorporates an expanding balloon around the top of your stomach. This technique is also known as an adjustable gastric band. This causes the stomach to be divided into two portions, and you are only able to consume enough food to fill the upper segment.

Dr. Erik P. Dutson, surgical director of the Center for Obesity and Metabolic Health at UCLA in Westwood, California, says bariatric surgeons and patients examine several aspects before choosing an option.

"Most U.S. bariatric surgery clinics do either gastric bypass or sleeve gastrectomy," he explains. "Most patients will perform well with either procedure, but others should not receive one due to medical issues. Larger individuals, those with advanced diabetes, and those with GERD (a disease in which stomach contents flow back up via the lower esophageal sphincter) perform better with gastric bypass."

Sleeve gastrectomy helps people with immunological suppression (such as organ transplant patients).

Dr. Judy Chen-Meekin, a surgeon and bariatric expert at the University of Washington School of Medicine, believes patients should be comfortable with the surgical choice, but medical factors typically drive the decision.

CHAPTER 2. BREAKFAST RECIPES

Recipe 1. Bacon and Cheese Cloud Eggs

Serving Size: 2

Preparation Time: 10 minutes

Cooking Time: 15 minutes

Ingredients:

- 4 eggs, yolks, and whites separated
- Black pepper and salt to taste
- 2 bacon slices
- 1 tablespoon chopped finely chopped chives
- 3 tbsp grated Pecorino cheese

Directions:

- A skillet is heated to a medium-high flame. Cook the bacon until it's actually crispy on all sides, approximately 5 minutes. Cool it down, and then slice it into pieces. Mix the egg yolks with salt with an electric mixer until stiff white peaks form. Add your Pecorino cheese as well as bacon.
- Divide the mixture into four mounds on a parchment-lined baking sheet. Make an indentation within each mound. Take care to spoon the egg yolk in each indentation Sprinkle by adding salt and seasoning with pepper. In the preheated oven at 400 F oven 3 mins or until the yolks have firm. Sprinkle with chives, and serve.

Nutritional Information:

- Cal 287
- Net Carbs 4.7g
- Fat 24g
- Protein 12g

Recipe 2. Bacon and Mushroom "Tacos"

Serving Size: 2

Preparation Time: 15 minutes

Cooking Time: 30 minutes

Ingredients:

- 1 egg that has been hard-boiled and then chopped
- 1 cup of mushrooms, cut into slices
- 3 oz mozzarella cheese, grated
- 3 oz bacon, chopped
- 1 shallot cut into slices
- 1 avocado, sliced
- 1 tbsp salsa
- 1 tbsp of sour cream

Directions:

- Preheat the oven to a heat of 350 degrees F. Set two heaps of mozzarella cheese in a baking dish lined with parchment, and gently flatten with your hands to make taco shells (circle tortillas). In the oven, bake for 10 to 12 minutes, or until the edges turn brown. Remove and let them cool.
- Cook your bacon inside a skillet on medium-high heat for four minutes until crisp; transfer to an oven-safe bowl. Saute the shallot and the mushrooms in the same oil over 5 mins. Transfer to the bowl with the bacon. Mix with the egg. Divide the mixture among taco shells. Top with avocado, salsa, and sour cream, and serve.

Nutritional Information:

- Cal 363
- Net Carbs 8g
- Fat 48g
- Protein 22g

Recipe 3. Broccoli Waffles

Serving Size: 4

Preparation Time: 10 minutes

Cooking Time: 8 minutes

Ingredients:

- ½ cup chopped broccoli
- 2 eggs
- ½ cup low-fat cheddar cheese, shredded
- 1 tsp. garlic powder
- 1 tsp. dried onion, minced
- Salt and black pepper, to taste

Directions:

- Preheat and grease waffle iron.
- Meanwhile, add broccoli, cheddar cheese, eggs, dried onion, garlic powder, salt, and pepper in a large bowl. Mix well.
- Pour the prepared batter on the waffle iron and cook for about 4 minutes.
- Take out and serve.
- Serve with green chili sauce.

Nutritional Information:

- Calories: 195
- Fat: 6.9 g
- Carbs: 1.7 g
- Protein: 6.7 g

Recipe 4. Canadian Bacon Eggs Benedict

Serving Size: 2

Preparation Time: 10 minutes

Cooking Time: 20 minutes

Ingredients:

- 1 teaspoon white wine vinegar
- 2 large eggs
- 4 Canadian bacon slices
- 1 tablespoon fresh parsley chopped

Directions:

- In a large skillet, heat it to medium heat. Cook the bacon for about 3-4 minutes on each side. Transfer to a towel to absorb any excess fat. Boil the vinegar and water in a pot on high heat. Then reduce it to simmer.
- Crack eggs into bowls and then gently place eggs into boiling water. Allow simmering for a couple of minutes. Utilize a spoon with a perforated hole to take the egg out of the water onto the cloth to air dry. Put the bacon on two plates. Each plate should be topped with an egg. Sprinkle with chopped parsley.

Nutritional Information:

- Cal 161
- Net Carbs 1.4g
- Fat 9g
- Protein 18g

Recipe 5. Cauliflower-Based Waffles

Serving Size: 2

Preparation Time: 15 minutes

Cooking Time: 25 minutes

Ingredients:

- 1 cup zucchini chopped and squeezed
- 2 green onions
- 1 tbsp olive oil
- 2 eggs
- 1/3 cup Parmesan cheese
- 1 cup mozzarella, grated
- Half head cauliflower
- 1 teaspoon garlic powder
- 1 tbsp sesame seeds
- 2 teaspoons thyme, chopped

Directions:

- Cut the cauliflower into florets. Mix the pieces in the food processor and then pulse until rice is created. Transfer to a dirty kitchen towel and press down to remove excess moisture. Return to your food processor, and add the zucchini, green onions and thyme. Pulse until smooth.
- Transfer into an empty bowl. Add all the other prepared ingredients and mix well. Allow sitting for 10 mins. Warm the waffle iron, then spread it all over the mixture. Cook until golden brown in about 5 minutes.

Nutritional Information:

- Cal 336
- Net Carbs 7.2g
- Fat 21g
- Protein 32g

Recipe 6. Cheese Waffles

Serving Size: 8

Preparation Time: 15 minutes

Cooking Time: 20 minutes

Ingredients:

- 2 garlic cloves, minced
- Salt and black pepper, to taste
- 1 cup frozen spinach
- 2 cups ricotta cheese, crumbled
- ½ cup low-fat parmesan cheese, grated
- 1 cup part-skim mozzarella cheese, shredded
- 2 eggs, beaten

Directions:

- Add eggs, garlic cloves, ricotta cheese, and spinach in a large bowl.
- Now, add mozzarella cheese, parmesan cheese, salt, and pepper.
- Whisk properly.
- Pour the prepared batter on the waffle iron and cook for about 5 minutes.
- Take out and serve hot.
- Serve with maple syrup on the top.

Nutritional Information:

- Calories: 119

- Fat: 7 g
- Carbs: 3.9 g
- Protein: 10.2 g

Recipe 7. Chorizo Frittata

Serving Size: 4

Preparation Time: 30 minutes

Cooking Time: 40 minutes

Ingredients:

- 1 chorizo sausage, sliced
- 1/2 cup of kale
- 1 tbsp butter
- 1/2 cup cheese from cotija shred
- Half red bell pepper chopped
- 4 eggs, salt, and black pepper to taste
- 1 tsp chipotle paste
- 1 green onion chopped

Directions:

- Oil and heat the pan and cook the onion. Add chorizo sausage, chipotle paste, and bell pepper. Cook for about 5-7 minutes. Mix the eggs in the bowl and then season with salt and black pepper.
- Put the kale in and boil for about 2 minutes. Incorporate eggs. Sprinkle the mixture evenly across the skillet, then place it in the oven. Cook for about 8 mins at 350 F until the top of the pan is cooked and golden. Sprinkle crumbled cotija cheese on top and bake for another 3 moments until cheese is completely melted. Cut and enjoy while warm.

Nutritional Information:

- Cal 335
- Net Carbs 7.3g
- Fat 31g
- Protein 24g

Recipe 8. Chili Omelet with Avocado

Serving Size: 2

Preparation Time: 5 minutes

Cooking Time: 15 minutes

Ingredients:

- 2 tsp olive oil
- 1 ripe avocado, chopped
- 2 spring onions chopped
- 2 spring garlic, chopped
- 4 eggs 1 cup buttermilk
- 2 tomatoes, sliced
- 1 pepper with green chili, chopped
- 2 tablespoons fresh cilantro, chopped
- black pepper, and salt to taste

Directions:

- Mix the buttermilk, eggs, salt, and black pepper. Oil and heat the pan and cook the garlic and onions until they are tender. Pour the dish into the pan, and employ a spatula for smoothing the surface.
- Include chili pepper, cilantro, avocado, tomatoes, and chili pepper on the other side of the egg dish. Fold it in half, then eventually cut it into pieces. Serve immediately.

Nutritional Information:

- Cal 322
- Net Carbs 11g
- Fat 32g
- Protein 19g

Recipe 9. Coconut Crepes with Vanilla Cream

Serving Size: 4

Preparation Time: 20 minutes

Cooking Time: 35 minutes

Ingredients:

- 5 large eggs
- ¼ coconut flour
- 1 tsp sugar-free cocoa powder
- ¼ cup flax milk
- 2 tbsp coconut oil, melted
- Vanilla cream
- ¼ cup butter
- 2 tbsp erythritol
- ½ tsp vanilla extract
- ½ cup coconut cream

Directions:

- Beat the prepared eggs with a whisk in a bowl. Add the flax milk, cocoa powder, coconut flour, and coconut oil and mix until well combined. Oil and heat the pan to spread the dough around the skillet and cook the crepe for 2-3 minutes.
- Melt the butter in a large-sized saucepan. Pour in the coconut cream and erythritol, reduce the heat to low, and let the sauce simmer for 8 minutes. Turn the heat

off and stir in the vanilla extract. Drizzle the sauce over the crepes and serve.

Nutritional Information:

- Cal 326
- Net Carbs 3g
- Fat 23g
- Protein 10g

Recipe 10. Crabmeat Frittata with Onion

Serving Size: 2

Preparation Time: 10 minutes

Cooking Time: 30 minutes

Ingredients:

- 1 tbsp olive oil
- 1/2 onion chopped
- Black pepper and salt to taste
- 3 oz crabmeat, chopped
- 4 large eggs, lightly beaten
- 1/2 cup sour cream

Directions:

- Set a pan on moderate heat and heat the oil to cook the onion. Add the crabmeat, and cook for 2 minutes. Add salt and pepper to taste.
- Mix the sour cream and the eggs. Transfer the egg mixture to the skillet. Place the pan in the oven to cook for about 17 mins at 350 F or until the eggs are cooked. Cut into wedges and serve.

Nutritional Information:

- Cal 345
- Net Carbs 6.5g
- Fat 26g
- Protein 23g

Recipe 11. Creamy Oatmeal

Serving Size: 4

Preparation Time: 15 minutes

Cooking Time: 10 minutes

Ingredients:

- 1 cup of berries of choice
- 2 cups oats, old fashioned
- 1 and one-third cup almonds, sliced
- 3 and one-fourth cups water
- 1 tablespoons. ground cinnamon

- 2 medium bananas

Directions:

- Crush the bananas thoroughly until smooth.
- Empty the water into a saucepan and incorporate the mashed banana.
- Combine the oats in the pan and heat until the water bubbles.
- Adjust the temperature of the burner to low and continue to warm for approximately 7 minutes.
- Remove from heat and top with the ground cinnamon, berries, and sliced almonds.
- Serve immediately and enjoy!

Nutritional Information:

- Calories: 368
- Sodium: 7 mg
- Protein: 18 g
- Fat: 21 g
- Sugar: 12 g

Recipe 12. Crespelle al Mascarpone

Serving Size: 2

Preparation Time: 20 minutes

Cooking Time: 35 minutes

Ingredients:

- 1 cup of almond flour
- 2 TSP liquid Stevia
- 1 tsp baking soda
- Half cup almond milk
- 1 tsp vanilla extract
- 1 large egg
- 1/4 cup olive oil
- Whole raspberries for garnish
- 1 cup mascarpone cheese
- 1 teaspoon mint
- 1 tsp mint, chopped

Directions:

- Make the egg beat in the bowl. Add the vanilla extract, almond milk, and half of the stevia, and mix to combine. Mix almond flour and the baking powder. Then, add eggs into almond flour. Place olive oil in an oven over medium-high heat. Pour in one teaspoon of batter.
- Transfer the pancake onto an oven-safe plate, and cook the pancake again until the butter is completely absorbed. Mix the mascarpone, the remaining mint,

and stevia in a small bowl. Make every mini pancake in mascarpone, and sprinkle the raspberry on top for serving.

Nutritional Information:

- Cal 369
- Net Carbs 3.2g
- Fat 32g
- Protein 29g

Recipe 13. Goat Cheese Frittata with Asparagus

Serving Size: 2

Preparation Time: 15 minutes

Cooking Time: 35 minutes

Ingredients:

- 1 tbsp olive oil
- 1/2 onion chopped
- 1 cup asparagus chopped
- 4 eggs, beaten
- 1/2 habanero pepper, minced
- Red pepper and salt, to taste
- 3/4 cup goat cheese, crumbled
- 1 tbsp chopped parsley

Directions:

- Preheat the oven to a heat of 350 F. Sauté the onion in olive oil at medium-high temperature until it is caramelized, about 6-8 minutes. In the asparagus, simmer until soft, around 5 minutes. Add habanero peppers and eggs. Season with salt and red pepper.
- Cook until eggs are cooked. Sprinkle the goat cheese and chopped parsley on top of the frittata. Bake for 20 minutes.

Nutritional Information:

- Cal 345
- Net Carbs 8.3g
- Fat 37g
- Protein 32g

Recipe 14. Ham and Egg Casserole

Serving Size: 4

Preparation Time: 5 minutes

Cooking Time: 25 minutes

Ingredients:

- 4 red potatoes, medium
- 1 cup chopped ham
- 10 huge eggs
- 1 teaspoon salt and pepper
- ½ diced onion
- 2 cups shredded cheese
- 1 cup skim milk

Directions:

- Spray inside of the prepared instant pot with cooking spray and in another dish then add eggs and milk till blended.
- Put the rest of the ingredients in there, mix it together, and then cover with foil.
- Add insert, and then casserole dish on top of there.
- Cook it on manual for 25 minutes with a natural pressure release.
- Serve immediately with toppings.

Nutritional Information:

- Calories: 310
- Fat: 10g
- Carbs: 15g
  - Protein: 22g

Recipe 15. Jackfruit Vegetable Fry

Serving Size: 6

Preparation Time: 5 minutes

Cooking Time: 5 minutes

Ingredients:

- 2 seeded and chopped red bell peppers
- 1/8 teaspoon. cayenne pepper
- 2 cups finely chopped cherry tomatoes
- Salt
- 1 tablespoon olive oil
- 3 cups seeded and chopped firm jackfruit
- 2 tablespoons. chopped fresh basil leaves
- 1/8 teaspoon. ground turmeric
- 2 finely chopped small onions

Directions:

- Oil and heat the pan to cook the onions, tomatoes and bell peppers for 5 minutes.
- Then add the salt, cayenne pepper, jackfruit, and turmeric, cook for 8 minutes.
- Garnish the meal with basil leaves.
- Serve warm.

Nutritional Information:

- Calories: 236
- Fat: 1.8 Gram

- Carbs: 5 Gram
- Protein: 7 Gram

Recipe 16. Mexican Eggs

Serving Size: 8

Preparation Time: 5 minutes

Cooking Time: 2 hours

Ingredients:

- 12 ounces low-fat cheese, shredded
- 1 garlic clove, minced
- 1 cup nonfat sour cream
- 10 eggs
- Olive oil cooking spray
- 5 ounces canned green chilies, drained
- 10 ounces tomato sauce, sodium-free
- ½ teaspoon chili powder
- Black pepper to the taste

Directions:

- In a bowl, mix the eggs with the cheese, sour cream, chili powder, black pepper, garlic, green chilies and tomato sauce, whisk, pour into your slow cooker after you've greased it with cooking oil, cover and cook on Low for 2 hours.
- Serve.

Nutritional Information:

- Calories 395
- Fat .27.5g
- Cholesterol 262mg
- Carbohydrate 18.8g
- Protein 20.9g

Recipe 17. Morning Herbed Eggs

Serving Size: 2

Preparation Time: 5 minutes

Cooking Time: 15 minutes

Ingredients:

- 1 spring onion finely chopped
- 2 Tbsp butter
- 1 teaspoon fresh thyme
- 4 eggs
- 1/2 tsp sesame seeds
- 2 cloves of garlic, chopped
- 1/2 cup chopped parsley
- 1/2 cup chopped sage
- 1/4 tsp cayenne pepper
- Black pepper and salt to taste

Directions:

- In a pan at medium temperature. Add garlic, parsley thyme, and sage and stir fry in 30-second intervals. Make sure to crack the eggs in the skillet.
- Serve the eggs with a drizzle of cayenne pepper and sesame seeds. Serve.

Nutritional Information:

- Cal 273
- Net Carbs 4g
- Fat 22g
- Protein 13g

Recipe 18. Mushroom and Cheese Cauliflower Risotto

Serving Size: 4

Preparation Time: 15 minutes

Cooking Time: 25 minutes

Ingredients:

- 3 tbsp olive oil
- 1 onion chopped
- 1/4 cup vegetable broth
- 1/3 cup Parmesan cheese
- 4 Tbsp heavy cream
- 3TBSP of chopped chives.
- 2 lbs mushrooms, sliced
- 1 large head cauliflower, break into florets
- 2 Tbsp chopped parsley, cut

Directions:

- In the food processor, blend the cauliflower florets until they achieve a rice-like texture. Heat 2 tbsp oil in a saucepan. Add the mushrooms, and cook on moderate heat for approximately 3 minutes.
- Mix in the broth and the cauliflower, then cook until the broth has been completely absorbed, about 7-8 minutes. Mix in the heavy cream as well as Parmesan cheese. Sprinkle with parsley and chives to serve.

Nutritional Information:

- Cal 255
- Net Carbs 5.3g
- Fat 21g
- Protein 10g

Recipe 19. Poached Eggs

Serving Size: 2

Preparation Time: 10 minutes

Cooking Time: 5 minutes

Ingredients:

- 2 eggs
- 2 slices of low-fat mozzarella
- 1 cup mayonnaise
- 1 bell pepper, halved
- 3 tablespoons sugar-free orange juice
- 1 teaspoon lemon juice
- 1 teaspoon turmeric powder
- 1 teaspoon mustard
- 1 tablespoon sugar
- 1 cup water

Directions:

- Crack eggs into the bell pepper cups and add mozzarella slice.
- Add water and then add the cups, and cover and cook on low for four minutes.
- In a bowl, mix the other ingredients, and then divide the poached eggs between plates, add the sauce over them, and then serve!

Nutritional Information:

- Calories: 200
- Fat: 5g
- Carbs: 21g
- Protein: 5g

Recipe 20. Rolled Smoked Salmon with Avocado

Serving Size: 2

Preparation Time: 10 minutes

Cooking Time: 10 minutes

Ingredients:

- 2 tbsp cream cheese, softened
- 1 lime, squeezed, zested, and juiced
- 1/2 avocado, pitted, peeled
- 1 tbsp mint and chopped
- Salt to taste
- 2 slices of smoked salmon

Directions:

- Mash the avocado using a fork in the bowl. Add the mint, lime juice zest, cream cheese, and salt, and mix until well-combined. Place each salmon piece onto a plastic wrap and fill with cream cheese mixture.
- Refrigerate the wrapped mixture for 2 minutes. Then take the plastic off, cut each wrap's sides, and cut pieces into the quarter-inch wheel. Serve.

Nutritional Information:

- Cal 320
- Net Carbs 3g
- Fat 31g
- Protein 50g

Recipe 21. Scrambled Eggs with Mushrooms and Spinach

Serving Size: 2

Preparation Time: 5 minutes

Cooking Time: 10 minutes

Ingredients:

- 2 egg whites
- 1 slice whole wheat toast
- ½ cup sliced fresh mushrooms
- 2 tablespoons Shredded
- Fat free American cheese
- Pepper
- 1 teaspoon olive oil
- 1 cup chopped fresh spinach
- 1 whole egg

Directions:

- Oil and heat the pan, add mushrooms, spinach. Cook for 2-3 minutes.
- Mix egg whites, and cheese. Season with pepper.
- Cook the egg mixture.
- Serve and enjoy with a piece of whole wheat toast.

Nutritional Information:

- Calories: 291
- Fat: 11.8 g
- Carbs: 21.8 g
- Protein: 24.3 g

Recipe 22. Serrano Ham Frittata with Salad

Serving Size: 2

Preparation Time: 15 minutes

Cooking Time: 25 minutes

Ingredients:

- 2 tbsp olive oil

- 3 slices serrano ham, chopped
- 1 tomato, cut into chunks
- 1 cucumber, sliced
- 1 small red onion cut into slices
- 1 tablespoon balsamic vinegar
- 4 eggs, beaten
- 1 cup Swiss Chard Chopped
- Black pepper and salt to taste
- 1 green onion cut into slices

Directions:

- Whisk together vinegar, one tablespoon of olive oil, and pepper into the salad bowl. Add the tomatoes and red onion, and the cucumber, and mix with olive oil to coat. Sprinkle with serrano ham. The remaining olive oil is heated in a skillet over medium-high temperatures. Cook onions and Swiss Chard for three minutes.
- Add salt and pepper, cooking for two minutes. Pour the eggs into the top, lower the heat to a simmer, cover, then simmer for four minutes. Serve the salad sliced and served alongside the salad.

Nutritional Information:

- Cal 354
- Net Carbs 7g
- Fat 26g
- Protein 20g

Recipe 23. Sesame and Poppy Seed Bagels

Serving Size: 4

Preparation Time: 20 minutes

Cooking Time: 30 minutes

Ingredients:

- 1/4 cup Coconut flour
- 6 eggs
- 1 cup meal of flaxseed
- 1/2 teaspoon onion powder
- 1/2 1 teaspoon garlic powder
- 1 teaspoon dried oregano
- 1 tsp sesame seeds
- 1 teaspoon poppy seeds

Directions:

- Combine the coconut flour eggs, 1 teaspoon of flaxseed meal, 1/2 cup water, garlic powder, onion powder, oregano, and onion powder.
- Pour the mix into a donut tray that has been greased. Sprinkle with sesame and poppy seeds. Baking the bread for about 20 minutes a 350 F. Cool for 5 minutes before serving.

Nutritional Information:

- Cal 352
- Net Carbs 3.3g
- Fat 24g
- Protein 20g

Recipe 24. Snazzy Baked Eggs

Serving Size: 4

Preparation Time: 5 minutes

Cooking Time: 8 minutes

Ingredients:

- 4 eggs
- 4 slices of meat, fish, or veggies of choice
- 4 slices of cheese or a shot of cream
- 4 garnishes of fresh herbs of choice
- Cooking oil

Directions:

- Add a cup of water, and then prepare your ramekins by setting olive oil on the bottom of it, and then the meat and veggies.
- Break an egg, and then add the cheese and creak of choice.
- Add it into the pressure cooker for low heat, 8 minutes.
- Remove, and put them into a little plate.

Nutritional Information:

- Calories: 175
- Fat: 4g
- Carbs: 8g
- Protein: 8g

Recipe 25. Soft Banana Bread

Serving Size: 4

Preparation Time: 10 minutes

Cooking Time: 4 hours

Ingredients:

- 2 eggs
- ½ teaspoon baking soda
- 3 bananas, peeled and mashed
- 2 cups whole wheat flour

- 1 teaspoon baking powder
- 2 tablespoons olive oil

Directions:

- In a bowl, mix the eggs with the oil, flour, baking powder and baking soda and whisk well.
- Add bananas, stir the batter, pour it into your greased slow cooker, cover and cook on Low for 4 hours.
- Slice the bread, divide it between plates and serve.

Nutritional Information:

- Calories 399
- Fat .10.1g
- Cholesterol 82mg
- Carbohydrate 68.7g
- Protein 10.2g

Recipe 26. Spinach Nests with Eggs and Cheese

Serving Size: 1

Preparation Time: 15 minutes

Cooking Time: 25 minutes

Ingredients:

- 1 tbsp olive oil
- 1 Tbsp dried dill
- 1 lb spinach, chopped
- 1 tbsp pine nuts
- Black pepper and salt to taste
- 1/4 cup feta cheese, crumbled
- 2 eggs

Directions:

- Sauté the spinach in the olive oil at medium-low temperatures for 5 minutes. Sprinkle with salt and pepper and put aside. Prepare a baking sheet by coating it with cooking spray, form two (firm and distinct) spinach nests on the baking sheet, and then crack an egg inside each nest.
- Sprinkle with feta, and then sprinkle with dill. Cook for about 15 mins a 350 F until the egg whites are settled and the yolks remain running. Serve the nests on plates decorated with pine nuts.

Nutritional Information:

- Cal 308
- Net Carbs 5.4g
- Fat 22g
- Protein 18g

Recipe 27. Sweet Chia Bowls

Serving Size: 4

Preparation Time: 10 minutes

Cooking Time: 2 hours

Ingredients:

- 1 teaspoon cinnamon powder
- 2 cups non-fat milk
- 1 tablespoon maple syrup
- 2 tablespoons chia seeds
- 2 bananas, peeled and sliced
- 1 teaspoon sugar
- 1 teaspoon vanilla extract
- 1 cup brown rice
- Directions:
- Mix the maple syrup, milk with the bananas, and the other ingredients, and cook for 2 hours.
- Serve.

Nutritional Information:

- Calories 321
- Fat .3.5g
- Cholesterol 3mg
- Carbohydrate 63.4g
- Protein 9.3g

Recipe 28. Tuna and Egg Salad with Chili Mayo

Serving Size: 4

Preparation Time: 10 minutes

Cooking Time: 20 minutes

Ingredients:

- 4 eggs
- 14 oz tuna in brine, drained
- 1/2 small head of lettuce Torn
- 2 spring onions chopped
- 1/4 cup ricotta, crumbled
- 2 tbsp sour cream
- 1/2 tbsp mustard powder
- 1/2 cup mayonnaise
- 1/2 tablespoon lemon juice
- 1/2 tbsp chili powder
- 2 pickles with dill, cut
- Black pepper and salt to taste

Directions:

- Boil eggs with salted water at moderate heat for about 8 minutes. Set them aside on an ice bath, allow them to cool, and then chop them into smaller pieces. Transfer them into an empty bowl. Put them in a bowl with the tuna, onions, and mustard powder.
- Add ricotta, lettuce, and sour cream. Mix together mayonnaise, lemon juice, and chili powder in a separate bowl. Season according to your taste. Mix in the tuna mix and mix thoroughly. Serve with slices of pickle.

Nutritional Information:

- Cal 391
- Net Carbs 4.5g
- Fat 22g
- Protein 35g

Recipe 29. Turkey Bacon and Spinach Crepes

Serving Size: 4

Preparation Time: 15 minutes

Cooking Time: 35 minutes

Ingredients:

- 3 eggs
- ½ cup cottage cheese
- 1 tbsp coconut flour
- ⅓ cup Parmesan, grated
- A pinch of xanthan gum
- 1 cup spinach
- 4 oz turkey bacon, cubed
- 4 oz mozzarella, shredded
- 1 garlic clove, minced
- ½ onion, chopped
- 2 tbsp butter
- ½ cup heavy cream
- Fresh parsley, chopped
- Salt and black pepper to taste

Directions:

- Combine cottage cheese, eggs, coconut flour, xanthan gum, and Parmesan cheese to obtain a crepe batter in a bowl. Grease a pan with cooking spray over medium heat, pour some of the batters, spread well into the pan, cook for 2 minutes, flip, and cook for 40 seconds more or until golden. Do the same actual procedure with the rest of the batter. Stack all the crepes on a serving plate.
- In the same medium-sized pan, melt the butter and stir in the onion and garlic; sauté for 3 minutes until tender. Stir in the spinach for 5 minutes. Add turkey bacon, heavy cream, mozzarella cheese, salt, pepper, and stir. Cook for 2-3 minutes. Fill each crepe with the mixture, roll up each, and arrange it on a serving plate. Top with parsley.

Nutritional Information:

- Cal 391
- Net Carbs 8.2g
- Fat 29g
- Protein 26g

Recipe 30. Western Omelet Quiche

Serving Size: 6

Preparation Time: 10 minutes

Cooking Time: 30 minutes

Ingredients:

- 6 beaten eggs
- 1/8 teaspoon of mineral salt and black pepper
- ¾ cup diced peppers
- ¾ spring onions, sliced
- ¾ cup shredded cheese
- ½ cup half and half
- 8 oz, chopped Canadian bacon
- ¼ cup shredded cheddar cheese to garnish

Directions:

- Add 2 cups of water to the very bottom of instant pot and then add trivet.
- Spray a souffle dish with butter or cooking spray, and then in a mixing bowl add the eggs, salt, milk, and pepper together.
- Put it in souffle dish, and from there, add to instant pot, cooking on high pressure for 30 minutes cook time.
- Open up lid and sprinkle the top of it with more cheese.

Nutritional Information:

- Calories: 365
- Fat: 15g
- Carbs: 6g
- Protein: 24g

Recipe 31. Zucchini and Pepper Caprese Gratin

Serving Size: 4

Preparation Time: 20 minutes

Cooking Time: 50 minutes

Ingredients:

- 2 zucchinis, sliced
- 1 red bell pepper chopped
- Salt and black pepper to taste
- 1 cup ricotta cheese, crumbled
- 4 oz fresh mozzarella, sliced
- 2 tomatoes, sliced
- 2 tablespoons butter
- 1/4 teaspoon of xanthan gum
- 1 cup of heavy whipped cream

Directions:

- Bake at 370 F. Creates an even layer of bell peppers and zucchinis in a baking dish that has been greased with the bell peppers and zucchinis overlapping. Sprinkle Ricotta cheese and salt and pepper on top.
- Mix butter, xanthan gum, and whipping cream in a microwave for two minutes, stir it until completely mixed and then sprinkle over the vegetables. Then, top with the remaining ricotta. The gratin is baked for 30 mins or until the top is golden brown. Layer eith tomato slices and fresh mozzarella. Bake for another 5-10 minutes. Slice into thin slices, and serve them warm.

Nutritional Information:

- Cal 283
- Net Carbs 5.6g
- Fat 22g
- Protein 16g

Recipe 32. Almond and Maple Quick Grits

Serving Size: 4

Preparation Time: 10 minutes

Cooking Time: 11 minutes

Ingredients:

- ¼ cup of slivered almonds
- 1 ½ cups of water
- ¼ cup of pure maple syrup
- Pinch sea salt
- ½ teaspoon of ground cinnamon
- ½ cup of unsweetened almond milk
- ½ cup of quick-cooking grits

Directions:

- Boil the water with salt and almond milk. Stir with a wooden spoon, slowly add the grits.
- Stir in the syrup, cinnamon, and almonds. Cook for 1 minute. Serve

Nutritional Information:

- Cal 151
- Net Carbs 10g
- Fat 12g
- Protein 15.4g

Recipe 33. Bacon Stuffed Mushrooms

Serving Size: 8

Preparation Time: 20 minutes

Cooking Time: 30 minutes

Ingredients:

- 1 tablespoon onion
- ¾ cup Cheddar cheese
- 8 cremini mushrooms
- 1 tablespoon butter
- 3 slices bacon

Directions:

- In a large-sized deep skillet, cook the bacon until brown.
- Add the vegetables and water, remove the stems from the mushrooms.
- Oil and heat the pan add the onion to cook
- Combine the mushroom stem combination, bacon, and ½ cups Cheddar in a medium mixing bowl. Mix everything thoroughly before scooping it into the mushroom caps.
- Bake until the cheese has melted. Take the cooked mushrooms out of the oven and top with the leftover cheese.

Nutritional Information:

- Cal 151
- Net Carbs 6.4g
- Fat 6.6g
- Protein 16.4g

Recipe 34. Bacon-Wrapped Chicken Wings

Serving Size: 12

Preparation Time: 30 minutes

Cooking Time: 1 hour 30 minutes

Ingredients:

- 6 drumette wings and 6 flat chicken wings
- 12 strips of bacon
- 1 tablespoon of kosher salt
- 1 tablespoon of freshly ground black pepper
- 1 tablespoon of loose brown sugar
- 1 teaspoon of fresh paprika
- 1 teaspoon of chili powder
- 1 teaspoon of oregano
- Some blue cheese dressing
- Some celery sticks

Directions:

- Preheat and prepare the oven at a temperature of 350°F. Mix salt with sugar, chili powder, paprika, some oregano, salt, and pepper.
- Scatter the wings after being patted and rubbed with the sauce.
- Wrap every single chicken wing piece with a good bacon strip tightly. Add the loose bacon end underneath the chicken wing to keep it intact after baking it.
- Add the chicken wings wrapped on top of a rack used for baking placed on a baking sheet lined with foil.
- Let the wings bake at a temperature of 350F for at least an hour before flipping it midway through cooking them. Cool them lightly before you serve them with a side of blue cheese as well as celery.

Nutritional Information:

- Cal 293
- Net Carbs 5.6g
- Fat 12g
- Protein 16g

Recipe 35. Baked Asparagus with Cheesy Sauce

Serving Size: 8

Preparation Time: 20 minutes

Cooking Time: 30 minutes

Ingredients:

- 1/2 teaspoon of ground mustard
- 2 teaspoons of cornstarch
- 1 cup of cream half-and-half
- 1 teaspoon of Italian seasoning
- 1/4 teaspoon of red pepper flakes
- 1/2 cup of grated Parmesan cheese
- 1 cup of shredded mozzarella cheese
- 1 pound of fresh asparagus trimmed
-

Directions:

- Arrange asparagus in a small-sized baking dish. In a mixing dish, combine the half-and-half, ground mustard, shredded mozzarella, red pepper flakes, cornstarch, & grated parmesan cheese.
- Preheat oven at 350°F and bake for approximately 10 minutes.

Nutritional Information:

- Cal 113
- Net Carbs 4.9g
- Fat 7.3g
- Protein 7.6g

Recipe 36. Baked Beans

Serving Size: 6

Preparation Time: 20 minutes

Cooking Time: 3 hours 20 minutes

Ingredients:

- ½ cup of chopped canned tomatoes
- ¾ cup of dry pinto beans
- 1 tablespoon of apple cider vinegar
- 1 medium onion peeled and halved
- 5 cups of low-sodium vegetable stock
- 1 tablespoon of Dijon mustard
- ¾ cup of dry navy beans
- 1 teaspoon of salt
- ¾ cup of dry red kidney beans
- 1/3 cup of molasses

Directions:

- Oil and heat the pan add the drained beans cook for 30 minutes.
- Place beans in a 2 ½ quart baking dish with onion.
- Mix remaining ingredients. Pour over beans, Bake for 3 hrs. Serve and enjoy.

Nutritional Information:

- Cal 250
- Net Carbs 49g
- Fat 1g
- Protein 13g

Recipe 37. Baked Chicken Thighs

Serving Size: 4

Preparation Time: 20 minutes

Cooking Time: 30 minutes

Ingredients:

- 1 and ½ pounds of chicken thighs, boneless and skinless
- 2 tablespoons of harissa paste
- ½ cup of Greek yogurt
- Salt and black pepper to taste
- 1 tablespoon of lemon juice
- 1 tablespoon of mint, finely chopped

Directions:

- Mix yoghurt and lemon juice, salt and pepper and stir. Add harissa, stir again and spread over chicken pieces.
- Marinate the chicken thighs and add salt and pepper to taste.
- Bake for 20 minutes. Serve after sprinkling mint on top.

Nutritional Information:

- Cal 250
- Net Carbs 2g
- Fat 12g
- Protein 31g

Recipe 38. Barley Porridge

Serving Size: 2

Preparation Time: 10 minutes

Cooking Time: 35 minutes

Ingredients:

- ½ cup hazelnuts, toasted and chopped
- 1 cup wheat berries
- ½ cup pomegranate seeds
- 2 cups unsweetened almond milk
- ½ cup blueberries
- 1 cup barley
- ¼ cup honey
- 2 cups water

Directions:

- Boil water to cook porridge as per the instructions.
- Divide amongst serving bowls and top each serving with 2 tablespoons blueberries, 2 tablespoons pomegranate seeds, 2 tablespoons hazelnuts, 1 tablespoon honey. Serve and enjoy!

Nutritional Information:

- Cal 295
- Net Carbs 16g
- Fat 8g
- Protein 6g

Recipe 39. Bite-Sized Baked Chicken

Serving Size: 4

Preparation Time: 20 minutes

Cooking Time: 25 minutes

Ingredients:

- 1 pound of chicken breast – cut into bite-size pieces
- 4 tablespoons of butter, melted
- 1 ¼ cup of Italian seasoned bread crumbs

Directions:

- Set your oven temperature for about 325 degrees before doing anything else.
- Get your margarine melted in a bowl and coat your chicken in it.
- Now dip the coated chicken in breadcrumbs.
- Cook the chicken in the oven for about 12 minutes, then flip them and cook for 8 to 10 more minutes.
- Enjoy your Bite-Sized Baked Chicken

Nutritional Information:

- Cal 381
- Net Carbs 7g
- Fat 10.4g
- Protein 12g

Recipe 40. Breakfast Quinoa

Serving Size: 4

Preparation Time: 15 minutes

Cooking Time: 26 minutes

Ingredients:

- 2 cups of water
- 1 cup of quinoa, rinsed
- ½ cup of dried apricots, chopped
- ½ teaspoon of nutmeg
- 1 teaspoon of cinnamon
- ½ cup of slivered almonds
- ⅓ cup of flax seeds

Directions:

- Boil water and quinoa in a pot for 8-12 minutes.

- Mix flax seeds, cinnamon, nutmeg, almonds and apricots and cook for 2-3 minutes. If sweetness is desired, add splash of honey.

Nutritional Information:

- Cal 287
- Net Carbs 35.2g
- Fat 11,7g
- Protein 10.5g

Recipe 41. Breakfast Sausage Pineapple Skewers

Serving Size: 6

Preparation Time: 25 minutes

Cooking Time: 1 hour 25 minutes

Ingredients:

- ½ cup of canned pineapple cubes
- ¼ lb. of cubed pancetta
- 1 cored and quartered red pepper
- ½ lb. of 2" cubed Italian sausage, sweet

Directions:

- Preheat oven to 375F. Thread sausage, pepper, pancetta and pineapple on skewers. Each will have two sets of these ingredients.
- Arrange the skewers on cookie sheet. Bake until lightly brown around edges. Pancetta should be fully cooked. Serve warm.

Nutritional Information:

- Cal 310
- Net Carbs 42g
- Fat 11g
- Protein 11g

Recipe 42. Buttered Carrot-Zucchini with Mayo

Serving Size: 4

Preparation Time: 30 minutes

Cooking Time: 40 minutes

Ingredients:

- 1 tablespoon grated onion
- 2 tablespoons butter, melted
- 1/2-pound carrots, sliced
- 1-1/2 zucchinis, sliced
- 1/4 cup water
- 1/4 cup mayonnaise
- 1/4 teaspoon prepared horseradish
- 1/4 teaspoon salt
- 1/4 teaspoon ground black pepper
- 1/4 cup Italian bread crumbs

Directions:

- Lighten skillet with cooking spray. Add the carrots. Cook for 360 minutes at 360oF. Put the zucchini and continue cooking for another five minutes. Meanwhile, whisk together the pepper, salt, horseradish, onion, mayonnaise, and water in a bowl.
- Pour into a vegetable skillet. Pull well over the coat. Cook for 10 minutes at 390 F until tops are lightly browned. Serve and enjoy.

Nutritional Information:

- Cal 223
- Net Carbs 13.8g
- Fat 17.4g
- Protein 2.7g

Recipe 43. Cauliflower Fried Rice with Bacon

Serving Size: 4

Preparation Time: 15 minutes

Cooking Time: 15 minutes

Ingredients:

- 4 slices of bacon
- 1 small onion
- 1 head of cauliflower
- 1 cup of frozen mixed vegetables
- 1 teaspoon of Bragg's Liquid Amino

Directions:

- In a wok or enormous sauté container over medium flame, cook bacon. Add the onions and pan-fried food until translucent. Set heat to high. Add the shredded cauliflower and pan-fried food for 1 moment.
- Add water and mixed vegetables, mix well, spread the dish and let the cauliflower blend steam for an additional 3 minutes or about just until tender. Add Bragg's Liquid Amino. Taste and add salt for extra flavoring as wanted.

Nutritional Information:

- Cal 492
- Net Carbs 28g
- Fat 22g

- Protein 38g

Recipe 44. Cheesy Sicillian Tortellini

Serving Size: 7

Preparation Time: 10 minutes

Cooking Time: 38 minutes

Ingredients:

- ½ pound of ground beef
- ½ pound of Italian sausage, casings removed
- 1 16-ounce jar of marinara sauce
- 1 4.5-ounce can of sliced mushrooms
- 1 14.5-ounce can of Italian-style diced tomatoes, undrained
- 1 9-ounce package of cheese tortellini
- 1 cup of shredded mozzarella cheese
- ½ cup of shredded cheddar cheese

Directions:

- Crumble the prepared Italian sausage and ground beef into a large skillet. Combine the ground meats, marinara sauce, mushrooms, and tomatoes in a slow cooker.
- Cook for 7 hours. Stir the tortellini in. Cook until the tortellini are tender.

Nutritional Information:

- Cal 132
- Net Carbs 10g
- Fat 14g
- Protein 8g

Recipe 45. Cheese Wraps

Serving Size: 5

Preparation Time: 20 minutes

Cooking Time: 35 minutes

Ingredients:

- 2 cups of shredded cheese
- 1 (16 ounce) package flour tortillas
- 2/3 cup of salsa or 2/3 cup of picante sauce
- 24-ounce of chicken breasts

Directions:

- Mix salsa and drained chicken in a mixing bowl.
- Get a spoonful and put it in the center of the tortillas.
- Add the cheese and spread out evenly and fold; and grill it for about 5 minutes.

Nutritional Information:

- Cal 201
- Net Carbs 10g
- Fat 14g
- Protein 9.9g

Recipe 46. Alfredo

Serving Size: 4

Preparation Time: 20 minutes

Cooking Time: 40 minutes

Ingredients:

- 6 cups cubed uncooked chicken
- 1 lb. fettuccini
- 3 cloves garlic, minced, divided
- ½ tsp. oregano
- ½ tsp. basil
- 5 tbsp. butter
- 1 onion, diced
- 3 minced garlic cloves
- 1 cup sliced mushrooms
- 2 cups heavy cream
- Salt and pepper to taste
- 1 ¼ cups shredded Italian blend cheese
- ¼ cup chopped basil

Directions:

- Heat 1 tbsp. Butter in a large-sized skillet and add the cubed chicken, basil, and oregano. Sauté for 5 minutes and set aside. Prepare the pasta in a large-sized pot of salted water for 10 minutes and drain. Heat 4 tbsp. Butter in the same large-sized skillet and sauté the onion, garlic, and mushrooms for 8 minutes.

    Add the cheese, blend the chopped basil, and stir until the cheese has melted.

- Pour the sauce over the prepared fettuccini.

Nutritional Information:

- Cal 149
- Net Carbs 9.9g
- Fat 10.3g
- Protein 13.2g

Recipe 47. Chickpea Fritters

Serving Size: 4

Preparation Time: 30 minutes

Cooking Time: 30 minutes

Ingredients:

- Two tablespoons of mix spice
- Half cup of chopped dill
- One cup of red onions
- One cup of gram flour
- A pinch of salt
- Half cup of chopped cilantro
- Vegetable oil
- One cup of parboiled chickpeas
- Water as required

Directions:

- To begin, get a big bowl. Put everything in the bowl, and make sure it's well combined. To create a new substance, pour some water into the bowl.
- Oil and heat the pan. Carefully dropping a tablespoon of batter into the pan, then cooking the items for a few minutes. When the fritters have reached the desired color, which is a light brown, serve it.

Nutritional Information:

- Cal 306
- Net Carbs 6.5g
- Fat 15.9g
- Protein 33.9g

Recipe 48. Glazed Carrots

Serving Size: 3

Preparation Time: 30 minutes

Cooking Time: 40 minutes

Ingredients:

- ½ teaspoon of coriander
- 2 tablespoons of fresh orange juice
- ½ pound of rainbow carrots, peeled
- Pinch of salt
- 1 tablespoon of honey

Directions:

- Mix the honey, coriander, orange juice, and salt in a small bowl.
- Spread the carrots in a baking dish in a single layer. Bake for 20 minutes. Serve and enjoy

Nutritional Information:

- Cal 184
- Net Carbs 20g
- Fat 11g
- Protein 9g

Recipe 49. Corn Meal Mush with Polish Sausage

Serving Size: 4

Preparation Time: 15 minutes

Cooking Time: 20 minutes

Ingredients:

- 1 (16-ounce) package refrigerated corn meal mush
- ½ (16-ounce) package skinless Polish sausage
- ½ tablespoon butter
- Stevia to taste

Directions:

- Set aside the mush and sausage pieces, which should be cut into 1-inch slices.
- Melt the prepared butter in a large pan over medium heat, then add the mush, arranging the pieces side by side.
- After flipping the mush over to brown the other side, add the sausage to the pan and distribute it around the borders of the skillet and between the mush pieces to keep everything warm (you may also use a separate skillet to heat sausage).
- Serve with maple syrup drizzled on top.

Nutritional Information:

- Cal 110
- Net Carbs 23.4g
- Fat 11g
- Protein 2.5g

Recipe 50. Chickpeas Bowls

Serving Size: 4

Preparation Time: 25 minutes

Cooking Time: 15 minutes

Ingredients:

- ½ teaspoon oregano, dried
- ½ cup Greek olives, pitted and chopped
- 1 yellow onion, chopped
- 1 tablespoon lemon juice
- 15 ounces canned chickpeas, drained and rinsed
- A pinch of salt and black pepper
- 1 cup water
- 2 garlic cloves, minced
- 15 ounces canned tomatoes, chopped
- 1 tablespoon olive oil
- ¾ cup whole wheat couscous

- 14 ounces canned artichokes, drained and chopped

Directions:

- Boil water and add the couscous, cook for 15 minutes.
- Cook the onions in a pan with oil.
- Add the couscous, toss, divide into bowls and serve for breakfast.

Nutritional Information:

- Cal 340
- Net Carbs 51g
- Fat 10g
- Protein 11g

Recipe 51. Fried Codfish

Serving Size: 4

Preparation Time: 25 minutes

Cooking Time: 15 minutes

Ingredients:

- 35.2 oz salted codfish
- 1 cup of flour
- 1 tablespoon extra virgin olive oil
- salt and pepper
- 1 cup beer
- 3 tablespoons chopped dill
- 3 tablespoons chopped parsley
- 2 tablespoons lemon juice
- oil for frying

Directions:

- Rinse the cod well under running water to remove the salt and place it in a bowl full of water for 2 days, changing it occasionally. On the second day, cut the cod into slices to improve the release of salt. After 48 hours, drain the fish and carefully remove the skin and all the bones, crumbling it.
- Put the flour, oil, salt, pepper and beer in a food processor. When the liquid is creamy, add the dill and parsley. Grind 3 seconds. Add the crumbled fish to the batter and mix well.
- Oil and heat the pan. Once hot, use a large tablespoon to take some of the fish and place it in the oil, occasionally turning until golden brown and crispy.
- Accompany with walnut skordalia.

Nutritional Information:

- Cal 199
- Net Carbs 6.6g
- Fat 10g
- Protein 18.3g

Recipe 52. Garlic and Tomato Bruschetta

Serving Size: 8

Preparation Time: 10 minutes

Cooking Time: 10 minutes

Ingredients:

- 8 slices of 1/2-inch thick of a French baguette
- 1 1/2 teaspoons of minced fresh garlic
- 1 1/4 cups of chopped plum tomatoes
- 1 teaspoon of extra-virgin olive oil
- 1 teaspoon of balsamic vinegar
- 1/2 teaspoon of dried basil
- 1/4 teaspoon of non-caloric sweetener
- 1/4 teaspoon of freshly ground pepper

Directions:

- Add olive oil to all sides of the baguette. Bake it for 5 minutes.
- Combine the rest of the remaining ingredients in a small bowl. Mix well. Add the mixture to the baguette.

Nutritional Information:

- Cal 157
- Net Carbs 11g
- Fat 10g
- Protein 9.2g

Recipe 53. Garlic Steamers

Serving Size: 5

Preparation Time: 30 minutes

Cooking Time: 30 minutes

Ingredients:

- 1/2 cup of white wine
- 1/4 cup of garlic, minced
- 2 tablespoons of chopped flat-leaf, italian parsley
- 3 pounds of soft shell clams
- salt to taste
- 1/4 cup of butter, melted

Directions:

- Butter and heat the pan. Sauté the garlic until it releases its fragrance but does not brown. Add the delicate shell clams to the saucepan and stir well to combine.
- Add the parsley and salt to taste as soon as each clam opens up. Serve right away.

Nutritional Information:

- Cal 401
- Net Carbs 44.1g
- Fat 13.3g
- Protein 38g

Recipe 54. Garlic Mashed Potatoes

Serving Size: 4

Preparation Time: 30 minutes

Cooking Time: 1 hour

Ingredients:

- 1 medium-sized garlic bulb, fresh
- 2 pounds red-skinned potatoes
- ½ cup milk
- ½ cup heavy cream
- ¼ cup butter
- Salt and pepper to taste

Directions:

- Preheat the oven to 400°F.
- Wrap the prepared whole garlic bulb in aluminum foil and bake for 45 minutes or until softened. Take it out of the oven. Then set it aside to cool in its wrapper.
- Once the garlic has cooled, take off the outer layer and squeeze off the cooked pulp. Then, remove it from the equation.
- Meanwhile, prepare the potatoes by cutting them, washing them, removing the skins, and placing them in a saucepan. Mash using your hands. Depending on your choice, lumps may be left. Serve.

Nutritional Information:

- Cal 204
- Net Carbs 24g
- Fat 10g
- Protein 7g

Recipe 55. Gazpacho with Melon and Ham

Serving Size: 6

Preparation Time: 5 minutes

Cooking Time: 5 minutes

Ingredients:

- 26 oz melon without peel
- 1 piece of fresh ginger root
- 1 pinch of salt
- 1 pinch of pepper
- 6 slices of Jamon Serrano
- 6 breadsticks

Directions:

- In a kitchen blender, blend the melon with the ginger root, salt and pepper.
- Add the ham and blend again.
- Transfer to a soup tureen and refrigerate for 2 hours.
- Remove from the fridge and serve accompanied by breadsticks that you will dip in the gazpacho.

Nutritional Information:

- Cal 129
- Net Carbs 18.3g
- Fat 3.1g
- Protein 7.2g

Recipe 56. Gnocchi in Cream Sauce

Serving Size: 4

Preparation Time: 10 minutes

Cooking Time: 10 minutes

Ingredients:

- 1 (12-ounce) package potato gnocchi
- ¼ teaspoon basil
- ⅔ cup half-and-half
- 2 ounces cream cheese, diced
- ½ teaspoon garlic powder
- ¼ teaspoon oregano
- ¼ teaspoon black pepper
- ½ teaspoon salt

Directions:

- Cook gnocchi according to package directions; drain.
- Meanwhile, in a saucepan add half-and-half, cream cheese, salt, garlic powder, oregano, basil and pepper; cook over medium heat until heated throughout and cream cheese is melted, about 10 minutes.
- Add ½ cup cooked soft vegetable, if desired.
- Place cooked gnocchi in serving dish; pour cream sauce over gnocchi.

Nutritional Information:

- Cal 361
- Net Carbs 56.8g
- Fat 10.9g
- Protein 9.5g

Recipe 57. Grouper with Wine Sauce

Serving Size: 4

Preparation Time: 5 minutes

Cooking Time: 20 minutes

Ingredients:

- 35 oz of cleaned grouper
- 2 garlic heads
- 10 peppercorns
- 1 glass of white wine
- 2 tablespoons of oil

Directions:

- Fry the grouper in a pan with the oil.
- Add the two garlic heads, the pepper and the wine. Cover the pan and simmer for approximately about 15 minutes or until the fish is cooked through.
- Remove from the heat, remove the heads of garlic, arrange the fillets on a serving plate, season with the remaining sauce and serve.

Nutritional Information:

- Cal 232
- Net Carbs 12g
- Fat 5.3g
- Protein 42.5g

Recipe 58. Ham and Sun-Dried Tomato Alfredo

Serving Size: 4

Preparation Time: 10 minutes

Cooking Time: 10 minutes

Ingredients:

- 8 oz. uncooked linguine
- 1/4 cup chopped oil-packed sun-dried tomatoes
- 1 cup heavy whipping cream
- 1/2 cup grated Parmesan cheese
- 1 cup cubed fully cooked ham

Directions:

- Cook the linguine following the package instructions.
- In the meantime, sauté tomatoes in a cooking-spray-coated big pan for a minute. Lower heat then mixes in cheese and cream. Boil gently on medium heat. Let it simmer for 5-7mins without cover until thick.
- Drain the linguine, then mix it into the sauce mixture. Put in ham, then heat thoroughly.

Nutritional Information:

- Cal 310
- Net Carbs 42g
- Fat 11g
- Protein 11g

Recipe 59. Honey Almond Ricotta Spread with Peaches

Serving Size: 4

Preparation Time: 5 minutes

Cooking Time: 8 minutes

Ingredients:

- 1/2 cup Fisher Sliced Almonds
- 1 cup whole milk ricotta
- extra honey for drizzling
- 1/4 teaspoon almond extract
- zest from an orange, optional
- 1 teaspoon honey
- hearty whole-grain toast
- English muffin or bagel
- extra Fisher sliced almonds
- sliced peaches

Directions:

- Place peaches cut side down onto the greased grill. Close lid cover and then just grill until the peaches have softened, approximately 6-10 minutes, depending on the size of the peaches.
- Then you will have to place peach halves onto a serving plate. Put a spoon of about 1 tablespoon of ricotta mixture into the cavity (you can also use a small scooper).
- Sprinkle it with slivered almonds, crushed amaretti cookies, and honey. Decorate with the mint leaves.

Nutritional Information:

- Cal 187
- Net Carbs 18g
- Fat 9g
- Protein 7g

Recipe 60. Lemon Parsley Swordfish

Serving Size: 5

Preparation Time: 15 minutes

Cooking Time: 30 minutes

Ingredients:

- 1 cup of fresh Italian parsley
- ¼ cup of lemon juice
- ¼ cup of extra-virgin olive oil
- ¼ cup of fresh thyme
- 1 clove of garlic
- ½ teaspoon of salt
- 2 swordfish steaks
- Olive oil spray

Directions:

- Preheat the oven to 450F. Grease a large pan with olive oil spray. Place the parsley, lemon juice, olive oil, thyme, garlic, and salt in a food processor and pulse until smoothly blended.
- Arrange the swordfish steaks in the greased baking dish and spoon the parsley mixture over the top. Bake for 18 minutes until flaky. Serve the fish among two plates and serve hot.

Nutritional Information:

- Cal 396
- Net Carbs 2.9g
- Fat 21.7g
- Protein 44.2g

Recipe 61. Mussels with Herbed Vinaigrette

Serving Size: 4

Preparation Time: 20 minutes

Cooking Time: 30 minutes

Ingredients:

- 1kg mussels
- Herb Vinaigrette
- 1 tablespoon chives
- 2 tablespoon parsley leaves
- 2 tablespoon basil leaves
- 1 teaspoon lemon thyme
- 4 tablespoon shallots
- 2 tomatoes
- ¼ teaspoon Maldon Sea salt
- Dash of black pepper
- 1 tablespoon sherry vinegar
- 1 tablespoon balsamic vinegar
- 1/3 cup olive oil

Directions:

- Mix the prepared ingredients for the vinaigrette. Heat a heavy-bottomed saucepan with a tight-fitting lid for one minute, then add the mussels without any water.
- Any mussels that have actually not opened should be discarded, and any liquid should be drained. Pour in the vinaigrette and mix well before serving.

Nutritional Information:

- Cal 158
- Net Carbs 5.9g
- Fat 12.1g
- Protein 8.3g

Recipe 62. Peppy Casserole

Serving Size: 5

Preparation Time: 30 minutes

Cooking Time: 60 minutes

Ingredients:

- 1-1/2 cups water
- 1-1/2 tsps. Italian seasoning
- 1 package scalloped potatoes
- 1/2 lb. ground beef
- 24 pepperoni slices
- 16 oz. tomato sauce
- 4 oz. sliced provolone cheese
- 1/2 cup shredded part-skim mozzarella cheese
- 1 tbsp. grated Parmesan cheese

Directions:

- Mix Italian seasoning, water, and tomato sauce together in a big saucepan; boil it. Add contents of sauce mix and potatoes. Remove into a non-oiled 2-quart baking dish.
- Oil and heat pan to cook beef and add to the potatoes, put pepperoni on top.
- Bake without a cover for 20 minutes at 400°. Put cheeses on top. Bake until the potatoes are soft, about another 15-20 minutes.

Nutritional Information:

- Cal 360
- Net Carbs 26g
- Fat 16g
- Protein 28g

Recipe 63. Pesto Fish Fillet

Serving Size: 2

Preparation Time: 15 minutes

Cooking Time: 18 minutes

Ingredients:

- 1/2 avocado, peeled and chopped
- 1/2 cup of water
- Salt and black pepper to taste
- 1/2 tablespoon of capers
- 1/2 tablespoon of garlic, chopped
- 1 tablespoon of lemon zest, grated
- 1/2 cup of basil, chopped
- 2 halibut fillets

Directions:

- Blend avocado, capers, garlic, lemon zest, pepper, basil, and salt. Place fish fillets on aluminum foil and spread the blended mixture on fish fillets. Fold foil around the fish fillets.
- Place the fish foil on the trivet. Cover the medium-sized pan with a lid and cook over high heat for 8 minutes. Once done, remove the lid. Serve and enjoy.

Nutritional Information:

- Cal 426
- Net Carbs 5.5g
- Fat 16.6g
- Protein 61.8g

Recipe 64. Pita with Greens, Fried Onions, and Bacon

Serving Size: 2

Preparation Time: 10 minutes

Cooking Time: 11 minutes

Ingredients:

- 3 ½ ounces of tomatoes
- 1 ½ ounces of red onion
- ½ lemon juiced
- Sea salt to taste
- Ground black pepper to taste
- 3 ½ ounces of bacon
- 2 garlic cloves
- 1 bunch of green salad
- 2 tablespoons of vegetable oil
- 2 pitas

Directions:

- Slice the garlic and onion and tomato into slices then oil and heat the pan to cook.
- Put the fried onions, the tomatoes, lettuce leaves on pita, and bacon on top. Before serving, sprinkle with lemon juice, salt, pepper to taste.

Nutritional Information:

- Cal 470
- Net Carbs 41.8g
- Fat 21g
- Protein 14.5g

Recipe 65. Pork Onions

Serving Size: 5

Preparation Time: 10 minutes

Cooking Time: 35 minutes

Ingredients:

- 1 ½ pound of Pork tenderloin (you can use chicken breasts or beef tenderloin)
- 1 teaspoon of Seasoning mix (or use a mixture of any onion, black pepper, garlic, salt, and parsley)

Directions:

- Marinate the tenderloin, heat and oil the pan to cook it, Cook each side for about 3 minutes, or until it turns brown.
- Transfer the tenderloins to the oven and allow them to cook for about 25 minutes
- Prepare the balsamic caramelize onions and serve with the sliced pork.

Nutritional Information:

- Cal 220
- Net Carbs 3.8g
- Fat 10g
- Protein 3.7g

Recipe 66. Rosemary Baked Chicken Drumsticks

Serving Size: 6

Preparation Time: 10 minutes

Cooking Time: 1 hour

Ingredients:

- 2 tablespoons chopped fresh rosemary leaves
- 1 teaspoon garlic powder
- ½ teaspoon sea salt
- 1/8 teaspoon freshly ground black pepper
- Zest of 1 lemon
- 12 chicken drumsticks

Directions:

- Preheat the oven to 350°F.
- Blend rosemary, garlic powder, sea salt, pepper, and lemon zest.
- Situate drumsticks in a 9-by-13-inch baking dish and sprinkle with the rosemary mixture. Bake for about 1 hour.

Nutritional Information:

- Cal 163
- Net Carbs 46g
- Fat 6g
- Protein 26g

Recipe 67. Shredded Beef

Serving Size: 8

Preparation Time: 15 minutes

Cooking Time: 30 minutes

Ingredients:

- 2 pounds of beef chuck roast
- 1 cup of onion, chopped
- 1 cup of mixed frozen vegetables (carrots, bell pepper), chopped
- 14 ounces of canned fire roasted tomatoes
- 2 tablespoons of red wine vinegar

Directions:

- Season the beef with salt. Add to the Instant Pot. Top with the onion and frozen vegetables. Pour the tomatoes and vinegar. Mix well. Seal the pot.
- . Let cool for 5 minutes. Shred the beef. Season with salt and pepper or Italian blend seasoning.

Nutritional Information:

- Cal 431
- Net Carbs 4.3g
- Fat 31.6g
- Protein 30.2g

Recipe 68. Smokey Spanish Garlic Shrimp

Serving Size: 4

Preparation Time: 20 minutes

Cooking Time: 20 minutes

Ingredients:

- 2 tablespoons dry sherry
- 1 tablespoon Italian parsley
- 1 teaspoon hot smoked paprika
- ¼ cup extra-virgin olive oil
- 1 pound shrimp
- 4 cloves garlic

Directions:

- Garlic minced. Paprika and salt season shrimp. Coat, mix.
- Cook garlic and oil over low heat.
- Cook until garlic becomes translucent, approximately 2 minutes.
- Extremely heat the shrimp.
- Toss and rotate the shrimp for two minutes, until they curl but are still raw.
- Add sherry. Stir for 1 minute, or until sauces boil and shrimp is cooked.
- Remove the pan from the heat. With a spoon, fold in the parsley.

Nutritional Information:

- Cal 151
- Net Carbs 6.4g
- Fat 6.6g
- Protein 16.4g

Recipe 69. Steamed Balsamic Artichokes

Serving Size: 4

Preparation Time: 10 minutes

Cooking Time: 15 minutes

Ingredients:

- 2 tbsp. of lemon juice, fresh-squeezed
- 4 artichokes, fresh
- 2 tbsp. of olive oil, extra virgin
- 1 tbsp. of vinegar, Balsamic
- 4 tbsp. of Italian dressing
- 1/2 tsp. of salt, kosher

Directions:

- Cut off stems and trim tops off artichokes. Clean them well. Place them in the steamer.
- Add some water to the steamer tank.
- Mix the rest of the ingredients. Pour that over the artichokes.
- Steam for 45 minutes – 1 hour until leaves are easy to pull out.
- Baste them every 10-15 minutes.
- Remove and serve.

Nutritional Information:

- Cal 213
- Net Carbs 13g
- Fat 12g
- Protein 17g

Recipe 70. Stewed Mussels and Clams with Tomatoes and Olives

Serving Size: 4

Preparation Time: 10 minutes

Cooking Time: 10 minutes

Ingredients:

- ¾ pound of fresh mussels, shell on
- ¾ pound of fresh clams, shell on
- 2 tablespoons of canola oil
- 3 cloves of garlic, smashed
- ¼ cup of white wine
- 1 tablespoon of lemon juice
- ½ cup of black olives, pitted
- 1 cup of fresh plum tomatoes, diced
- 1 cup of low-sodium vegetable or seafood stock
- Zest of 1 lemon
- 1/8 teaspoon of red chili flakes
- 5 tablespoons of fresh parsley, chopped

Directions:

- Soak clams and mussels in cold running water to clean. Discard any open or broken shells.
- Heat oil in the prepared sauté pan over medium heat, add garlic and chili flakes. Cook 1 minute and increase heat to high.
- Add remaining ingredients except parsley and cover. Steam for 5 to 8 minutes until shellfish are open.
- Pour into bowl, add parsley, and serve with crusty bread.

Nutritional Information:

- Cal 250
- Net Carbs 10g
- Fat 12g
- Protein 23g

Recipe 71. Tahini Pine Nuts Toast

Serving Size: 4

Preparation Time: 10 minutes

Cooking Time: 10 minutes

Ingredients:

- 2 whole wheat bread slices, toasted
- 1 teaspoon water
- 1 tablespoon tahini paste
- 2 teaspoons feta cheese, crumbled
- Juice of ½ lemon
- 2 teaspoons pine nuts
- A pinch of black pepper

Directions:

- In a large-sized bowl, mix the tahini with the water and the lemon juice, whisk really well and spread over the toasted bread slices.
- Top each serving with the remaining ingredients and serve for breakfast.

Nutritional Information:

- Cal 142
- Net Carbs 13.7g
- Fat 7.6g
- Protein 5.8g

Recipe 72. Toasted Baguette with Tomatoes and Anchovies

Serving Size: 8

Preparation Time: 20 minutes

Cooking Time: 20 minutes

Ingredients:

- 1/3 cup extra-virgin olive oil
- 1 16-oz. French-bread baguette
- 3 garlic cloves
- 4-inch-long pieces, lightly toasted
- 2 1/4 lbs. vine-ripened tomatoes
- 12 to 20 anchovy fillets

Directions:

- Grate tomatoes down to its skin with coarse grater placed on medium-sized bowl. Throw the skin away. To grated tomatoes, all garlic and 1/3 cup of olive oil. Season the prepared mixture with pepper and salt to taste. You may prepare tomatoes 2 hours in advance. Allow to rest at room temperature.
- Put the pieces of toast onto a platter. Sprinkle with more oil. Put the anchovies in one small bowl. Serve the toast, passing the anchovies and tomatoes on the side.

Nutritional Information:

- Cal 300
- Net Carbs 35g

- Fat 14g
- Protein 10g

Recipe 73. Tomato-Basil Poached Cod

Serving Size: 4

Preparation Time: 10 minutes

Cooking Time: 4 hours 20 minutes

Ingredients:

- ¼ cup of extra-virgin olive oil
- 1 tablespoon of minced garlic
- 1-pound of grape tomatoes halved
- ¼ cup of dry white wine
- Zest and juice of 1 lemon
- 1 cup of minced fresh basil
- 4 (6-ounce) cod fillets
- Sea salt
- Freshly ground black pepper

Directions:

- Heat a prepared large-sized skillet over medium heat until hot, then pour in the oil, and tilt to coat the bottom. Add the tomatoes, garlic, and cook for 5 minutes, or until the tomatoes soften.
- Increase the heat to medium-high, and add the white wine. Simmer for 2 minutes to cook off some of the alcohol.
- Season the cod fillets with salt and pepper, and nestle them into the tomato mixture—Cook for about 3 minutes.
- Flip, and cook for approximately about 3 minutes, or until the cod flakes easily with a fork.

Nutritional Information:

- Cal 252
- Net Carbs 31g
- Fat 4g
- Protein 27.8g

Recipe 74. Tortellini in Chicken Broth

Serving Size: 6

Preparation Time: 30 minutes

Cooking Time: 1 hour 20 minutes

Ingredients:

- 3-4 pounds chicken parts on bone
- 2 cups fresh celery tops, chopped
- 12 cups water (or chicken stock)
- 2 teaspoons dried thyme
- 2 teaspoons dried sage
- 3 cloves garlic, minced
- ¾ cup carrot, sliced
- ¾ cup celery, diced
- ¼ cup green onions, diced
- 3 tablespoons fresh parsley, minced
- Sea salt and freshly ground pepper
- 2 bay leaves
- 1 package cheese tortellini

Directions:

- Combine chicken, celery tops, thyme, and sage in 12 cups water in a large stockpot. Bring to a boil, and reduce heat. Cook for at least approximately about half an hour or so, just until the chicken is well done.
- Measure 6 cups of strained broth into another stockpot (store remaining chicken and broth.). Add the following 8 remaining ingredients. Cover and simmer over a heat of medium heat until vegetables are tender, about 15 minutes.
- Add tortellini and cook per pasta directions. Remove bay leaves. Taste and season with the prepared salt and ground pepper as needed.

Nutritional Information:

- Cal 374
- Net Carbs 7.1g
- Fat 22.6g
- Protein 38g

Recipe 75. Tuna with Lemon Butter Sauce

Serving Size: 4

Preparation Time: 10 minutes

Cooking Time: 5 minutes

Ingredients:

- 4 tuna fillets
- 1/4 cup lemon juice
- 1 tablespoon fresh dill
- 1 tablespoon butter

Directions:

- Pour 1 cup water and lemon juice into the Instant Pot.
- Add the steamer basket.
- Put the tuna fillet on top of the basket.
- Season with salt and pepper and dill.

- Seal the pot.
- Choose the manual setting.
- Cook at high pressure for 5 minutes.
- Release the pressure quickly.
- Remove from the pot.
- Place the butter on top.
- Let it melt, and then serve.

Nutritional Information:

- Cal 213
- Net Carbs 9g
- Fat 18.5g
- Protein 10.8g

Recipe 76. Vanilla-Cream Morning Oatmeal

Serving Size: 4

Preparation Time: 20 minutes

Cooking Time: 45 minutes

Ingredients:

- 4 cups of water
- Pinch of sea salt
- 1 cup of steel-cut oats
- ¾ cup of unsweetened almond milk
- 2 teaspoons of pure vanilla extract

Directions:

- Add the water and salt to a large saucepan over high heat and bring to a boil. Once its actually boiling, reduce the heat to low and add the oats. Mix well and cook for 30 minutes, stirring occasionally.
- Fold in the almond milk and vanilla and whisk to combine. Continue cooking for about 10 minutes, or until the oats are thick and creamy. Ladle the oatmeal into bowls and serve warm.

Nutritional Information:

- Cal 116
- Net Carbs 19g
- Fat 21g
- Protein 14.2g

Recipe 77. Fruit and Nuts

Serving Size: 8

Preparation Time: 20 minutes

Cooking Time: 30 minutes

Ingredients:

- 2 cups of almond milk
- 1 cup of dried mixed fruit
- ¼ teaspoon of salt
- 16 ounces of farro
- ½ cup of chopped toasted mixed nuts
- ¼ cup of maple syrup
- 4 ½ cups of water

Directions:

- Mix maple syrup, water, lace farro, and salt.
- Set the pot to cook for 30 minutes. Press the Cancel button, open lid, and add dried fruit. Warm setting for 20 minutes. Serve warm with nuts and almond milk.

Nutritional Information:

- Cal 347
- Net Carbs 65g
- Fat 7g
- Protein 9g

Recipe 78. Pumpkin and Cinnamon Cream

Serving Size: 4

Preparation Time: 10 minutes

Cooking Time: 30 minutes

Ingredients:

- 17.6 oz diced squash
- 1 ½ cups vegetable stock
- 1 oz extra virgin olive oil
- 1 shallot
- 2 cinnamon sticks
- 1 pinch of salt
- 1 pinch cinnamon powder

Directions:

- Slice the shallot.
- Put the pumpkin, broth, extra virgin olive oil, shallot, cinnamon sticks and salt in a large pot and cook for 30 minutes.
- At the end of the actual cooking time remove the cinnamon sticks and blend the soup with an immersion blender.
- Serve sprinkled with cinnamon powder.

Nutritional Information:

- Cal 195
- Net Carbs 10.5g
- Fat 7.8g
- Protein 1.8g

Recipe 79. Tomato and Prosciutto Sandwiches

Serving Size: 4

Preparation Time: 10 minutes

Cooking Time: 10 minutes

Ingredients:

- 8 thin prosciutto slices
- Salt and black pepper to taste
- 1 avocado, halved and pitted
- 8 whole-wheat bread slices
- 1 tablespoon of cilantro, chopped
- 1 large, ripe tomato, sliced into 8 rounds
- 8 romaine lettuce leaves

Directions:

- Toast the bread and place on a large platter. Scoop the avocado flesh out of the skin into a small bowl. Season with pepper and salt. With a fork, gently mash the avocado until it resembles a creamy spread.
- Smear 4 bread slices with the avocado mix. Top with a layer of lettuce leaves, tomato slices, and prosciutto slices. Repeat the layers one more time, sprinkle with cilantro, then cover with the remaining bread slices. Serve and enjoy!

Nutritional Information:

- Cal 262
- Net Carbs 35g
- Fat 12.2g
- Protein 8g

Recipe 80. Vegetarian Spanish Toast with Escalivada

Serving Size: 4

Preparation Time: 15 minutes

Cooking Time: 15 minutes

Ingredients:

- Flat-leaf parsley
- Sea salt
- 80g soft goat's cheese
- 1 slice Serrano ham
- ½ jar of Escalivada
- Green olives
- Extra virgin olive oil
- 1 large bruschetta bread

Directions:

- After toasting one side, drizzle olive oil on the uncooked side.
- Fork-drain escalivada.
- Top with olives and goat cheese.
- Reheat the toast.
- Sprinkling Spicy salami on top.
- Serve hot with chopped flat-leaf parsley and sea salt.

Nutritional Information:

- Cal 174
- Net Carbs 7g
- Fat 8.2g
- Protein 18g

CHAPTER 3. LUNCH RECIPES

Recipe 81. Asparagus and Beef Shirataki

Serving Size: 4

Preparation Time: 20 minutes

Cooking Time: 35 minutes

Ingredients:

- 1 lb of fresh asparagus cut into
- 1-inch pieces
- 2. (8 8 oz) boxes angel hair Shirataki
- 3 tbsp olive oil
- 2 shallots finely chopped
- 3 cloves of garlic, minced
- 1/2 lb ground beef
- 1 cup of grated Parmesan cheese
- Black pepper and salt to taste

Directions:

- In a large-sized pot, bring 2 cups of water boiling. Then strain the shirataki and rinse it well under hot, running water. Transfer the pasta to boiling water. Cook until 3 mins, then strain. Put a dry skillet in the oven and cook the shirataki pasta until dry, 2 to 3 minutes. Set aside.
- In an oven and put in the beef. Cook for 10 minutes. Transfer onto a plate. In the same pan, sauté asparagus for 7 mins. Add shallots and garlic to the same skillet and simmer until about 2 minutes. Sprinkle with salt and pepper. Mix in the Shirataki and beef, then toss until mixed. Serve the dish with Parmesan cheese before serving.

Nutritional Information:

- Cal 398
- Net Carbs 6.9g
- Fat 25g
- Protein 31g

Recipe 82. Baked Chicken

Serving Size: 4

Preparation Time: 15 minutes

Cooking Time: 35 minutes

Ingredients:

- 2 pounds chicken tenders
- 3 dill sprigs
- 1 large zucchini
- 1 cup grape tomatoes
- 2 tablespoons olive oil

  For topping:

- 1 tablespoon fresh lemon juice
- 1 tablespoon olive oil
- 2 tablespoons feta cheese, crumbled
- 1 tablespoon fresh dill, chopped

Directions:

- Warm oven to 200 C/ 400 F. Drizzle the olive oil on a baking tray, then place chicken, zucchini, dill, and tomatoes on the tray. Season with salt. Bake chicken within 30 minutes.
- Place chicken on the serving tray, then top with veggies and discard dill sprigs. Sprinkle topping mixture on top of chicken and vegetables. Serve and enjoy.

Nutritional Information:

- Calories: 557
- Fat: 28.6g
- Protein: 67.9g
- Carbs: 5.2g

Recipe 83. Baked Chicken Nuggets

Serving Size: 2

Preparation Time: 15 minutes

Cooking Time: 30 minutes

Ingredients:

- 2 tbsp ranch dressing
- 1 cup of almond flour
- 1 egg
- 2 tbsp garlic powder
- 2 chicken breasts cubed
- Black pepper and salt to taste
- 1 tbsp butter, melt

Directions:

- Preheat the oven up to a heat of 400 F. Grease a baking dish with butter. A bowl mix of salt and powdered garlic, almond flour, and black pepper. Mix. Separately, beat eggs. Dip the prepared chicken cubes in the egg and then into the flour mixture.

- Bake for about 18-20 minutes, turning halfway through, until golden and crispy. Transfer to paper towels, remove any grease accumulated and then serve it with ranch dressing.

Nutritional Information:

- Cal 373
- Net Carbs 7.6g
- Fat 37g
- Protein 31g

Recipe 84. Barbecued Pork Chops

Serving Size: 2

Preparation Time: 15 minutes

Cooking Time: 20 minutes

Ingredients:

- 2 pork loin chops, boneless
- 1/2 cup BBQ sauce, sugar-free
- Black pepper and salt to taste
- 1/2 tsp ginger powder
- 1/2 1 teaspoon onion powder
- 1/2 1 teaspoon garlic powder
- 1 teaspoon red pepper flakes
- 2 thyme sprigs chopped

Directions:

- Mix salt, black pepper ginger powder, salt powder, garlic powder, and red pepper flakes in one small bowl. Rub the spice mixture on the chops of pork. The grill should be heated too high.
- Lower the temperature to moderate, then apply the BBQ sauce over the meat, cover and cook for five minutes. Unlock the lid, rotate the meat, and brush it using barbecue sauce. Continue cooking, covered, for five minutes. Serve sprinkled with Thyme.

Nutritional Information:

- Cal 342
- Net Carbs 1g
- Fat 18g
- Protein 40g

Recipe 85. BBQ Beef Sliders

Serving Size: 4

Preparation Time: 1 hour 30 minutes

Cooking Time: 4 hours 15 minutes

Ingredients:

- 2 lb of chuck roast boneless
- 1 teaspoon onion powder
- 2 1 tsp garlic powder
- 1 tbsp smoked paprika
- 2 tbsp tomato paste
- 1 cup of white vinegar
- 2 tbsp tamari sauce
- 1 cup of bone broth
- 1/4 cup of butter that is melted
- 4 zero carb buns, halved
- Black pepper and salt to taste
- 1/4 cup baby spinach
- 4 slices of cheddar cheese

Directions:

- Mix salt, pepper, onion, and garlic powders in one small bowl. Add paprika and. Slice the meat into 2 pieces. Rub the rub on the beef before placing it in the slow cooker.
- Mix vinegar, tomato paste, Tamari sauce, broth, and butter in a separate bowl. Pour this mixture over the steak, then cook it for four hours. After the beef is cooked then, shred it with two forks. Divide the spinach among buns, place the beef on top, and add the cheddar cheese slice. Serve.

Nutritional Information:

- Cal 400
- Net Carbs 5.6g
- Fat 32g
- Protein 55g

Recipe 86. BBQ Pulled Chicken

Serving Size: 6

Preparation Time: 20 minutes

Cooking Time: 35 minutes

Ingredients:

- 1 tablespoon canola oil
- 1 large yellow onion, chopped
- 3 cloves garlic, minced
- 2½ cups low-sodium ketchup
- ¼ cup tomato paste
- ½ cup Diet Coke
- 1/3 cup apple cider vinegar
- ¼ cup molasses
- ¼ teaspoon black pepper
- 2 tablespoons dry mustard
- ½ teaspoon liquid smoke

- 1 (3-pound) roasted chicken, meat pulled off and shredded, skin removed

Directions:

- Oil and heat the pan add onions, and cook until soft (about 5 minutes), then add garlic and cook 1 minute.
- Add ketchup, tomato paste, Coke, vinegar, molasses, pepper, mustard, and liquid smoke and bring to a boil, then reduce heat and allow to simmer for 15 minutes.
- Add shredded chicken and cook for 10 more minutes, then place on your favorite toasted bun and enjoy.

Nutritional Information:

- Calories: 410
- Fat: 9g
- Protein: 48g
- Carbohydrates: 32g

Recipe 87. Beef and Cheese Avocado Boats

Serving Size: 4

Preparation Time: 15 minutes

Cooking Time: 30 minutes

Ingredients:

- 7 tbsp of shredded Monterey Jack cheese
- 2 avocados, half-cut and pitted
- 2 tbsp avocado oil
- Black pepper and salt to taste
- 1 teaspoon garlic powder
- 1 teaspoon onion powder
- 1/4 cup iceberg lettuce, torn
- 1 teaspoon cumin powder
- 2 tsp taco seasoning
- 4 tbsp sour cream
- 2 tsp smoked paprika
- 1 cup raw pecans, chopped
- 1 tbsp hemp seeds, hulled
- 1 medium tomato, sliced
- 1 2 lb ground beef

Directions:

- Heat one-half of the avocado oil inside a large skillet and cook the beef for 10 minutes. Sprinkle with salt pepper, chili powder and onions powder, cumin taco seasoning, and smokey chili powder.
- Add the hemp seeds, and stir fry over 10 mins. Mix in 3 tbsp Monterey Jack cheese to melt. Pour the filling into avocado holes, then top with a couple of slices of tomato and some lettuce, 1 tablespoon of sour cream, and the rest of the Monterey Jack cheese, and serve immediately.

Nutritional Information:

- Cal 400
- Net Carbs 6g
- Fat 69g
- Protein 39g

Recipe 88. Beef, Bell Pepper and Mushroom Kebabs

Serving Size: 4

Preparation Time: 10 minutes

Cooking Time: 15 minutes

Ingredients:

- 1 lb cremini mushrooms, halved
- 2 lbs of beef tri-tip steak cubed
- 2 tablespoons coconut oil
- 2 bell peppers of yellow
- 1 tbsp tamari sauce
- 1 lime Juiced
- 1 tbsp ginger powder
- 1/2 teaspoon ground cumin

Directions:

- Peel the bell peppers, then cut them into squares. In a bowl, combine coconut oil with tamari sauce, ginger, lime juice, and cumin. In the bowl, add the mushrooms, beef, and bell peppers.
- Remove the wrapper and put the beef, mushrooms, and bell peppers in this order onto skewers until all ingredients are used up. Grill the skewers for approximately about 5 minutes on each side. Transfer them to serving plates for serving warm. Serve with steamed cauliflower rice or asparagus braised.

Nutritional Information:

- Cal 379
- Net Carbs 4.2g
- Fat 23g
- Protein 49g

Recipe 89. Beef Burgers with Lettuce and Avocado

Serving Size: 2

Preparation Time: 10 minutes

Cooking Time: 15 minutes

Ingredients:

- 1/2 lb ground beef
- 1 green onion chopped
- 1/2 1 teaspoon garlic powder
- 1 Tbsp butter
- Black pepper and salt to taste
- 1 tbsp olive oil
- 1/2 tsp Dijon mustard
- 2 zero carb buns, halved
- 2 tbsp mayonnaise
- 1/2 tsp balsamic vinegar
- 2 tbsp iceberg lettuce, torn
- 1 avocado, sliced

Directions:

- Mix ground beef and green onions, mustard, garlic powder, salt, and pepper in a bowl. Create two hamburgers.
- Warm the olive oil and butter in a pan and cook the burgers for three minutes on each side.
- The buns are filled with mayonnaise, lettuce, balsamic vinegar, burgers, and avocado slices for serving.

Nutritional Information:

- Cal 400
- Net Carbs 4.6g
- Fat 52g
- Protein 34g

Recipe 90. Beef Cheese and Egg Casserole

Serving Size: 4

Preparation Time: 15 minutes

Cooking Time: 25 minutes

Ingredients:

- 2 tbsp olive oil
- 2 zucchinis, sliced
- 1/2 tsp nutmeg
- 1/2 lb ground beef
- Black pepper and salt to taste
- 5 eggs, beaten
- 1 cup Gouda cheese, grated
- 2 cups tomatoes cut into pieces
- 1 cup of heavy cream
- 1 Banana pepper cut into pieces
- 1 yellow onion cut into pieces
- 2 cloves of garlic to be chopped

Directions:

- Stir fry the garlic, banana pepper, and onions for 2 minutes until they are tender. Incorporate the ground beef and cook for about 4-6 minutes, stirring frequently. Sprinkle with salt, nutmeg, and pepper. Transfer the mix to an oven dish.
- Layer the tomatoes on top and place the zucchini slices over the top. Then bake for 30 minutes. Within a bowl, combine the eggs, cheese, and heavy cream. Add the salt and black pepper. Remove the baking dish and spread the cheese mixture on top. Bake for 10 minutes. Enjoy!

Nutritional Information:

- Cal 400
- Net Carbs 6.4g
- Fat 46g
- Protein 56g

Recipe 91. Beef Patties Topped with Broccoli Mash

Serving Size: 4

Preparation Time: 30 minutes

Cooking Time: 40 minutes

Ingredients:

- 1 Lb ground beef
- 1 egg
- 1/2 white onion chopped
- 2 tbsp olive oil
- 1 lb. broccoli
- 5 TBSP butter, softened
- 2 oz grated Parmesan
- 2 1 tbsp lemon juice
- Black pepper and salt to taste

Directions:

- Combine ground beef, egg, onion, salt, and pepper in a bowl. Mix well and form 6-8 cakes from the mix. Heat an olive oil pan and cook your patties for 6-8 mins on each side.
- Transfer them to the plate. Place lightly salted water in the pot on medium heat. Boil the Broccoli. Drain and place in the bowl. Add 2 tablespoons of butter as well as Parmesan cheese.
- Make use of the immersion blender to blend all the ingredients till smooth and creamy. Set aside. To make lemon butter make a mixture of the butter with lemon juice and salt and pepper in an ice-cold bowl. The cakes are served with broccoli Mash as well as lemon butter.

Nutritional Information:

- Cal 400
- Net Carbs 1.6g
- Fat 41g
- Protein 33g

Recipe 92. Beef Sausage and Okra Casserole

Serving Size: 4

Preparation Time: 20 minutes

Cooking Time: 35 minutes

Ingredients:

- 1/2 cup marinara sauce, sugar-free
- 1/2 cup okra, trimmed
- 1 tbsp olive oil
- 1 celery stalk cut into pieces
- 3/4 cup almond flour
- 1 egg
- 1 lb beef sausage chopped
- Black pepper and salt to taste
- 1/2 tbsp dried parsley
- 1/4 TSP red pepper flakes
- 1 cup Parmesan cheese grated
- 2 green onions cut into pieces
- 1/2 1 teaspoon garlic powder
- 1/4 teaspoon dried oregano
- 1/2 cup ricotta cheese
- 1 cup cheddar cheese grated

Directions:

- A bowl is used to mix with the peppers, sausage, flakes, oregano, Parmesan cheese, green onions, almond flour, salt parsley, celery, and garlic powder. Form balls, place them on a parchment-lined baking sheet, then place them on the baking sheet, bake at 390 F, then bake them for about 15 mins.
- Remove the baking sheets from the preheated oven and then cover with half the marinara sauce and Okra. Sprinkle the ricotta over, then the remaining marinara sauce. Sprinkle the cheddar cheese on top after baking for 10 minutes. Let it cool before serving.

Nutritional Information:

- Cal 400
- Net Carbs 7.3g
- Fat 33g
- Protein 33g

Recipe 93. Braised Chicken with Tomato and Garlic

Serving Size: 4

Preparation Time: 10 minutes

Cooking Time: 30 minutes

Ingredients:

- 2 tbsp butter
- 1 lb of chicken thighs
- Black pepper and salt to taste
- 3 cloves garlic, minced
- 2 cups tomatoes cut into pieces
- 1 eggplant cut into pieces
- 2 tablespoons basil leaves, chopped

Directions:

- In a pot at medium temperature. Add salt and black pepper, and cook for four minutes each aspect until the chicken is golden. Transfer to the plate. In the same pot, cook the garlic for one minute, pour in the tomatoes, and cook for about 8 minutes.
- Add the eggplant, then cook it for four minutes. Adjust the seasoning before returning the chicken to the pan. Add fresh basil leaves, then serve.

Nutritional Information:

- Cal 353
- Net Carbs 6.3g
- Fat 32g
- Protein 25g

Recipe 94. Broccoli and Carrot Turkey Bake

Serving Size: 4

Preparation Time: 20 minutes

Cooking Time: 45 minutes

Ingredients:

- 1 lb turkey breasts cooked and shredded
- 2 tbsp olive oil
- 1 carrot chopped, then shred
- 10 oz broccoli florets
- Half cup almond milk
- Half cup thick cream
- 1 cup cheddar cheese grated
- 4 tbsp pork rinds, crushed
- Black pepper and salt to taste

- 1/2 1 tsp of paprika
- 1 teaspoon oregano

Directions:

- Preheat the oven to a heat of 350 F and spray baking pans using cooking spray. Place the turkey in a large bowl, including almond milk, olive oil, broccoli, paprika oregano, paprika salt, and black pepper. Stir to mix.
- Transfer the mix onto the baking sheet. The heavy cream should be poured on top of the dish and then sprinkled the dish with cheddar cheese and pork rinds. Put it in the oven to simmer until bubbling for 20 to 25 minutes. Serve.

Nutritional Information:

- Cal 385
- Net Carbs 6g
- Fat 42g
- Protein 39g

Recipe 95. Buffalo Chicken Salad Wrap

Serving Size: 4

Preparation Time: 10 minutes

Cooking Time: 10 minutes

Ingredients:

- 3-4 ounces chicken breasts
- 2 whole-grain tortillas (12-inch diameter)
- 2 whole chipotle peppers
- 1/2 cup thinly sliced rutabaga
- 1/4 cup low-calorie mayonnaise
- 2 stalks celery, diced
- 2 carrots, cut into matchsticks
- 1 small yellow onion, diced
- 1/4 cup white wine vinegar
- 4 ounces spinach, cut into strips

Directions:

- Bake the chicken first for 10 minutes per side. Blend chipotle peppers with mayonnaise and wine vinegar in the blender. Dice the baked chicken into cubes or small chunks.
- Mix the chipotle mixture with all the ingredients except tortillas and spinach. Spread 2 ounces of spinach over the tortilla and scoop the stuffing on top. Wrap the tortilla and cut it into half. Serve.

Nutritional Information:

- Calories 300
- Fat 16.4 g
- Carbs 8.7 g
- Protein 38.5 g

Recipe 96. Burgundy Beef with Mushrooms

Serving Size: 4

Preparation Time: 30 minutes

Cooking Time: 1 hour 5 minutes

Ingredients:

- 1 Tbsp chopped parsley, chopped
- 1 Cup Burgundy red wine
- 1 Tbsp dried thyme
- Black pepper and salt to taste
- 1 leaf of a bay
- 1 cup beef stock
- 1 Lb of stewed beef cubed
- Twelve pearl onions cut in half
- 1 tomato cut into pieces
- 4 oz pancetta, chopped
- 2 cloves of garlic, minced
- 1/2 lb. of mushrooms and chopped

Directions:

- Affix a skillet to high heat. Stir in pancetta and beef. Let them cook until lightly browned. Set aside. Add the prepared mushrooms, onions, and garlic and cook for five minutes.
- Pour into the wine to make the pan's bottom, and add the cattle stock, bay leaves, and tomatoes. Add salt and pepper, and add thyme. Add the pancetta and meat covered, and cook for about 50 minutes. Serve with fresh parsley.

Nutritional Information:

- Cal 367
- Net Carbs 5g
- Fat 24g
- Protein 33g

Recipe 97. Cabbage and Broccoli Chicken Casserole

Serving Size: 4

Preparation Time: 15 minutes

Cooking Time: 55 minutes

Ingredients:

- 1 tablespoon coconut oil melt
- 2 cups mozzarella, grated
- 1/2 head of cabbage, shredded
- 1 head broccoli, cut into florets
- 1-lb breasts of chicken
- cubed 1 cup mayonnaise
- 1/3 cup chicken stock
- Black pepper and salt to taste
- Juice from 1 lemon
- 1 tbsp of cilantro, chopped

Directions:

- Cover a baking dish with coconut oil. Set chicken pieces on the bottom. Add the broccoli and the green cabbage, and then sprinkle with half of the mozzarella cheese. A bowl mixes the mayonnaise, black pepper, lemon juice, stock, and salt. Spread the mix over the chicken, top with the remaining mozzarella cheese, and then wrap in aluminum foil.
- In the oven for 30-minutes at 350 F. Open aluminum foil and cook for an additional 20 minutes. Add cilantro to the dish and enjoy.

Nutritional Information:

- Cal 333
- Net Carbs 6.4g
- Fat 32g
- Protein 52g

Recipe 98. Cauliflower and Beef Casserole

Serving Size: 4

Preparation Time: 15 minutes

Cooking Time: 40 minutes

Ingredients:

- 2 tbsp olive oil
- 1 2 lb ground beef
- Black pepper and salt to taste
- 1/2 cup cauli rice
- 1 tbsp chopped parsley
- 1 cup kohlrabi, chopped
- 5 oz can diced tomatoes
- 1/2 cup mozzarella cheese, grated

Directions:

- The olive oil is actually heated in a saucepan at medium temperature. Grill the meat for 5-6 mins until it's no longer pink. Breaking it up with a wooden spatula. Include kohlrabi, cauli rice tomatoes, kohlrabi, and 1/4 cup of water. Stir well and cook and cover with a cover for about 5 mins to make the sauce thicker.
- Add Black pepper and salt. Pour the prepared beef mixture into the baking dish, spreading it all over. Sprinkle with mozzarella cheese. Bake in the oven for approximately about 15 minutes, at 338 F, till the cheese melts and the crust is golden brown. Take it out and let it cool for four minutes. Serve with sprinkles of parsley.

Nutritional Information:

- Cal 391
- Net Carbs 6.3g
- Fat 23g
- Protein 30g

Recipe 99. Chicken and Brussels Sprout Bake

Serving Size: 4

Preparation Time: 20 minutes

Cooking Time: 30 minutes

Ingredients:

- 1 1/2 lb chopped Brussels sprouts
- 1-lb breasts of chicken cubed
- 3 tablespoons butter
- 5 cloves of garlic, minced
- 1 1/4 cup coconut cream
- 2 cups of grated Cheese
- 3/4 cup chopped Parmesan
- Black pepper and salt to taste

Directions:

- Preheat the oven to a heat of 400 F. Sprinkle the chicken by adding salt and black pepper. Melt butter in a large-sized pan and sauté the chicken cubes for 6 minutes, then transfer to an oven-safe plate. Add the Brussels sprouts and garlic to the skillet and cook until an attractive color appears. Add coconut cream to the mix and cook for 4 minutes.
- Mix with chicken cubes. Put the sauté in a baking dish, then add cheddar and Parmesan cheeses. Cook for about 10 minutes. Serve warm and have a blast!

Nutritional Information:

- Cal 318
- Net Carbs 7g

- Fat 34g
- Protein 13g

Recipe 100. Chicken Curry

Serving Size: 2

Preparation Time: 10 minutes

Cooking Time: 30 minutes

Ingredients:

- 2 chicken breasts
- 1 garlic clove
- 1 small onion
- 1 zucchini
- 2 carrots
- 1 box of bamboo shoots or sprouts
- 1 cup coconut milk
- 1 Tablespoon. tomato paste
- 2 tablespoons. yellow curry paste

Directions:

- Mince the onion and sauté in a pan with a little oil for a few minutes.
- Add chicken cut in large cubes and crushed garlic, salt, pepper and sauté quickly over high heat until meat begins to color.
- Pour zucchini and carrots in thick slices into the pan.
- Sear over high heat for a few minutes, then add the coconut milk, tomato sauce, bamboo shoots and one to two tablespoons curry paste, depending on your taste.
- Cook over low heat and cover for 30 to 45 minutes, stirring occasionally
- Once cooked, divide the chicken curry between 2 containers
- Store the containers in the refrigerator

Nutritional Information:

- Calories: 626
- Fat: 53.2 g
- Carbs: 9 g
- Protein 27.8 g

Recipe 101. Chicken with Noodles

Serving Size: 6

Preparation Time: 15 minutes

Cooking Time: 30 minutes

Ingredients:

- 4 chicken breasts, skinless, boneless
- 1-pound pasta (angel hair, or linguine, or ramen)
- ½ teaspoon sesame oil
- 1 Tablespoon canola oil
- 2 Tablespoons chili paste
- 1 onion, diced
- 2 garlic cloves, chopped coarsely
- ½ cup of soy sauce
- ½ medium cabbage, sliced
- 2 carrots, chopped coarsely

Directions:

- Cook your pasta in a large pot. Mix the canola oil, sesame oil, and chili paste and heat for 25 seconds in a large pot. Add the onion, cook for 2 minutes. Put the garlic and fry within 20 seconds. Add the chicken, cook on each side 5 - 7 minutes, until cooked through.
- Remove the mix from the pan, set aside. Add the cabbage, carrots, cook until the vegetables are tender. Pour everything back into the pan. Add the noodles. Pour in the soy sauce and combine thoroughly. Heat for 5 minutes. Serve immediately.

Nutritional Information:

- Calories - 210
- Protein - 30g
- Carbohydrates - 32g
- Fat - 18g

Recipe 102. Cilantro Beef Balls stuffed with Mascarpone

Serving Size: 4

Preparation Time: 20 minutes

Cooking Time: 45 minutes

Ingredients:

- 1 clove of garlic, chopped
- 1 2 lb ground beef
- A small, small onion that has been chopped
- 1 jalapeno pepper, chopped
- 2 tsp cilantro
- 1/2 tsp allspice
- 1 teaspoon cumin
- Black pepper and salt to taste
- 1 tbsp butter and 1 1/2 tbsp of melted
- 1/2 cup mascarpone cheese
- 1/4 tsp turmeric
- 1/4 tsp baking soda
- 1 cup flax meal
- 3/4 cup Coconut flour

Directions:

- Puree onions with jalapeno, garlic, and 1/4 cup of liquid in the blender. Put 1 tbsp of butter in a large-sized skillet at medium-low temperature. The beef is cooked for three minutes. Add the onion mix, then cook it for two minutes. Add cilantro and salt, cumin, turmeric, allspice, and pepper, and cook until 3 mins.
- A bowl is used to mix Flax meal, coconut flour, and baking soda. In another medium-sized bowl, mix the melted butter and the Mascarpone cheese. Mix the two ingredients to form a dough. Make balls of the mixture, place the balls on parchment and roll each one into circles. Divide the beef mixture into half of the dough circle, cover with the second half, seal the edges, and place on a sheet lined with. Bake for approximately about 25 to 30 minutes at 350 F.

Nutritional Information:

- Cal 374
- Net Carbs 9g
- Fat 26g
- Protein 33g

Recipe 103. Coconut-Olive Beef with Mushrooms

Serving Size: 4

Preparation Time: 15 minutes

Cooking Time: 30 minutes

Ingredients:

- 1 cup of button mushroom, cut into slices
- 4 ribeye steaks
- 3 Tbsp butter
- 1 yellow onion cut into pieces
- 1/3 cup coconut milk
- 2 Tbsp coconut cream
- 1/2 1 tsp dried thyme
- 2 TBSP chopped parsley
- 3 tbsp black olives, sliced

Directions:

- Make 2 tablespoons of butter and warm it in a large pan at medium-low temperature. Add the mushrooms and sauté for about 4 minutes until they are tender. Add the onion and cook for an additional 3 minutes. Remove and set aside.
- Melt the butter remaining into the hot pan, and fry the steak in the skillet for about 10 minutes. Return the prepared onions and mushrooms to the pan and add coconut cream, milk, and thyme, 1 tablespoon of chopped parsley. Stir and simmer for two minutes. Add black olives, mix and turn off the heat. Serve with the rest of the parsley.

Nutritional Information:

- Cal 400
- Net Carbs 2.9g
- Fat 48g
- Protein 71g

Recipe 104. Country Spare Ribs with White Beans

Serving Size: 8

Preparation Time: 20 minutes

Cooking Time: 2 hours 20 minutes

Ingredients:

- 2 pounds lean country pork ribs
- ¼ cup canola oil
- ½ cup red peppers, diced
- 1 cup diced onion
- ½ cup celery, diced
- 2 tablespoons flour
- 1 tablespoon diced garlic
- 1 cup canned diced plum tomatoes
- ½ cup dried navy beans
- 4 cups vegetable stock
- 1 tablespoon Dijon mustard
- 1 tablespoon garlic powder
- 2 tablespoons Worcestershire sauce
- 1 tablespoon dried oregano
- 2 sprigs fresh thyme
- 1 bay leaf 1 teaspoon salt
- 1 teaspoon fresh ground black pepper
- Steamed brown rice

Directions:

- Preheat oven to 350°F.
- Place ribs on sheet pan in oven and cook 10 minutes per side to render fat and brown.
- Heat Dutch oven. Add oil, peppers, onions, and celery. Cook about 6–7 minutes or until onions are clear.
- Add flour and stir. Add garlic and beans, place ribs on top. Pour stock, tomatoes, mustard, garlic powder, Worcestershire, oregano, thyme, bay leaf, salt, and pepper over ribs.
- Place Dutch oven in oven and simmer ribs and beans for 1½–2 hours, stirring every 15 minutes.
- Serve over brown rice.

Nutritional Information:

- Calories: 390
- Fat: 18g
- Protein: 30g
- Carbohydrates: 30g

Recipe 105. Creamy Chicken with Caramelized Leeks

Serving Size: 4

Preparation Time: 20 minutes

Cooking Time: 55 minutes

Ingredients:

- 1 lb chopped leeks, 1 inch sliced
- 1/2 teaspoon onion powder
- 1/2 1 teaspoon garlic powder
- 2 tbsp Lard
- 2 tbsp olive oil
- Half cup thick cream
- 1/2 teaspoon yellow mustard
- 1 tbsp rosemary chopped,
- 1 lb of chicken thighs
- Black pepper and salt to taste

Directions:

- Preheat the oven to 360 F. Mix in a bowl black pepper, salt, garlic powder, and onion powder. Rub the mix on the chicken. Heat the oil with olives in a pan to cook the chicken till golden. About 6-8 minutes. Transfer the chicken to a baking dish, and add 1 cup of water. Roast for approximately about 20 minutes or until the skin turns crispy and golden.
- Combine the thick cream, salt, mustard, and pepper, then pour it into your chicken recipe. Bake for five more minutes. In the skillet, then add the leeks. Then cook for 8-10 minutes, or until they are lightly caramelized. Sprinkle with Black pepper and salt. Sprinkle your chicken off with rosemary, and serve it with leeks served on the side.

Nutritional Information:

- Cal 359
- Net Carbs 4.2g
- Fat 28g
- Protein 35g

Recipe 106. Eggplant Beef Lasagna

Serving Size: 4

Preparation Time: 30 minutes

Cooking Time: 1 hour 5 minutes

Ingredients:

- 2 large, ripe eggplants cut lengthwise
- 2 tbsp olive oil
- 1/2 red chili chopped
- 1/2 lb ground beef
- 2 cloves of garlic, minced
- 1 shallot chopped
- 1 cup tomato sauce
- Black pepper and salt to taste
- 2 tsp sweet paprika
- 1 Tbsp dried thyme
- 1 teaspoon dried basil
- 1 cup mozzarella cheese, grated
- 1 cup chicken broth

Directions:

- The oil should be heated in a skillet. Cook the beef for about 4 minutes, breaking up any lumps you find as you stir. Add shallot, garlic chili tomato sauce salt, paprika, salt, and black pepper. Cook for 5 minutes. Place 1/3 of the slices of eggplant in a baking dish that has been greased.
- Then, top with 1/3 of the beef mix and repeat the layering two times more using the same amount. Add thyme and basil to the dish. Incorporate your chicken broth. Add the cheese over the top and place the baking dish into the oven. The lasagna is baked for about 35 minutes at the temperature of 380 F. Take the lasagna out and allow it to rest for 10 minutes before serving.

Nutritional Information:

- Cal 399
- Net Carbs 9.8g
- Fat 20g
- Protein 41g

Recipe 107. Feta and Kale Chicken Bake

Serving Size: 6

Preparation Time: 20 minutes

Cooking Time: 35 minutes

Ingredients:

- 1/4 cup of shredded
- Monterey Jack cheese

- 4 chicken breasts to be cut into strips
- 2 tbsp olive oil
- 1 small onion chopped
- 2 cloves of garlic, minced
- 1/2 1 tbsp red wine vinegar
- 1 1/2 crushed tomatoes
- 2 tbsp tomato paste
- 1 teaspoon Italian seasoning
- 2 medium zucchinis, chopped
- 1 cup of baby Kale
- 1/4 cup of crumbled cheese feta
- 1 cup of grated Parmesan
- Black pepper and salt to taste

Directions:

- Preheat the oven to a heat of 400 F. Warm the olive oil inside a pan, add the chicken, sprinkle with salt and pepper, and cook for 8 mins to remove from the heat. In the skillet, add sauté garlic and onions for 3 minutes. Mix in tomatoes and vinegar along with tomato paste. Cook until 8 minutes.
- Add salt and pepper along with Italian seasoning. Mix in zucchinis, chicken, kale, feta, and salt. Put the mix in an oven-proof dish. Sprinkle it with Monterey Jack cheese. It should bake for around 15 minutes until it melts and turns golden. Serve the Cheese with Parmesan, and then enjoy.

Nutritional Information:

- Cal 359
- Net Carbs 3.6g
- Fat 28g
- Protein 46g

Recipe 108. Green Bean and Broccoli Chicken Stir Fry

Serving Size: 2

Preparation Time: 15 minutes

Cooking Time: 45 minutes

Ingredients:

- 2 breasts of chicken Cut into strips
- 2 tbsp olive oil
- 1 teaspoon red pepper flakes
- 1 teaspoon onion powder
- Fresh ginger 1 tbsp grated
- 1/4 cup tamari sauce
- 1/2 1 teaspoon garlic powder
- 1/2 cup of water
- 1/2 cup 1/2 cup xylitol
- 4 oz green beans, chopped
- 1/2 tsp of xanthan gum
- 1/2 cup chopped green onions chopped
- 10 oz broccoli florets

Directions:

- Steam the broccoli and green beans for 5-6 minutes until the broccoli is a tender, crisp, and still vibrant green. Put aside. Heat the olive oil inside a saucepan on medium heat. Cook both the ginger and chicken for four minutes.
- Mix the rest of the ingredients, and let it cook down for fifteen minutes. Add the broccoli and green beans and cook for six minutes. Serve.

Nutritional Information:

- Cal 311
- Net Carbs 6.2g
- Fat 25g
- Protein 28g

Recipe 109. Grilled Beef Steaks and Vegetable Medley

Serving Size: 2

Preparation Time: 15 minutes

Cooking Time: 30 minutes

Ingredients:

- One red bell pepper seeded to cut into strips
- 2 sirloin beef steaks
- Black pepper and salt to taste
- 2 tbsp olive oil
- 1 1/2 tbsp balsamic vinegar
- 1/4 lb asparagus, cut
- 1/2 cup of mushrooms, cut into slices
- Half cup Snow Peas
- 1-small onion cut into quarters
- 1 garlic clove, cut in half

Directions:

- Put in a bowl and add asparagus and mushrooms, snow peas, bell pepper, onions, and garlic. Mix salt, pepper, salt, and olive oil with balsamic vinegar together in small bowls and then pour half the mix over the vegetables and stir until it is all combined. In the remaining oil mixture, add the beef and mix to coat.
- Grill pans are heated to high temperatures. Place the prepared steaks on the grill pan, and cook for 6-8 minutes on both sides. Remove the steaks and place

them aside. Place the marinade and vegetables into the pan and simmer for five minutes before turning every so often. Divide the vegetables onto plates. Add beef on top and drizzle the sauce from the pan and serve.

Nutritional Information:

- Cal 400
- Net Carbs 7g
- Fat 31g
- Protein 37g

Recipe 110. Ground Pork Stuffed Mushrooms

Serving Size: 4

Preparation Time: 20 minutes

Cooking Time: 30 minutes

Ingredients:

- 1/4 cup of shredded Parmesan
- 12 portobello mushroom caps
- 1/2 lb ground pig
- 2 tbsp butter
- 1 tsp paprika
- 7 oz cream cheese
- 3 tablespoons chopped Chives, chopped
- Salt and pepper as desired

Directions:

- Preheat the oven to 390 F. Make batter by melting it in a pan, add the ground pork, and sprinkle with salt, paprika, and pepper. Stir-fry until golden brown, about 10 minutes. Mix in 2/3 of the cream cheese and chives until evenly mixed.
- Pour the mixture into the mushrooms and then transfer them to an oven-proof baking sheet that has been greased. Then, top with the Parmesan cheese and bake until the mushrooms become golden, and the cheese is melted about 10 minutes. Sprinkle with remaining chopped chives, and serve.

Nutritional Information:

- Cal 382
- Net Carbs 4.2g
- Fat 29g
- Protein 21g

Recipe 111. Ham and Cheese Stuffed Chicken

Serving Size: 4

Preparation Time: 25 minutes

Cooking Time: 40 minutes

Ingredients:

- 2 tbsp olive oil
- 1/4 cup Ham chopped
- 1 cup spinach
- 2 tbsp mozzarella, shredded
- 1/3 cup tomato-basil sauce
- 1 2 lb chicken breasts

Directions:

- Preheat the oven up to a heat of 400 F and spray the baking dish with olive oil in half. Mix the mozzarella cheese, the chopped ham with spinach, and ham in a dish, and mix thoroughly. Cut pockets in the side of chicken breasts.
- Put the chicken breasts in the pockets with the mix you prepared. Then, brush your tops with oil. Place the dish on the baking tray and bake for about 25 minutes. Pour the tomato-basil sauce on top and bake in the oven. Cook for 5 more minutes. Serve.

Nutritional Information:

- Cal 343
- Net Carbs 4.7g
- Fat 3g
- Protein 36g

Recipe 112. Herby Veggies and Chicken Casserole

Serving Size: 4

Preparation Time: 25 minutes

Cooking Time: 35 minutes

Ingredients:

- 2 chicken breasts cubed
- 3/4 lb Brussels sprouts,
- halved 2 large zucchinis, chopped
- 2 bell peppers, red quartered
- 1/4 cup olive oil
- 1 tablespoon balsamic vinegar
- 1 teaspoon chopped thyme leaves
- 1 teaspoon chopped
- rosemary 1/2 cup
- Toasted walnuts
- Black pepper and salt to taste

Directions:

- Bake at 400 F. Scatter Brussels sprouts and bell peppers, zucchinis, and chicken on baking sheets. Sprinkle with the prepared salt and pepper and drizzle olive oil.
- Combine with balsamic vinegar. Sprinkle with rosemary and thyme. Then bake for 25 minutes, shaking every so often. Sprinkle with walnuts. Serve.

Nutritional Information:

- Cal 391
- Net Carbs 6.7g
- Fat 34g
- Protein 35g

Recipe 113. Honey Spiced Cajun Chicken

Serving Size: 4

Preparation Time: 15 minutes

Cooking Time: 20 minutes

Ingredients:

- 2 chicken breasts, skinless, boneless
- 1 Tablespoon butter or margarine
- 1 pound of linguini
- 3 large mushrooms, sliced
- 1 large tomato, diced
- 2 Tablespoons regular mustard
- 4 Tablespoons honey
- 3 ounces low-fat table cream
- Parsley, roughly chopped

Directions:

- Wash and dry the chicken breasts. Warm 1 tablespoon of butter or margarine in a large pan. Add the chicken breasts. Season with salt and pepper. Cook on each side 6 – 10 minutes, until cooked thoroughly. Pull the chicken breasts from the pan. Set aside.
- Cook the linguine as stated to instructions on the package in a large pot. Save 1 cup of the pasta water. Drain the linguine. Add the mushrooms, tomatoes to the pan from cooking the chicken. Heat until they are tender.
- Add the honey, mustard, and cream. Combine thoroughly. Add the chicken and linguine to the pan. Stir until coated. Garnish with parsley. Serve immediately.

Nutritional Information:

- Calories - 312
- Protein - 12g
- Carbohydrates - 56g
- Fat - 20g

Recipe 114. Juicy Beef Meatballs

Serving Size: 4

Preparation Time: 20 minutes

Cooking Time: 30 minutes

Ingredients:

- 1 2 lb ground beef
- Black pepper and salt to taste
- 1/2 1 teaspoon garlic powder
- 1 1/4 tbsp of coconut aminos
- 1 cup of beef broth
- 1/4 cup of almond flour
- 1 tbsp fresh parsley chopped
- 1 onion, cut into slices
- 2 Tbsp butter
- 1 tbsp olive oil
- 1/4 cup sour cream

Directions:

- Preheat the oven to a heat of 390 F and grease the baking dish. A bowl mix of beef, salt and cinnamon powder, garlic powder parsley, 1 tablespoon of coconut aminos black pepper, and 1/2 cup beef stock. Make patties and place them on the baking pan. Cook for about 18 mins.
- Place a pan with butter and olive oil on moderate heat. Add the onion, then cook it for three minutes. Mix in the remaining beef stock, sour cream, and coconut aminos remaining, and then bring it to a boil. Adjust the seasoning by adding salt and black pepper. Serve the meatballs with onions sauce.

Nutritional Information:

- Cal 398
- Net Carbs 4.7g
- Fat 24g
- Protein 31g

Recipe 115. Juicy Chicken with Broccoli and Pine Nuts

Serving Size: 4

Preparation Time: 20 minutes

Cooking Time: 25 minutes

Ingredients:

- 2 tbsp olive oil
- 2 breasts of chicken that have been cut into strips
- 2 tbsp Worcestershire sauce
- 2 tsp balsamic vinegar
- 2 tsp 2 tsp
- 1 lemon juiced
- 1 cup of pine nuts
- 2 cups of broccoli.
- One onion, finely cut
- Black pepper and salt to taste
- 1 tbsp chopped cilantro, cut

Directions:

- In a dry pan at moderate temperature, roast your pine nuts for two mins until the nuts are golden. Then set aside. In the same pan, heat olive oil and cook the onion for four minutes until it is soft and brown before transferring it from the nuts. A bowl is used to mix together the balsamic vinegar, Worcestershire sauce, lemon juice, and xanthan gum; keep aside.
- Add the chicken to the skillet and cook for four minutes. In the meantime, add the broccoli and salt, and black pepper. Stir fry, and then add the mixture of lemons. Let the mixture cook for four minutes, then add the onion and pine nuts. Stir again and cook for a minute. Serve the stir-fry chicken with cilantro.

Nutritional Information:

- Cal 386
- Net Carbs 6.4g
- Fat 30g
- Protein 20g

Recipe 116. Lemongrass Prawns

Serving Size: 2

Preparation Time: 10 minutes

Cooking Time: 15 minutes

Ingredients:

- ½ red chili pepper, seeded and chopped
- 2 lemongrass stalks
- ½ lb. prawns, deveined and peeled
- 6 tbsp. butter
- ¼ tsp. smoked paprika

Directions:

- Preheat the oven to a heat of 390° F and grease a baking dish.
- Mix together red chili pepper, butter, smoked paprika, and prawns in a bowl.
- Marinate for about 2 hours and then thread the prawns on the lemongrass stalks.
- Arrange the threaded prawns on the baking dish and transfer them to the oven.
- Bake for about 15 minutes and dish out to serve immediately.
- Place the prawns in a dish and set them aside to cool for meal prepping.
- Divide it into the prepared 2 containers and close the lid. Refrigerate for about 4 days and reheat in microwave before serving.

Nutritional Information:

- Calories: 322
- Fat: 18 g
- Carbs: 3.8 g
- Protein: 34.8 g

Recipe 117. Marinated Fried Chicken

Serving Size: 2

Preparation Time: 15 minutes

Cooking Time: 15 minutes

Ingredients:

- 2 tbsp olive oil
- 2 breasts of chicken Cut into strips
- 1/2 cup pork rinds, crushed
- 8 oz jarred pickle juice
- 1 egg

Directions:

- Cover the chicken with the juice of a pickle in a bowl. Refrigerate for 12 hours while covered. Whisk eggs in a bowl and put the pork rinds in an additional bowl. In a bowl, dip the chicken pieces into the egg, and then dip them in the pork rinds. Be sure to coat them thoroughly.
- Set the pan on moderate heat, and then warm your olive oil. Cook the chicken for 3 minutes per side. Transfer to paper towels and then rinse off the grease. Serve warm, topped with homemade Ketchup if you wish.

Nutritional Information:

- Cal 389
- Net Carbs 2g
- Fat 46g
- Protein 45g

Recipe 118. Oaxacan Chicken

Serving Size: 2

Preparation Time: 15 minutes

Cooking Time: 28 minutes

Ingredients:

- 1 4-ounce chicken breast, skinned and halved
- ½ cup uncooked long-grain rice
- 1 teaspoon of extra-virgin olive oil
- ½ cup low-sodium salsa
- ½ cup chicken stock, mixed with 2 Tablespoons water
- ¾ cup baby carrots
- 2 tablespoons green olives, pitted and chopped
- 2 Tablespoons dark raisins
- ½ teaspoon ground Cinnamon
- 2 Tablespoons fresh cilantro or parsley, coarsely chopped

Directions:

- Warm oven to 350 F. In a large saucepan that can go in the oven, heat the olive oil. Add the rice. Sauté the rice until it begins to pop, approximately 2 minutes.
- Add the salsa, baby carrots, green olives, dark raisins, halved chicken breast, chicken stock, and ground cinnamon. Bring the mix to a simmer, stir once.
- Cover the mixture tightly, bake in the oven until the chicken stock has been completely absorbed, approximately 25 minutes. Sprinkle fresh cilantro or parsley, mix. Serve immediately.

Nutritional Information:

- Calories - 343
- Protein - 102g
- Carbohydrates - 66g
- Fat - 18g

Recipe 119. Olive Capers Chicken

Serving Size: 4

Preparation Time: 15 minutes

Cooking Time: 16 minutes

Ingredients:

- 2 pounds chicken
- 1/3 cup chicken stock
- 3.5 ounces Capers
- 6 ounces olives
- 1/4 cup fresh basil
- 1 tablespoon olive oil
- 1 teaspoon oregano
- 2 garlic cloves, minced
- 2 tablespoons red wine vinegar
- 1/8 teaspoon pepper
- 1/4 teaspoon salt

Directions:

- Put olive oil in your instant pot and set the pot on sauté mode.
- Add chicken to the pot and sauté for 3-4 minutes. Add remaining ingredients and stir well. Seal pot with the lid and select manual and set timer for 12 minutes.
- Serve and enjoy.

Nutritional Information:

- Calories: 433
- Fat: 15.2g
- Protein: 66.9g
- Carbs: 4.8g

Recipe 120. Oregano Chicken Thighs

Serving Size: 6

Preparation Time: 15 minutes

Cooking Time: 20 minutes

Ingredients:

- 12 chicken thighs
- 1 teaspoon dried parsley
- ¼ teaspoon pepper and salt.
- ½ cup extra virgin essential olive oil
- 4 minced garlic cloves
- 1 cup chopped oregano
- ¼ cup low-sodium veggie stock

Directions:

- In your food processor, mix parsley with oregano, garlic, salt, pepper, and stock and pulse. Put chicken thighs within the bowl, add oregano paste, toss, cover, and then leave aside within the fridge for 10 minutes.
- Heat the kitchen grill over medium heat, add chicken pieces, close the lid and cook for twenty or so minutes with them. Divide between plates and serve!

Nutritional Information:

- Calories: 254
- Fat:3 g
- Carbs:7 g
- Protein:17 g

Recipe 121. Pan-Fried Chicken with Anchovy Tapenade

Serving Size: 2

Preparation Time: 15 minutes

Cooking Time: 20 minutes

Ingredients:

- 1 breast of chicken, divided into four pieces
- 2 tbsp olive oil
- 1 clove of garlic, minced
- Tapenade 2 tbsp olive oil 1 cup black olives
- 1 oz of anchovy fillets cleaned
- 1 clove of garlic crushed
- Black pepper and salt to taste
- 1 cup of fresh basil chopped
- 1 2 tbsp lemon juice

Directions:

- Place a pan on medium-high heat. Add olive oil. Mix in the garlic for 2 minutes and then cook. Put the chicken pieces in and cook for about 4 minutes. Transfer to a plate for serving.
- Chop the anchovy and black olives and place them in the food processor. Add olive oil and basil and the juice of a lemon, salt, and black pepper. Mix thoroughly. Pour the tapenade on top of the chicken, and serve.

Nutritional Information:

- Cal 392
- Net Carbs 3.3g
- Fat 47g
- Protein 35g

Recipe 122. Pancetta and Cheese Stuffed Chicken

Serving Size: 2

Preparation Time: 15 minutes

Cooking Time: 35 minutes

Ingredients:

- 4 slices pancetta
- 2 tbsp olive oil
- 2 chicken breasts
- 1 clove of garlic, chopped
- 1 shallot finely chopped
- 2 tbsp dried oregano
- 4 oz mascarpone cheese
- 1 lemon, zested
- Black pepper and salt to taste

Directions:

- In an oven-proof skillet. Sauté the shallots and garlic for three minutes. Add black pepper, salt as well as lemon zest. Transfer the mixture to a bowl and allow it to cool. Mix in the mascarpone cheese and oregano. Create a pocket inside the breasts of each chicken.
- Fill the pockets with the cheese mixture, then cover them with the chicken cut-out. The breasts are then wrapped with two pancetta slices and tied to the ends using toothpicks. Place the chicken on a baking sheet that has been greased. In the oven, cook for about 20 minutes at 350 F. Warm it up.

Nutritional Information:

- Cal 336
- Net Carbs 8.2g
- Fat 45g
- Protein 45g

Recipe 123. Parmesan Chicken Meatballs

Serving Size: 4

Preparation Time: 10 minutes

Cooking Time: 15 minutes

Ingredients:

- 4 tomatoes sundried, chopped
- 1/2 cup passata tomato sauce
- 1 lb of ground chicken
- 2 tbsp basil chopped
- 1/2 teaspoon garlic powder
- 1 egg
- Black pepper and salt to taste
- 3/4 cup almond flour
- 2 tbsp olive oil
- 3 tablespoons Parmesan cheese grated

Directions:

- Combine everything but the basil and oil in the bowl to make meatballs.
- Sprinkle the sauce over them to cook the meatballs for four minutes. Serve with basil.

Nutritional Information:

- Cal 363
- Net Carbs 5g

- Fat 27g
- Protein 22g

Recipe 124. Peanut-Crusted Chicken

Serving Size: 4

Preparation Time: 10 minutes

Cooking Time: 25 minutes

Ingredients:

- 1 egg, beaten
- Black pepper and salt to taste
- 3 tablespoons of canola oil
- 1/4 cup ground peanuts
- 2 breast halves of a chicken
- Lemon slices to garnish

Directions:

- Sprinkle your chicken seasoning with pepper and salt. Dip it in the egg, then dip in the ground peanuts. Heat the oil from the canola in a skillet over moderate heat.
- Brown the chicken for two minutes on each side. Transfer the chicken to a baking tray and place it in the preheated 350 F oven to bake in the oven for 10 mins. Serve with slices of lemon.

Nutritional Information:

- Cal 354
- Net Carbs 4.7g
- Fat 52g
- Protein 46g

Recipe 125. Pesto Chicken Cacciatore

Serving Size: 4

Preparation Time: 20 minutes

Cooking Time: 50 minutes

Ingredients:

- Chicken breasts 2 pounds cubed
- 3 tbsp butter
- 1/2 lemon juiced
- 3 tbsp basil pesto
- 3/4 cup heavy cream
- 1/2 cup cream cheese, softened
- 1 celery chopped
- 1/2 cup diced tomatoes
- 1 lb of radishes cut into slices
- 1/2 cup of shredded Pepper Jack

Directions:

- Preheat the oven to 400 F. Mix pesto, lemon juice, heavy cream, and cream cheese in a bowl. Set aside. In a skillet, melt butter to cook your chicken until it is no more pink, about 8 minutes. Transfer the chicken to a casserole that has been greased with the pesto mixture over the top.
- Add tomatoes, celery, and radishes. Add Pepper Jack cheese on top. Serve warm and have a blast!

Nutritional Information:

- Cal 371
- Net Carbs 5.8g
- Fat 47g
- Protein 49g

Recipe 126. Pimiento Cheese Pork Meatballs

Serving Size: 4

Preparation Time: 10 minutes

Cooking Time: 20 minutes

Ingredients:

- 1 1/2 1 lb ground pork
- 1 large egg
- 2 tbsp olive oil
- 1/4 cup chopped pimientos
- 1/3 cup mayonnaise
- 3 tbsp softened cream cheese
- 1 teaspoon 1 tsp
- 1 pinch of cayenne pepper
- 1 tbsp Dijon mustard
- 4 oz grated Parmesan cheese

Directions:

- A bowl mixes the pimientos with mayonnaise, cream cheese, cayenne pepper, paprika mustard, Parmesan cheddar, pork ground, and egg.
- Mix the ingredients and create large meatballs. Make sure to heat olive oil in an oven-proof skillet. Fry your meatballs in small batches, turning them over until golden brown, about 10 minutes total. Serve with a salad if you wish.

Nutritional Information:

- Cal 393
- Net Carbs 4.5g
- Fat 69g

- Protein 37g

Recipe 127. Pork Chops with Nutmeg

Serving Size: 3

Preparation Time: 10 minutes

Cooking Time: 40 minutes

Ingredients:

- 8 ounces mushrooms, sliced
- ¼ cup coconut milk
- 1 teaspoon garlic powder
- 1 yellow onion, chopped
- 3 pork chops, boneless
- 2 teaspoons nutmeg, ground
- 1 tablespoon balsamic vinegar
- ½ cup olive oil

Directions:

- Heat up a large-sized pan with the oil over medium heat, add mushrooms and onions, stir, and cook for 5 minutes.
- Add pork chops, nutmeg and garlic powder and cook for 5 minutes more.
- Add vinegar and coconut milk, toss, introduce in the oven and bake at 350 degrees F and bake for 30 minutes.
- Divide between plates and serve.
- Enjoy!

Nutritional Information:

- Calories 260
- Fat 10
- Carbs 8
- Protein 22

Recipe 128. Pork with Apple Sauce

Serving Size: 6

Preparation Time: 10 minutes

Cooking Time: 1 hour 30 minutes

Ingredients:

- 1 tablespoon lemon juice
- 2 cups low-sodium veggie stock
- 17 ounces apples, cored and cut into wedges
- 2 pounds pork belly, trimmed and scored
- 1 teaspoon sweet paprika
- Black pepper to the taste
- A drizzle of olive oil

Directions:

- In your blender, mix the stock with apples and lemon juice and pulse very well.
- Put pork belly in a roasting pan, add apple sauce, also add the oil, paprika and black pepper, toss well, introduce in the oven, and bake at 380 degrees F for 1 hour and 30 minutes.
- Slice the pork belly, divide it between plates, drizzle the sauce all over and serve.
- Enjoy!

Nutritional Information:

- Calories 356
- Fat 14
- Carbs 10
- Protein 27

Recipe 129. Pork with Scallions and Peanuts

Serving Size: 4

Preparation Time: 10 minutes

Cooking Time: 16 minutes

Ingredients:

- 2 tablespoons lime juice
- 2 tablespoons coconut aminos
- 1 and ½ tablespoons brown sugar
- 5 garlic cloves, minced
- 3 tablespoons olive oil
- Black pepper to the taste
- 1 yellow onion, cut into wedges
- 1 and ½ pound pork tenderloin, cubed
- 3 tablespoons peanuts, chopped
- 2 scallions, chopped

Directions:

- In a bowl, mix lime juice with aminos and sugar and stir very well.
- In another bowl, mix garlic with 1 and ½ teaspoon oil and some black pepper and stir.
- Heat up a pan with the rest of the oil over medium-high heat, add meat, cook for 3 minutes on each side and transfer to a bowl.
- Heat up the same pan over medium-high heat, add onion, stir, and cook for 3 minutes.
- Add the garlic mix, return the pork, also add the aminos mix, toss, cook for 6 minutes, divide between plates, sprinkle scallions and peanuts on top and serve.

- Enjoy!

Nutritional Information:

- Calories 273
- Fat 4
- Carbs 12
- Protein 18

Recipe 130. Prosciutto Broccoli Chicken Stew

Serving Size: 4

Preparation Time: 10 minutes

Cooking Time: 20 minutes

Ingredients:

- 4 chicken breasts cubed
- 6 slices prosciutto cut into slices, chopped
- 2 tbsp butter
- 4 cloves of garlic chopped and minced
- 1 cup baby Kale Chopped
- 1 head broccoli, cut into florets
- 1 1/2 cups heavy cream
- 1/4 cup of shredded Parmesan

Directions:

- Place the prosciutto in a pan and fry it until it is crispy and golden about 5 minutes. Set aside. In the same pan, cook the chicken until it's the chicken is no longer pink. Add garlic, and sauté for one minute.
- Mix with prosciutto, heavy cream, and kale. Let simmer for approximately about 5 minutes until the sauce begins to thicken. Put the prepared broccoli in a microwave-safe bowl, cover with water, and then microwave for 2 minutes until the broccoli becomes soft. In the skillet, add Parmesan Stir, then cook until the cheese is melted. Serve.

Nutritional Information:

- Cal 399
- Net Carbs 5.5g
- Fat 48g
- Protein 69g

Recipe 131. Risotto with Green Beans, Sweet Potatoes, and Peas

Serving Size: 8

Preparation Time: 30 minutes

Cooking Time: 4 hours

Ingredients:

- 1 large, sweet potato, peeled and chopped
- 1 onion, chopped
- 5 garlic cloves, minced
- 2 cups short-grain brown rice
- 1 tsp. dried thyme leaves
- 7 cups low-sodium vegetable broth
- 2 cups green beans, cut in half crosswise
- 2 cups frozen baby peas
- 3 tbsp. unsalted butter
- ½ cup grated Parmesan cheese

Directions:

- In a 6-quart slow cooker, mix the sweet potato, onion, garlic, rice, thyme, and broth. Cover and cook on low for 3 to 4 hours, or until the rice is tender.
- Stir in the prepared green beans and frozen peas. Cover and cook on low for 30 to 40 minutes or until the vegetables are tender.
- Stir in the butter and cheese. Cover and cook on low for 20 minutes, then stir and serve.

Nutritional Information:

- Calories: 385
- Fat: 10 g
- Carbs: 50 g

Recipe 132. Roasted Pork Stuffed with Ham and Cheese

Serving Size: 2

Preparation Time: 15 minutes

Cooking Time: 40 minutes

Ingredients:

- 2 tablespoons Olive oil and zest of
- 1 lime 1 clove of garlic minced
- 2 tablespoons fresh cilantro, chopped
- 2 1 tbsp fresh mints and chopped
- Black pepper and salt to taste
- 1 teaspoon cumin
- 2 pork loin steaks
- 1 pickle that has been chopped
- 2 oz smoked ham, sliced
- 2 oz Gruyere cheese sliced
- 1 tbsp mustard

Directions:

- Mix the zest of lime and the oil, black pepper, cilantro, cumin, lime juice, mint, garlic, and salt in the food

processor. Transfer the mixture into an empty bowl. Put the steaks in the marinade and stir to coat.
- The steaks should be laid out on a work surface. Divide the pickles, cheese, mustard, and ham, then roll them up and tie using toothpicks. In a skillet, heat the temperature, then add the pork rolls. Cook each side for two minutes before transferring them to a baking tray and bake for 35 minutes. Serve and have fun!

Nutritional Information:

- Cal 387
- Net Carbs 6.2g
- Fat 44g
- Protein 61g

Recipe 133. Rosemary Buttered Pork Chops

Serving Size:

Preparation Time: minutes

Cooking Time: minutes

Ingredients:

- 1/2 tbsp olive oil
- 2 tbsp butter
- 1 tbsp rosemary
- 2 pork chops
- Black pepper and salt to taste
- A little the spice paprika
- 1/2 tsp chili powder

Directions:

- Make sure to rub the chops in olive oil, salt, pepper chili powder, and paprika. Cook on medium-high heat and add the pork chops to cook them for about 10 minutes, turning every so often.
- Transfer to a plate for serving. In a saucepan set over low heat, cook butter till it becomes a nutty brown. Pour it over the chops, add rosemary, then serve.

Nutritional Information:

- Cal 363
- Net Carbs 1.8g
- Fat 32g
- Protein 38g

Recipe 134. Saffron Shrimp

Serving Size: 4

Preparation Time: 10 minutes

Cooking Time: 30 minutes

Ingredients:

- 1 teaspoon lemon juice
- Black pepper to the taste
- ½ cup avocado mayo
- ½ teaspoon sweet paprika
- 3 tablespoons olive oil
- 1 fennel bulb, chopped
- 1 yellow onion, chopped
- 2 garlic cloves, minced
- 1 cup canned tomatoes, no-salt-added and chopped
- 1 and ½ pounds big shrimp, peeled and deveined
- ¼ teaspoon saffron powder

Directions:

- In a bowl, combine the garlic with lemon juice, black pepper, mayo and paprika and whisk.
- Add the shrimp and toss.
- Heat up a pan with the oil over medium-high heat, add the shrimp, fennel, onion, and garlic mix, toss and cook for 4 minutes.
- Add tomatoes and saffron, toss, divide into bowls and serve.
- Enjoy!

Nutritional Information:

- Calories 210
- Fat 2
- Carbs 8
- Protein 4

Recipe 135. Salmon Casserole

Serving Size: 4

Preparation Time: 10 minutes

Cooking Time: 1 hour

Ingredients:

- 8 sweet potatoes, sliced
- 4 cups salmon, cooked and flaked
- 1 red onion, chopped
- 2 carrots, chopped
- Black pepper to the taste
- 1 celery stalk, chopped
- 2 cups coconut milk
- 3 tablespoons olive oil
- 2 tablespoons chives, chopped
- 2 garlic cloves, minced

Directions:

- Heat up a pan with the oil over medium heat, add garlic, stir and cook for 1 minute.
- Add coconut milk, black pepper, carrots, celery, chives, onion and salmon, stir and take off heat.
- Arrange a layer of potatoes in a baking dish, add the salmon mix, top with the rest of the potatoes, introduce in the oven and bake at 375 degrees F for 1 hour.
- Slice, divide between plates and serve.
- Enjoy!

Nutritional Information:

- Calories 220
- Fat 9
- Carbs 8
- Protein 12

Recipe 136. Salmon Meatballs with Garlic

Serving Size: 4

Preparation Time: 10 minutes

Cooking Time: 30 minutes

Ingredients:

- Cooking spray
- 2 garlic cloves, minced
- 1 yellow onion, chopped
- 1-pound wild salmon, boneless and minced
- ¼ cup chives, chopped
- 1 egg
- 2 tablespoons Dijon mustard
- 1 tablespoon coconut flour
- A pinch of salt and black pepper

Directions:

- In a bowl, mix onion with garlic, salmon, chives, coconut flour, salt, pepper, mustard and egg, stir well, shape medium meatballs, arrange them on a baking sheet, grease them with cooking spray, introduce in the oven at 350 degrees F and bake for 25 minutes.
- Divide the meatballs between plates and serve with a side salad.
- Enjoy!

Nutritional Information:

- Calories 211
- Fat 4
- Carbs 6
- Protein 13

Recipe 137. Salmon with Mushroom

Serving Size: 4

Preparation Time: 30 minutes

Cooking Time: 10 minutes

Ingredients:

- 8 ounces salmon fillets, boneless
- 2 tablespoons olive oil
- Black pepper to the taste
- 2 ounces white mushrooms, sliced
- ½ shallot, chopped
- 2 tablespoons balsamic vinegar
- 2 teaspoons mustard
- 3 tablespoons parsley, chopped

Directions:

- Brush salmon fillets with 1 tablespoon olive oil, season with black pepper, place on preheated grill over medium heat, cook for 4 minutes on each side and divide between plates.
- Heat up a pan with the rest of the oil over medium-high heat, add mushrooms, shallot and some black pepper, stir and cook for 5 minutes.
- Add the mustard, the vinegar and the parsley, stir, cook for 2-3 minutes more, add over the salmon and serve.
- Enjoy!

Nutritional Information:

- Calories 220
- Fat 4
- Carbs 6
- Protein 12

Recipe 138. Salsa Chicken

Serving Size: 4

Preparation Time: 50 minutes

Cooking Time: 5 minutes

Ingredients:

- 1 pound chicken breast, boneless and skinless
- 16-ounce scanned salsa Verde
- Black pepper to the taste
- A pinch of sea salt
- 1 tablespoon olive oil
- 1 and ½ cups fat free Montereyjack cheese, shredded
- ¼ cup cilantro, chopped

- Wild rice, cooked for serving
- Juice from 1 lime

Directions:

- Mix chicken with salt, pepper, and oil and toss to coat.
- Spread salsa in a baking dish, add chicken on top, introduce in the oven at 400 degrees F and bake for 40 minutes.
- Take chicken out of the oven, add cheese, introduce everything in preheated broiler and broil for 3 minutes.
- Add lime juice, divide between plates, sprinkle cilantro and serve with white rice.

Nutritional Information:

- Calories 150
- Fat 1
- Fiber 4
- Carbs 20

Recipe 139. Seared Scallops with Apricot Orzo Salad

Serving Size: 3

Preparation Time: 15 minutes

Cooking Time: 20 minutes

Ingredients:

- 1 ½ cups cooked orzo
- 3 tablespoons dried cherries
- ¼ cup chopped dried apricots
- 2 tablespoons toasted pine nuts Salt and pepper, to taste
- 1 teaspoon canola oil
- 6 large U/10 dry-packed scallops

Directions:

- Place cherries and apricots in a strainer and pour boiling water from orzo over them to soften and drain.
- Once drained, combine with pine nuts and salt and pepper to taste.
- Heat skillet over high heat and add canola oil, heating until smoking.
- Season the prepared scallops with salt and pepper, place in hot oil, cook 2 minutes and turn, cooking an additional 2 minutes over medium-high heat.
- Place on plate and serve with orzo salad.

Nutritional Information:

- Calories: 380

- Fat: 16g
- Protein: 13g
- Carbohydrates: 48g

Recipe 140. Shrimp and Orzo

Serving Size: 4

Preparation Time: 10 minutes

Cooking Time: 30 minutes

Ingredients:

- 1 pound shrimp, peeled and deveined
- Black pepper to the taste
- 3 garlic cloves, minced
- 1 tablespoon olive oil
- ½ teaspoon oregano, dried
- 1 yellow onion, chopped
- 2 cups low-sodium chicken stock
- 2 ounces orzo
- ½ cup water
- 4 ounces canned tomatoes, no-salt-added and chopped
- Juice of 1 lemon

Directions:

- Heat up a large-sized pan with the oil over medium-high heat, add onion, garlic, and oregano, stir and cook for 4 minutes.
- Add orzo, stir, and cook for 2 more minutes.
- Add stock and the water, bring to a boil, cover, reduce heat to low and cook for 12 minutes.
- Add lemon juice, tomatoes, black pepper, and shrimp, introduce in the oven and bake at 400 degrees F for 15 minutes.
- Divide between plates and serve.
- Enjoy!

Nutritional Information:

- Calories 328
- Fat 4
- Carbs 7
- Protein 8

Recipe 141. Shrimp Quesadillas

Serving Size: 2

Preparation Time: 16 minutes

Cooking Time: 5 minutes

Ingredients:

- 2 whole wheat tortillas

- ½ tsp. ground cumin
- 4 cilantro leaves
- 3 oz. diced cooked shrimp
- 1 de-seeded plump tomato
- ¾ c. grated non-fat mozzarella cheese
- ¼ c. diced red onion

Directions:

- In medium bowl, combine the grated mozzarella cheese and the warm, cooked shrimp. Add the ground cumin, red onion, and tomato. Mix together. Spread the mixture evenly on the tortillas.
- Heat a non-stick frying pan. Place the tortillas in the pan, then heat until they crisp.
- Add the cilantro leaves. Fold over the tortillas.
- Press down for 1 – 2 minutes. Slice the tortillas into wedges.
- Serve immediately.

Nutritional Information:

- Calories: 299
- Fat: 9 g
- Carbs: 7.2 g
- Protein: 59 g

Recipe 142. Spinach Chicken

Serving Size: 2

Preparation Time: 10 minutes

Cooking Time: 10 minutes

Ingredients:

- 2 garlic cloves, minced
- 2 tablespoons unsalted butter, divided
- ¼ cup parmesan cheese, shredded
- ¾ pound chicken tenders
- ¼ cup heavy cream
- 10 ounces frozen spinach, chopped
- Salt and black pepper, to taste

Directions:

- Heat 1 tablespoon of butter in a large skillet and add chicken, salt, and black pepper.
- Cook for about 3 minutes on both sides and remove the chicken to a bowl.
- Melt remaining butter in the skillet and add garlic, cheese, heavy cream, and spinach.
- Cook for about 2 minutes and add the chicken.
- Cook for approximately about 5 minutes on low heat and dish out to immediately serve.

- Place chicken in a dish and set aside to cool for meal prepping. Divide it in 2 containers and cover them. Refrigerate for about 3 days and reheat in microwave before serving.

Nutritional Information:

- Calories: 288
- Carbs: 3.6g
- Protein: 27.7g
- Fat: 18.3g

Recipe 143. Stewed Pork with Cauliflower and Broccoli

Serving Size: 4

Preparation Time: 20 minutes

Cooking Time: 40 minutes

Ingredients:

- 2 tbsp olive oil
- One red bell pepper cut into pieces
- 1 lb stewed pork, cubed
- Black pepper and salt to taste
- 2 cups cauliflower, florets
- 2 cups broccoli with florets
- 1 onion cut into pieces
- 14 OZ canned diced tomatoes
- 1/4 teaspoon garlic powder
- 1 tbsp tomato puree
- 1 1/2 cups of water
- 2 tbsp chopped parsley

Directions:

- In the pan where you heat olive oil, cook the pork on moderate heat for 5 minutes or until cooked. Put in the bell pepper and onions to cook for 4 mins.
- Mix in the water and broccoli, tomatoes, tomatoes, cauliflower, and garlic powder. Bring to a boil and allow to cook for 20 minutes, being covered. Sprinkle with parsley.

Nutritional Information:

- Cal 456
- Net Carbs 5.7g
- Fat 28g
- Protein 22g

Recipe 144. Stir Fry Ground Pork

Serving Size: 10

Preparation Time: 10 minutes

Cooking Time: 25 minutes

Ingredients:

- 3 garlic cloves, minced
- 1 pound pork, ground
- ½ cup tomato sauce, no-salt-added
- 1 yellow onion, chopped
- 2 habanero peppers, chopped
- 1 teaspoon curry powder
- 1 teaspoon thyme, dried
- 2 teaspoons coriander, ground
- ½ teaspoon allspice, ground
- 2 teaspoons cumin, ground
- ½ teaspoon turmeric powder
- Black pepper to the taste
- 1 teaspoon garlic powder
- 2 tablespoons olive oil

Directions:

- Heat up a large-sized pan with the oil over medium-high heat, add the onion and the garlic, stir, and cook for 5 minutes.
- Add habanero peppers, curry powder, thyme, coriander, allspice, cumin, turmeric, black pepper, and garlic powder, stir and cook for 5 minutes more.
- Add the pork and the tomato sauce, toss, cook for 15 minutes more, divide everything into bowls and serve.
- Enjoy!

Nutritional Information:

- Calories 267
- Fat 23
- Carbs 12
- Protein 22

Recipe 145. Taco Casserole

Serving Size: 8

Preparation Time: 35 minutes

Cooking Time: 55 minutes

Ingredients:

- 1 lb. ground turkey
- 1 cauliflower, small & chopped into florets
- 1 jalapeno diced
- ¼ cup red peppers, diced
- ¼ cup onion, diced
- 1 tsp. cumin
- 1 tsp. parsley
- 1 tsp. garlic minced
- 1 tsp. turmeric
- 1 tsp. oregano
- 1 ½ cups cheddar cheese, shredded
- 1 cup sour cream

Directions:

- Put your minced meat and cauliflower in a bowl before adding all your herbs and spices. Stir in your red peppers, jalapenos, and onions together, mixing in a cup of your cheese.
- Pour into a casserole dish before topping with remaining cheese.
- Bake at 350° F for an hour and serve with sour cream.

Nutritional Information:

- Calories: 240
- Fat: 17 g
- Carbs: 4 g
- Protein: 16 g

Recipe 146. Tamari Chicken Thighs and Capers

Serving Size: 4

Preparation Time: 15 minutes

Cooking Time: 25 minutes

Ingredients:

- 1 1/2 lb of chicken thighs
- 2 tbsp butter
- 2 cups heavy bream
- 8 oz cream cheese
- 1/3 capers in a cup
- 1 tbsp tamari sauce

Directions:

- Bake at 350 F. Melt butter in a skillet, then fry in the oven until chicken is golden brown. Approximately 8 minutes. Transfer the prepared chicken to a greased baking sheet, and wrap in aluminum foil to bake for 8 mins. Save the butter that was that is used for cooking the chicken. Remove the chicken from the oven. Take off the foil and then pour the drippings into a pan with the fried butter.
- Place the chicken in a warm place to be served later. Place the saucepan on the stove at a low temperature and mix in the heavy cream and cream cheese. Let the sauce simmer until it becomes thicker. Mix in the capers and tamari sauce, and cook further for one minute. Divide the chicken between plates and pour the sauce all over.

Nutritional Information:

- Cal 329
- Net Carbs 5.9g
- Fat 33g
- Protein 36g

Recipe 147. Teriyaki Chicken Wings

Serving Size: 6

Preparation Time: 15 minutes

Cooking Time: 30 minutes

Ingredients:

- 3 pounds of chicken wings (15 – 20)
- 1/3 cup lemon juice
- ¼ cup of soy sauce
- ¼ cup of vegetable oil
- 3 tablespoons chili sauce
- 1 garlic clove, finely chopped
- ¼ teaspoon fresh ground pepper
- ¼ teaspoon celery seed
- Dash liquid mustard

Directions:

- Prepare the marinade. Combine lemon juice, soy sauce, chili sauce, oil, celery seed, garlic, pepper, and mustard. Stir well, set aside. Rinse and dry the chicken wings.
- Pour marinade over the chicken wings. Coat thoroughly. Refrigerate for 2 hours. After 2 hours. Preheat the broiler in the oven. Drain off the excess sauce.
- Place the wings on a cookie sheet with parchment paper. Broil on each side for 10 minutes. Serve immediately.

Nutritional Information:

- Calories - 296
- Protein - 15g
- Carbohydrates - 63g
- Fat - 15g

Recipe 148. Thyme Chicken with Mushrooms and Turnip

Serving Size: 4

Preparation Time: 25 minutes

Cooking Time: 50 minutes

Ingredients:

- 3 cups mixed mushrooms teared up
- 2 tbsp olive oil
- 4 tbsp butter, melt
- 1.25 lbs chicken breasts cut into slices
- White wine 4 tablespoons
- 1 turnip cut in half, then sliced
- 2 cloves garlic, minced
- 4 sprigs of thyme chopped
- 1 lemon juiced
- Black pepper and salt to taste
- 2 tbsp Dijon mustard

Directions:

- Preheat the oven to 420 F. Place the turnips on a baking tray, sprinkle with a bit of oil, and bake for 15 minutes. In the bowl, combine the chicken, the roasted turnips, mushrooms, garlic lemon juice, thyme, salt pepper, salt, and mustard.
- Divide the chicken mixture among four large sheets of aluminum foil and sprinkle with olive oil, white wine, and butter. The edges should be sealed to create packets. Set the packets on a baking sheet and bake for about 25 minutes. Serve it warm.

Nutritional Information:

- Cal 394
- Net Carbs 4.6g
- Fat 29g
- Protein 25g

Recipe 149. Tilapia Broccoli Platter

Serving Size: 2

Preparation Time: 4 minutes

Cooking Time: 14 minutes

Ingredients:

- 6-ounce tilapia, frozen
- 1 tablespoon almond butter
- 1 tablespoon garlic, minced
- 1 teaspoon lemon pepper seasoning
- 1 cup broccoli florets, fresh

Directions:

- Preheat your oven to 350 degrees F.
- Add fish in aluminum foil packets.
- Arrange broccoli around fish.
- Sprinkle lemon pepper on top.
- Close the packets and seal.
- Bake for 14 minutes.

- Take a bowl and add garlic and almond butter, mix well and keep the mixture on the side.
- Remove the packet from oven and transfer to platter.
- Place almond butter on top of the fish and broccoli, serve and enjoy!

Nutritional Information:

- Calories: 362
- Fat: 25g
- Carbohydrates: 2g
- Protein: 29g

Recipe 150. Turkey and Vegetable Casserole

Serving Size: 2

Preparation Time: 15 minutes

Cooking Time: 25 minutes

Ingredients:

- 2 tablespoons coconut oil
- 1 Turkey breast cut into slices
- 2 zucchinis, sliced
- 1 onion cut into pieces
- 1 carrot chopped
- 1 cup of mushrooms, cut into slices
- 1 bell pepper with a green color chopped
- 1 clove of garlic, minced
- Black pepper and salt to taste
- 2 tbsp chopped parsley

Directions:

- Place a pan on moderate heat. Add coconut oil. Grill the turkey pieces for 3 minutes on each side. Reserve. In the same pan, add the garlic and onion for 3 mins.
- Add bell peppers, zucchinis, mushrooms, peppers, salt, and carrots, and cook for 6-8 minutes. Add the turkey back in and cook for another 3 minutes. Serve with a sprinkle of parsley.

Nutritional Information:

- Cal 364
- Net Carbs 8.6g
- Fat 23g
- Protein 53g

Recipe 151. Turkey Bacon-Wrapped Beef Tenderloin

Serving Size: 2

Preparation Time: 25 minutes

Cooking Time: 40 minutes

Ingredients:

- Cooking spray
- 4 strips turkey bacon
- 2 (4-ounce) beef tenderloins
- 1 tablespoon crushed peppercorns
- 1 cup sliced mushrooms
- 1 clove garlic, smashed
- 1 teaspoon dry thyme
- 1 tablespoon flour
- 3 ounces red wine
- 3 ounces low-sodium beef stock

Directions:

- Spray medium-sized sauce pan with cooking spray, then heat over medium heat until hot.
- Wrap bacon around tenderloin and secure with a toothpick.
- Roll tenderloins (bacon side out) in peppercorns and sear for 3 minutes per side for medium doneness.
- Remove meat from pan and cook mushrooms and garlic in the pan for 3 minutes.
- Add flour and red wine and thyme, and simmer for 3–4 minutes until reduced by ¾.
- Add stock and simmer 3–4 minutes until thickened.
- Add tenderloins back to sauce for 1 minute and serve hot.

Nutritional Information:

- Calories: 400
- Fat: 25g
- Protein: 29g
- Carbohydrates: 8g

Recipe 152. Turnip and Pork Packets with Grilled Halloumi

Serving Size: 4

Preparation Time: 10 minutes

Cooking Time: 30 minutes

Ingredients:

- 3 tbsp olive oil
- 4 oz halloumi cheese, cubed
- 1 lb turnips, cubed
- 1/2 cup salsa verde
- 2 tsp chili powder
- 1 teaspoon cumin powder

- Pork chops with boneless bones
- Black pepper and salt to taste

Directions:

- The grill should be heated too high. Cut four 18x12-inch sheets made of heavy-duty aluminum foil. The sheets should be sprayed by spraying them with cooking oil. A bowl is used to mix the turnips with salsa verde chili and cumin.
- Sprinkle with salt and pepper. Place the pork chops on the foil sheets, spoon the turnip mixture onto the meat, and sprinkle halloumi and olive oil cheese on the top. Wrap the foil around the meat and put it on the grill in the oven for about 10 minutes. Flip the foil over and cook for another 8 minutes. Transfer the foil packs to platters and serve. Enjoy!

Nutritional Information:

- Cal 399
- Net Carbs 6.1g
- Fat 28g
- Protein 49g

Recipe 153. Zucchini and Bell Pepper Chicken Gratin

Serving Size: 2

Preparation Time: 15 minutes

Cooking Time: 40 minutes

Ingredients:

- 1 bell pepper red cut into slices
- 1 zucchini, chopped
- Black pepper and salt to taste
- 1 teaspoon garlic powder
- 1 tbsp olive oil
- Two chicken breasts cut
- 1 tomato that has been chopped
- 1/2 1 tsp dried oregano
- 1/2 tsp dried, chopped basil
- 1/2 cup mozzarella, shredded

Directions:

- Salt the chicken with black pepper, garlic, and salt powder. Heat the oil with olives in a pan on medium heat, then add the chicken pieces. Cook until golden before transferring to the baking dish. Add the tomatoes, zucchini bell pepper, zucchini oregano, and salt to the same skillet, and cook for two minutes.
- Sprinkle the mix on top of the chicken. Roast in the oven to the temperature of 360 F for 20 minutes. Sprinkle the prepared mozzarella on top of the chicken, return to the oven, and then bake for 5 mins until the cheese melts and is bubbling. Serve.

Nutritional Information:

- Cal 397
- Net Carbs 6.2g
- Fat 23g
- Protein 45g

Recipe 154. Zucchini Beef Lasagna

Serving Size: 4

Preparation Time: 20 minutes

Cooking Time: 45 minutes

Ingredients:

- 1/2 cup Pecorino Romano cheese
- 4 yellow zucchinis, sliced
- 1/2 lb ground beef
- 1 1/2 cups grated mozzarella
- 2 cups goat cheese that has been crumbled
- 1 2 tablespoons Lard
- 1 teaspoon garlic powder
- 1 teaspoon onion powder
- 2 tablespoons coconut flour
- 1 large egg
- 2 cups marinara sauce
- 1 tbsp Italian herb seasoning
- Red chili flakes 1/4 teaspoon
- Fresh basil leaves, 1/4 cup
- Black pepper and salt to taste

Directions:

- Preheat the oven to 350 F. Then, melt the lard in a pan and cook the beef for 10 minutes. Set aside. In a bowl, mix the onion powders, garlic, coconut flour, salt, pepper, mozzarella cheese, the half Pecorino cheese goat cheese, a pinch of salt, and an egg. Combine Italian herb seasoning and chili flakes in marinara sauce.
- Create an even layer of zucchini in a well-greased baking dish, then spread 14 of egg mix over and 1/4 of marinara sauce. Repeat this process and finish with the rest of the Pecorino cheese. Then bake in the oven for at least 20 minutes. Sprinkle with basil leaves, cut, and serve.

Nutritional Information:

- Cal 399
- Net Carbs 7.5g

- Fat 37g
- Protein 49g

Recipe 155. Cabbage Roll Casserole with Veal

Serving Size: 6

Preparation Time: 5 minutes

Cooking Time: 4 hours

Ingredients:

- 1-pound raw ground veal
- 1 head of cabbage
- 1 medium green pepper
- 1 medium onion, chopped
- 1 (15-ounce) can of tomatoes
- 2 (15-ounce) cans tomato sauce
- 1 teaspoon minced garlic
- 1 tablespoon Worcestershire sauce
- 1 tablespoon beef bouillon
- ½ teaspoon salt
- ½ teaspoon pepper
- 1 cup uncooked brown rice

Directions:

- Situate all the ingredients to your slow cooker
- Stir well to combine.
- Adjust your slow cooker to high and cook for 4 hours, or cook for 8 hours on low.

Nutritional Information:

- Cal 335
- Net Carbs 34g
- Fat 18g
- Protein 22.9g

Recipe 156. Chicken Stir-Fry

Serving Size: 2

Preparation Time: 15 minutes

Cooking Time: 10 minutes

Ingredients:

- 1/2 cup chicken broth, low sodium
- 12 ounces skinless chicken breasts, cut into strips
- 1 cup red bell pepper, seeded and chopped
- 8 ounces (1 cup) broccoli, cut into florets
- 1 teaspoon crushed red pepper

Directions:

- Place a small amount of chicken broth in a saucepan. Heat over medium flame and stir in the chicken. Water sautés the chicken for at least 5 minutes while stirring constantly.
- Place the rest of the ingredients and stir.
- Cover the pan with the lid and cook for another 5 minutes.

Nutritional Information:

- Cal 237
- Net Carbs 15.4g
- Fat 12g
- Protein 15g

Recipe 157. Chicken with Zucchini Noodles

Serving Size: 2

Preparation Time: 10 minutes

Cooking Time: 20 minutes

Ingredients:

- 2 package zucchini noodles
- 1 tsp fine sea salt
- 1lb/0.45kg boneless chicken breast
- 2 tsp oil
- ½ tsp ground black pepper
- 4 minced garlic clove
- 2 tsp lemon zest
- 2 tbsp butter
- 2 tsp dried oregano
- 1/3 cup parmesan
- 2/3 cup broth
- Lemon slices and parsley for garnishing

Directions:

- Cook the zucchini noodles according to the package instruction, then drain well.
- In a large skillet, heat the oil. Salt and pepper the chicken, then brown it in the pan for 3-4 minutes on each side, depending on thickness. Remove chicken from the heat and set aside.
- Sauté the garlic in the remaining oil in the skillet for about 30 seconds.
- Add butter, lemon zest, and oregano. Pour the chicken broth to deglaze.
- Bring the chicken and sauce to a boil. Reduce the heat to low and continuously whisk in the parmesan cheese. Continue to simmer for 3-4 minutes, or until the sauce has reduced and thickened.

- Serve warm over zucchini noodles garnish with lemon slices and parsley.

Nutritional Information:

- Cal 433
- Net Carbs 5g
- Fat 14g
- Protein 7.9g

Recipe 158. Falafel Salad with Lemon-Tahini Dressing

Serving Size: 4

Preparation Time: 10 minutes

Cooking Time: 20 minutes

Ingredients:

- 1 cup dried chickpeas
- 5 tbsp tahini
- 2 cup sliced cucumbers
- ¼ cup chopped red onion
- 3 tbsp lemon juice
- 2 cup flat-leaf parsley
- 2 cloves garlic
- 1 tbsp ground cumin
- 6 cups sliced romaine lettuce
- 20oz/570g quartered grape tomatoes
- 1 tsp salt
- 5 tbsp extra virgin oil
- 5 tbsp warm water

Directions:

- Before preparing this dish, soak the chickpea in cold water for 12 to 24 hours.
- Transfer the chickpea to a blender. Add a cup of parsley, chopped garlic and onions, 1 tbsp of oil, 1 tbsp of lemon juice, ½ tsp of salt, and cumin. Blend until evenly ground and fine. Shape into 12 patties about 1 ½ inch wide.
- Place a nonstick skillet over medium-high heat to warm 2 tbsp of oil. Reduce the heat to medium and cook the falafel until golden brown, about 3 to 5 minutes.
- While the falafel is cooking, whisk the tahini, water, and remaining 2 tbsp of lemon juice, ½ teaspoon of salt, and 1 tbsp of oil in a large bowl. Transfer a quarter cup of the mixture to a small bowl before tossing the romaine and remaining 1 cup of parsley around in the big dish to coat.
- Place the cucumber, sliced onion, falafel, and tomatoes on a dish and drizzle with the reserved cup of dressing.

Nutritional Information:

- Cal 499
- Net Carbs 44.8g
- Fat 11g
- Protein 15.7g

Recipe 159. Glazed Ribs

Serving Size: 4

Preparation Time: 10 minutes

Cooking Time: 1 hour 20 minutes

Ingredients:

- 1 rack of pork ribs, ribs separated
- 1 and ¼ cups of tomato sauce
- ¼ cup of white vinegar
- 3 tablespoons of spicy mustard
- 2 tablespoons of coconut sugar
- 3 tablespoons of water
- ¼ teaspoon of hot sauce
- 1 teaspoon of onion powder
- Cooking spray

Directions:

- Cover the ribs with foil and bake for 1 hour at 400°F.
- Combine the tomato sauce, mustard, sugar, vinegar, water, onion powder, and hot sauce in a skillet, swirl to combine, and simmer for 10 minutes.
- Brush half of the sauce over the ribs put them on a prepared grill over medium-high heat, spray with cooking spray, cook for 4 minutes on each side, split into plates, and serve with the remaining sauce on the side.
- Enjoy!

Nutritional Information:

- Cal 287
- Net Carbs 16g
- Fat 5g
- Protein 15g

Recipe 160. Kale and Ground Beef Casserole

Serving Size: 4

Preparation Time: 10 minutes

Cooking Time: 16 minutes

Ingredients:

- 4-ounces mozzarella, shredded
- 2 cups marinara sauce
- 10-ounces kale, fresh
- 1 teaspoon oregano
- 1 teaspoon onion powder
- ½ teaspoon sea salt
- 1 lb. lean ground beef
- 2 tablespoons olive oil

Directions:

- In a deep skillet, heat the olive oil for 2-minutes, add in the ground beef, and cook for an additional 8-minutes or until meat is browned.
- In a mixing dish, combine the salt and pepper.
- In batches, stir the kale into beef mixture, cooking for another 2-minutes.
- Add the marinara sauce and simmer for another 2 minutes.
- Mix in half the cheese into the mixture.
- Transfer mixture into the air fryer baking dish.
- Sprinkle the remaining cheese on top.
- Broil in the air fryer at 400° Fahrenheit for 2-minutes.
- Allow resting for 5-minutes before serving.

Nutritional Information:

- Cal 312
- Net Carbs 9.2g
- Fat 13.2g
- Protein 13.2g

Recipe 161. Lemon Garlic Thighs with Asparagus

Serving Size: 4

Preparation Time: 5 minutes

Cooking Time: 40 minutes

Ingredients:

- 1 ¾ pounds (794 g) bone-in, skinless chicken thighs
- 2 tablespoons lemon juice
- 2 tablespoons minced fresh oregano
- 2 cloves garlic, minced
- 1/4 teaspoon pepper
- 1/4 teaspoon salt
- 2 pounds (907 g) asparagus, trimmed

Directions:

- Preheat the oven to 350°F.
- Toss all the ingredients except the asparagus in a mixing bowl until combined.
- Roast the chicken thighs in the preheated oven for about 40 minutes or until it reaches an internal temperature of 165°F.
- When cooked, remove the chicken thighs from the oven and set them aside to cool.
- Meanwhile, steam the asparagus in the microwave to the desired doneness.
- Serve the asparagus with roasted chicken thighs.

Nutritional Information:

- Cal 197
- Net Carbs 14g
- Fat 14g
- Protein 9g

Recipe 162. Pork and Peppers Chili

Serving Size: 4

Preparation Time: 5 minutes

Cooking Time: 8 hours 5 minutes

Ingredients:

- 1 red onion, chopped
- 2 pounds' pork, ground
- 4 garlic cloves, minced
- 2 red bell peppers, chopped
- 1 celery stalk, chopped
- 25 ounces' fresh tomatoes, peeled, crushed
- 1/4 cup green chilies, chopped
- 2 tablespoons fresh oregano, chopped
- 2 tablespoons chili powder
- A pinch of salt and black pepper
- A drizzle of olive oil

Directions:

- Heat the oil in a sauté pan with the onion, garlic, and meat. After 5 minutes of mixing and browning, add to your slow cooker.
- Toss in the other ingredients, cover, and simmer for 8 hours on low.
- Divide everything into bowls and serve.

Nutritional Information:

- Cal 448
- Net Carbs 20.2g
- Fat 13g
- Protein 23g

Recipe 163. Pork Chops and Tomato Sauce

Serving Size: 4

Preparation Time: 10 minutes

Cooking Time: 20 minutes

Ingredients:

- 4 pork chops, boneless
- 1 tablespoon soy sauce
- ¼ teaspoon sesame oil
- 1 and ½ cups tomato paste
- 1 yellow onion
- 8 mushrooms, sliced

Directions:

- Toss pork chops in a dish with soy sauce and sesame oil, then set aside for 10 minutes. Set your instant pot to sauté mode, add the pork chops, and brown them on all sides for 5 minutes.
- Stir in onion, and cook for 1-2 minutes more. Toss in the tomato paste and mushrooms, cover, and simmer for 8-9 minutes on high. Divide everything between plates and serve. Enjoy!

Nutritional Information:

- Cal 300
- Net Carbs 18g
- Fat 7g
- Protein 4g

Recipe 164. Rosemary Baked Chicken Drumsticks

Serving Size: 6

Preparation Time: 5 minutes

Cooking Time: 1 hour

Ingredients:

- 2 tablespoons chopped fresh rosemary leaves
- 1 teaspoon garlic powder
- ½ teaspoon sea salt
- 1/8 teaspoon freshly ground black pepper
- Zest of 1 lemon
- 12 chicken drumsticks

Directions:

- Preheat the oven to 350°F.
- Blend rosemary, garlic powder, sea salt, pepper, and lemon zest.
- Situate drumsticks in a 9-by-13-inch baking dish and sprinkle with the rosemary mixture. Bake for about 1 hour.

Nutritional Information:

- Cal 263
- Net Carbs 16g
- Fat 6g
- Protein 26g

Recipe 165. Shrimp Lunch Rolls

Serving Size: 4

Preparation Time: 10 minutes

Cooking Time: 0 minutes

Ingredients:

- 12 rice paper sheets, soaked in warm water and drained
- 1 cup of cilantro, chopped
- 12 basil leaves
- 12 baby lettuce leaves
- 1 small cucumber, sliced
- 1 cup of carrots, shredded
- 20 ounces of shrimp, cooked, peeled, and deveined

Directions:

- Arrange all rice papers on a working surface, divide cilantro, bay leaves, baby lettuce leaves, cucumber, carrots, and shrimp, wrap, seal edges, and serve lunch.
- Enjoy!

Nutritional Information:

- Cal 200
- Net Carbs 14g
- Fat 4g
- Protein 8g

CHAPTER 4. DINNER RECIPES

Recipe 166. Almond-Crusted Zucchini Chicken Stacks

Serving Size: 4

Preparation Time: 20 minutes

Cooking Time: 30 minutes

Ingredients:

- 1 1/2 lbs of chicken thighs Skinless and boneless cut into strips
- 2 large zucchinis, sliced
- 4 tbsp olive oil
- 3 tablespoons almond flour
- 2 tsp Italian herb blend
- 1/2 cup chicken broth
- Black pepper and salt to taste

Directions:

- Preheat the oven up to 350 F. Put the almond flour, salt, and pepper in the zipper bag. Mix well, and then put the pieces of chicken in the bag. Close the bag and shake it to coat. Place the zucchinis on a baking tray that is greased. Sprinkle with salt and pepper, and drizzle with olive oil.
- Take the chicken out of the mixture made with almonds, rub out the excess, and place 3-4 chicken pieces on each zucchini. Add the Italian herb mixture and drizzle the remainder of the olive oil. The oven should be set for eight minutes, and then add broth. Then bake for 10 mins. Serve.

Nutritional Information:

- Cal 308
- Net Carbs 1.2g
- Fat 39g
- Protein 31g

Recipe 167. Artichoke and Spinach Chicken

Serving Size: 4

Preparation Time: 15 minutes

Cooking Time: 5 minutes

Ingredients:

- 10 oz baby spinach
- ½ tsp. crushed red pepper flakes
- 14 oz. chopped artichoke hearts
- 28 oz. no-salt-added tomato sauce
- 2 tbsps. Essential olive oil
- 4 boneless and skinless chicken breasts

Directions:

- Heat-up a pan with the oil over medium-high heat, add chicken and red pepper flakes and cook for 5 minutes on them.
- Add the prepared spinach, artichokes, and tomato sauce, toss, cook for ten minutes more, divide between plates, and serve. Enjoy!

Nutritional Information:

- Calories: 312
- Fat:3 g
- Carbs:16 g
- Protein:20 g

Recipe 168. Asparagus and Lemon Salmon

Serving Size: 3

Preparation Time: 5 minutes

Cooking Time: 15 minutes

Ingredients:

- 2 salmon fillets, 6 ounces each, skin on
- Sunflower seeds to taste
- 1 pound asparagus, trimmed
- 2 cloves garlic, minced
- 3 tablespoons almond butter
- ¼ cup cashew cheese

Directions:

- Preheat your oven to 400 degrees F.
- Line a baking sheet with oil.
- Take a kitchen towel and pat your salmon dry, season as needed.
- Put salmon onto the baking sheet and arrange asparagus around it.
- Place a pan over medium heat and melt almond butter.
- Add garlic and cook for 3 minutes until garlic browns slightly.
- Drizzle sauce over salmon.
- Sprinkle salmon with cheese and bake for 12 minutes until salmon looks cooked all the way and is flaky.

- Serve and enjoy!

Nutritional Information:

- Calories: 434
- Fat: 26g
- Carbohydrates: 6g
- Protein: 42g

Recipe 169. Bacon and Parsnip Chicken Bake

Serving Size: 4

Preparation Time: 25 minutes

Cooking Time: 55 minutes

Ingredients:

- 1/2 lb parsnips, diced
- 6 bacon slices cut into pieces
- 2 tbsp butter
- 1 lb ground turkey
- 1 cup of heavy cream
- 2 oz cream cheese, softened
- 1 1/4 cup grated
- Pepper Jack
- 1 cup chopped up scallions

Directions:

- Preheat oven to 390 F. Place bacon in a skillet, cook it until golden and crispy, about 6 minutes, and then put aside. Melt butter and sauté parsnips in the skillet until soft and lightly brown. Cook the chicken until it is no longer pink, around 8 minutes. Set aside too. Incorporate heavy cream, cream cheese, and two-thirds of Pepper Jack cheese into the skillet.
- Mix the ingredients on moderate heat, frequently stirring, for 7 minutes. Spread the mixture onto an oven dish, pour the heavy cream mixture over it, and sprinkle bacon and scallions. Sprinkle with the rest of the cheese and bake until the cheese is melted for about 30 minutes. Serve.

Nutritional Information:

- Cal 351
- Net Carbs 9g
- Fat 56g
- Protein 30g

Recipe 170. Bacon Topped Turkey Meatloaf

Serving Size: 3

Preparation Time: 10 minutes

Cooking Time: 15 minutes

Ingredients:

- 3 tbsp olive oil
- 2 cloves of garlic, minced
- 1 yellow onion chopped
- 6 bacon slices, slices
- 1 1/2 1 lb ground turkey
- 1 small zucchini, minced
- 2 tablespoons coconut aminos
- 1 tbsp tomato paste
- 2 large eggs
- Black pepper and salt to taste
- 2 tbsp Dijon mustard
- 1/4 tsp Worcestershire sauce

Directions:

- Set the oven temperature to 350 F. The olive oil should be warm in a pan at medium temperature. Add the onion and garlic for 3 minutes and let cook or until soft. Transfer the mixture to a bowl and allow it to cool for approximately 4-5 minutes. Mix the turkey ground and coconut aminos, zucchini egg yolks, tomato paste, Worcestershire sauce, mustard, salt, and pepper.
- Combine with your hands until well-integrated. Make an unbaked loaf that has been greased. The loaf should bake for about 35 mins or until it is no longer pink. Remove the loaf from the oven and then cover the loaf in bacon slices. Return to bake for another 10 minutes. Let it cool for a couple of minutes. Cut and serve.

Nutritional Information:

- Cal 326
- Net Carbs 2.7g
- Fat 29g
- Protein 31g

Recipe 171. Baked Cheesy Chicken Tenders

Serving Size: 4

Preparation Time: 20 minutes

Cooking Time: 45 minutes

Ingredients:

- 1 tbsp olive oil
- 2 eggs

- 3 cups crushed cheddar cheese
- 1/2 cup pork rinds, crushed
- 1 1 lb chicken tenders
- Add salt to your taste Lemon wedges to garnish

Directions:

- Preheat the oven to a heat of 350 F. Line a baking sheet with parchment paper. Beat eggs in a bowl. Combine the cheese with pork rinds together in another bowl. Sprinkle chicken with salt, dip it in the egg mixture, and cover well with cheese and rind mixture.
- Set the chicken on the baking tray Cover with aluminum foil and cook for about 25 minutes. Remove foil, apply olive oil, and bake for another 10 minutes, until the chicken is golden brown. Serve the chicken along with wedges of lemon.

Nutritional Information:

- Cal 312
- Fat 43g
- Net Carbs 2.2g
- Protein 35g

Recipe 172. Baked Chicken Legs with Tomato Sauce

Serving Size: 4

Preparation Time: 30 minutes

Cooking Time: 1 hour 35 minutes

Ingredients:

- 1 (14 1 oz) can tomato sauce without sugar
- 2 bell peppers with greens, chopped into pieces
- 2 tbsp olive oil
- 1 lb chicken legs
- Two chopped green onions
- 1/2 parsnip chopped
- 1 chopped carrot
- 2 cloves of garlic, minced
- 1/4 cup coconut flour
- 2 cups chicken broth
- 2 tablespoons Italian seasoning
- Black pepper and salt to be taste

Directions:

- Salt the legs and pepper. The oil should be actually heated in an oven-proof skillet over medium-high heat. Fry the prepared chicken until golden brown on both sides for about 10 minutes. Transfer the chicken to an oven dish. In the same skillet, cook the parsnips, green onions, bell peppers, parsnips, carrots, and garlic for about 10 minutes.
- A bowl combines coconut flour, broth, tomatoes, and Italian seasoning. Then, sprinkle it over all the veggies in the skillet. Stir it in and cook for about 4 minutes. Serve the sauce over the chicken in the baking dish, then bake for one an hour in the oven at 390 F. Serve warm.

Nutritional Information:

- Cal 385
- Net Carbs 9.5g
- Fat 18g
- Protein 25g

Recipe 173. Baked Chicken Wrapped in Smoked Salmon

Serving Size: 2

Preparation Time: 15 minutes

Cooking Time: 40 minutes

Ingredients:

- 1/2 lb chicken breasts
- 1 tbsp olive oil
- 1 tbsp fresh parsley chopped
- 1 tsp garlic paste chopped
- 1/2 teaspoon sage Salt and black pepper according to your preference
- 1/2 tsp smoked paprika
- 2 oz smoked bacon, sliced

Directions:

- Mix the garlic paste with sage, smoked paprika, sage salt, and the black pepper into a bowl. Rub on chicken, then roll fillets into the bacon slices.
- Lay them out on the baking dish with olive oil to bake for 30 mins at a temperature of 390 F. Serve the chicken and sprinkle with fresh parsley.

Nutritional Information:

- Cal 356
- Net Carbs 2.3g
- Fat 38g
- Protein 51g

Recipe 174. Baked Zucchini with Cheese and Chicken

Serving Size: 4

Preparation Time: 15 minutes

Cooking Time: 45 minutes

Ingredients:

- 1-lb breasts of chicken cubed
- 1 tbsp butter
- 1 tbsp olive oil
- 1 Red Bell Pepper, chopped
- 1 shallot, sliced
- 2 zucchinis, cubed
- 1 clove of garlic, chopped
- Black pepper and salt to taste
- 1/2 cup cream cheese, softened
- 1/4 cup mayonnaise
- 1 tbsp Worcestershire sauce
- 1 cup mozzarella, shredded

Directions:

- The oven should be set to a heat of 350 F. Warm the butter, olive oil, and the skillet at medium-high heat, then add to the chicken. Cook until lightly golden in about 5 minutes. In the dish, add shallots and zucchini cubes. Add garlic, black pepper bell peppers, salt, and thyme. Cook in a 5-minute cook, or until soft; then set aside.
- A bowl mixes together the mayonnaise and cream cheese along with Worcestershire sauce. Mix in cooked chicken, as well as veggies. Put the mix in a baking dish coated with oil, then bake it for 20 minutes. Sprinkle the mixture with mozzarella cheese and bake until golden, about 5 minutes.

Nutritional Information:

- Cal 348
- Net Carbs 5.2g
- Fat 31g
- Protein 35g

Recipe 175. Balsamic Chili Roast

Serving Size: 6

Preparation Time: 10 minutes

Cooking Time: 4 hours

Ingredients:

- 4-pound pork roast
- 6 garlic cloves, minced
- 1 yellow onion, chopped
- ½ cup balsamic vinegar
- 1 cup low-sodium chicken stock
- 2 tablespoons coconut aminos
- Black pepper to the taste
- A pinch of red chili pepper flakes

Directions:

- Put the roast in a baking dish, add garlic, onion, vinegar, stock, aminos, black pepper and chili flakes, cover, introduce in the oven and cook at 325 degrees F for 4 hours.
- Slice, divide between plates and serve with a side salad.
- Enjoy!

Nutritional Information:

- Calories 265
- Fat 7
- Carbs 15
- Protein 32

Recipe 176. Beef and Bell Pepper Frittata

Serving Size: 4

Preparation Time: 30 minutes

Cooking Time: 55 minutes

Ingredients:

- 1 Tbsp butter
- 12 OZ ground sausage made from beef
- 1/4 cup shredded cheddar
- 12 whole eggs
- 1 cup sour cream
- 2 bell peppers red cut into pieces
- Black pepper and salt to taste

Directions:

- Preheat the oven to 350 F. Crack eggs in a blender. Add the salt, sour cream, and pepper. Then, at a low speed, blend the ingredients. Set aside. In a large skillet at medium-high temperature. Add bell peppers, and cook until soft, 6 mins to put aside. Add the beef sausage, and cook until golden brown, continually stirring and breaking the lumps into tiny pieces for 10 minutes.
- The beef is then flattened on the bottom of the skillet. Sprinkle bell peppers on top, pour the egg mixture all over, and sprinkle top cheddar cheese. Place the skillet in the oven for at least 30 mins or so until the eggs are set, and the cheese melts. Take the frittata out, cut it into slices and serve warm with salad.

Nutritional Information:

- Cal 321
- Net Carbs 6.5g
- Fat 49g
- Protein 33g

Recipe 177. Beef and Mushroom Meatloaf

Serving Size: 4

Preparation Time: 30 minutes

Cooking Time: 1 hour 10 minutes

Ingredients:

- 1/2 lb ground beef
- 1/2 onion chopped
- 1 Tbsp almond milk
- 1 tablespoon almond flour
- 1 clove of garlic, minced
- 1 cup chopped mushrooms
- 1 small egg
- Black pepper and salt to taste
- 1 Tbsp chopped parsley, chopped
- 1/3 cup Parmesan cheese, grated Glaze
- 1/3 cup balsamic vinegar
- 1/4 tbsp of the xylitol
- 1/4 tbsp tomato paste
- 1/4 teaspoon garlic powder
- 1/4 teaspoon onion powder
- 1 tbsp of ketchup Sugar-free

Directions:

- Ensure to grease a loaf pan with cooking spray, and then set it aside. Preheat the oven up to 390 F. Mix the meatloaf ingredients into one large bowl. Then, press the mixture into the loaf pan that you have prepared.
- Bake the loaf in the oven for around 30 minutes. For the glaze to be made, mix all the ingredients together in the bowl. The glaze should be drizzled onto the meatloaf. Return the meatloaf to the oven for another 20 minutes. Let meatloaf sit for 10 minutes before slicing. Serve and have fun!

Nutritional Information:

- Cal 311
- Net Carbs 5.5g
- Fat 21g
- Protein 24g

Recipe 178. Brown Basmati Rice Pilaf

Serving Size: 2

Preparation Time: 10 minutes

Cooking Time: 3 minutes

Ingredients:

- ½ tablespoon vegan butter
- ½ cup mushrooms, chopped
- ½ cup brown basmati rice
- 2-3 tablespoons water
- 1/8 teaspoon dried thyme
- Ground pepper to taste
- ½ tablespoon olive oil
- ¼ cup green onion, chopped
- 1 cup vegetable broth
- ¼ teaspoon salt
- ¼ cup chopped, toasted pecans

Directions:

- Place a saucepan over medium-low heat. Add butter and oil.
- When it melts, add mushrooms, and cook until slightly tender.
- Stir in the green onion and brown rice. Cook for 3 minutes. Stir constantly.
- Stir in the broth, water, salt, and thyme.
- When it begins to boil, lower the heat and cover with a lid. Simmer until rice is cooked. Add more water or broth if required.
- Stir in the pecans and pepper.
- Serve.

Nutritional Information:

- Calories 189
- Fats 11 g
- Carbohydrates 19 g
- Proteins 4 g

Recipe 179. Cabbage and Beef Steaks

Serving Size: 4

Preparation Time: 25 minutes

Cooking Time: 55 minutes

Ingredients:

- 1 lb. chuck steak
- 1 headcanon cabbage, grated
- 1/4 cup olive oil
- 3 tablespoons coconut flour
- 1 tsp Italian mixed herb blend

- 1 cup of bone broth

Directions:

- Preheat the oven to a heat of 380 F. Cut the steak into thin strips across the grain using an abrasive knife. Put in the coconut flour and the steak slices in a zipper bag. Close the bag and shake it to coat. Create little mounds of cabbage in a well-greased baking dish. Serve with olive oil.
- Then, remove the meat strips made of coconut flour Shake off any excess flour, and place 3-4 beef strips on each cabbage mound. Sprinkle with the Italian herb mix and drizzle it with the olive oil remaining. Roast for about 30 minutes. Take the pan off and add the broth. Place back in the oven and cook for another 10 minutes, or until the meat is cooked. Serve and enjoy!

Nutritional Information:

- Cal 331
- Net Carbs 4.5g
- Fat 20g
- Protein 23g

Recipe 180. Chicken and Cheese Stuffed Peppers

Serving Size: 6

Preparation Time: 25 minutes

Cooking Time: 55 minutes

Ingredients:

- 2 tbsp olive oil
- 3 Tbsp butter
- 4 bell peppers of yellow
- 3 cloves of garlic, minced
- 1 large white onion chopped
- 2 lb. ground chicken
- 1 teaspoon chili powder
- 10-ounce canned tomatoes chopped
- 1 1/2 cups cheddar grated
- Black pepper and salt to taste
- 1 1/2 cups mayonnaise
- 10 oz green leafy leaves

Directions:

- Bake at 350 F. Slice the bell peppers in half in length and remove the seeds. Sprinkle in olive oil. In a saucepan and cook garlic and onions for three minutes. Mix in the chili powder, chicken salt, and pepper. Cook for up to 8 minutes.
- Mix in the tomatoes and sauté for another 3-4 minutes. Scoop the tomato mixture into the bell peppers. Then top with cheddar cheese and put it in a greased baking dish. Bake until cheese melts and becomes bubbly about 25-30 minutes. Serve with mayonnaise and greens to serve.

Nutritional Information:

- Cal 335
- Net Carbs 10g
- Fat 57g
- Protein 38g

Recipe 181. Chicken and Chorizo Traybake

Serving Size: 4

Preparation Time: 10 minutes

Cooking Time: 50 minutes

Ingredients:

- 1 bell pepper red broken into pieces
- 1/2 cup of mushrooms, chopped
- 1 lb chorizo sausages, sliced
- 4 tbsp olive oil
- 1 teaspoon dried rosemary
- 4 cherry peppers cut into pieces
- 1 red onion Cut into wedges
- 2 garlic cloves, chopped
- 2 cups tomatoes cut into pieces
- 1 lb of chicken thighs
- Black pepper and salt to taste
- 1/2 cup chicken stock
- 2 tbsp capers
- 1 tbsp chopped parsley

Directions:

- Set the oven temperature up to 390 F. In a small bowl, mix your garlic, two tablespoons of olive oil, dried rosemary, salt, and pepper. Stir it until the ingredients are well blended. Rub the mixture on the chicken.
- On a baking tray, mix the bell pepper, mushrooms, chorizo, red onions, capers, cherry peppers, tomatoes, the remaining olive oil, salt, and pepper. Lay the chicken thighs skin-side up on top of each other, then pour them into the chicken broth. Roast for 40-50 minutes, or until the skin of the chicken is crisp, and the veggies have been softened. Add parsley to the chicken and enjoy the warmth.

Nutritional Information:

- Cal 305
- Net Carbs 8.3g
- Fat 56g
- Protein 42g

Recipe 182. Chicken and Sausage Gumbo

Serving Size: 4

Preparation Time: 25 minutes

Cooking Time: 40 minutes

Ingredients:

- 1 sausage, sliced
- 2 chicken breasts cubed
- 1 stick of celery chopped
- 1 leaf of a bay
- 1 bell pepper cut into pieces
- 1 onion chopped
- 1 cup chopped tomatoes, 1
- 4 cups chicken broth
- 2 tbsp garlic powder
- 2 1 tbsp dry mustard
- 1 2 tbsp chili powder
- Black pepper and salt to taste
- 2 tbsp Cajun seasoning
- 3 tbsp olive oil
- 1 tablespoon sage cut into pieces

Directions:

- The olive oil is heated in an oven at medium temperature. Add the chicken and sausage and cook for five minutes.
- Add the other ingredients, except the sage, and bring to the boiling point. Simmer for 25 minutes. Serve with sage sprinkled.

Nutritional Information:

- Cal 303
- Net Carbs 8.7g
- Fat 23g
- Protein 36g

Recipe 183. Chicken Cacciatore

Serving Size: 6

Preparation Time: 5 minutes

Cooking Time: 45 minutes

Ingredients:

- 2 tablespoons extra virgin olive oil
- 6 chicken thighs
- 1 sweet onion, chopped
- 2 garlic cloves, minced
- 2 red bell peppers, cored and diced
- 2 carrots, diced
- 1 rosemary sprig
- 1 thyme sprig
- 4 tomatoes, peeled and diced
- ½ cup tomato juice
- ¼ cup dry white wine
- 1 cup chicken stock
- 1 bay leaf
- Salt and pepper to taste

Directions:

- Heat the oil in a heavy sauce skillet.
- Cook chicken on all sides until golden.
- Add the mixture of garlic and onion and cook for 2 minutes.
- Stir in the rest of the ingredients and season with salt and pepper.
- Cook on low heat for 30 minutes.
- Serve the chicken cacciatore warm and fresh.

Nutritional Information:

- Calories: 363
- Fat: 14 Gram
- Carbs: 7 Gram
- Protein: 42 Gram

Recipe 184. Chicken Relleno Casserole

Serving Size: 6

Preparation Time: 19 minutes

Cooking Time: 29 minutes

Ingredients:

- 6 Tortilla Factory low-carb whole wheat tortillas, torn into small pieces
- 1 ½ cups hand-shredded cheese, Mexican
- 1 beaten egg
- 1 cup milk
- 2 cups cooked chicken, shredded
- 1 can Ro-tel
- ½ cup salsa verde

Directions:

- Grease an 8 x 8 glass baking dish
- Heat oven to 375 degrees

- Combine everything together, but reserve ½ cup of the cheese
- Bake it for 29 minutes
- Take it out of oven and add ½ cup cheese
- Broil for about 2 minutes to melt the cheese

Nutritional Information:

- Calories: 265
- Total Fat: 16g
- Protein: 20g
- Total Carbs: 18g

Recipe 185. Chicken Tikka

Serving Size: 6

Preparation Time: 15 minutes

Cooking Time: 20 minutes

Ingredients:

- 4 chicken breasts, skinless, boneless; cubed
- 2 large onions, cubed
- 10 Cherry tomatoes
- 1/3 cup plain non-fat yogurt
- 4 garlic cloves, crushed
- 1 ½ inch fresh ginger, peeled and chopped
- 1 small onion, grated
- 1 ½ teaspoon chili powder
- 1 Tablespoon ground coriander
- 1 teaspoon salt
- 2 tablespoons of coriander leaves

Directions:

- In a large bowl, combine the non-fat yogurt, crushed garlic, ginger, chili powder, coriander, salt, and pepper. Add the cubed chicken, stir until the chicken is coated. Cover with plastic film, place in the fridge. Marinate 2 – 4 hours. Heat the broiler or barbecue.
- After marinating the chicken, get some skewers ready. Alternate pieces of chicken cubes, cherry tomatoes, and cubed onions onto the skewers.
- Grill within 6 – 8 minutes on each side. Once the chicken is cooked through, pull the meat and vegetables off the skewers onto plates. Garnish with coriander. Serve immediately.

Nutritional Information:

- Calories - 417
- Protein - 19g
- Carbohydrates - 59g
- Fat - 19g

Recipe 186. Chicken, Tomato and Green Beans

Serving Size: 4

Preparation Time: 15 minutes

Cooking Time: 25 minutes

Ingredients:

- 6 oz. low-sodium canned tomato paste
- 2 tbsps. Olive oil
- ¼ tsp. black pepper
- 2 lbs. trimmed green beans
- 2 tbsps. Chopped parsley
- 1 ½ lbs. boneless, skinless, and cubed chicken breasts
- 25 oz. no-salt-added canned tomato sauce

Directions:

- Heat a pan with 50 % with the oil over medium heat, add chicken, stir, cover, cook within 5 minutes on both sides and transfer to a bowl. Heat inside the same pan while using rest through the oil over medium heat, add green beans, stir, and cook for 10 minutes.
- Return chicken for that pan, add black pepper, tomato sauce, tomato paste, and parsley, stir, cover, cook for 10 minutes more, divide between plates, and serve. Enjoy!

Nutritional Information:

- Calories: 290
- Fat:4 g
- Carbs:12 g
- Protein:9 g

Recipe 187. Chicken with Garlic and Fennel

Serving Size: 4

Preparation Time: 10 minutes

Cooking Time: 45 minutes

Ingredients:

- 2 yellow onions, chopped
- 2 pounds chicken breast, skinless, boneless, and roughly cubed
- 2 fennel bulbs, shredded
- 4 garlic cloves, minced
- 2 tablespoons olive oil
- 1 cup chicken stock
- A pinch of sea salt and black pepper

- 2 tablespoons parsley, chopped

Directions:

- Heat up a pan with the oil over medium heat, add the onions and the garlic and sauté for 5 minutes.
- Add the fennel and the meat and brown for 5 minutes more.
- Add the rest of the ingredients, toss, bring to a simmer and cook over medium heat for 35 minutes.
- Divide everything between plates and serve.

Nutritional Information:

- Calories 200
- Fat 4
- Carbs 10
- Protein 16

Recipe 188. Chicken with Potatoes Olives and Sprouts

Serving Size: 4

Preparation Time: 15 minutes

Cooking Time: 35 minutes

Ingredients:

- 1 pound chicken breasts, skinless, boneless, and cut into pieces
- ¼ cup olives, quartered
- 1 teaspoon oregano
- 1 ½ teaspoon Dijon mustard
- 1 lemon juice
- 1/3 cup vinaigrette dressing
- 1 medium onion, diced
- 3 cups potatoes cut into pieces
- 4 cups Brussels sprouts, trimmed and quartered
- ¼ teaspoon pepper
- ¼ teaspoon salt

Directions:

- Warm-up oven to 400 F. Place chicken in the center of the baking tray, then place potatoes, sprouts, and onions around the chicken.
- In a small bowl, mix vinaigrette, oregano, mustard, lemon juice, and salt and pour over chicken and veggies. Sprinkle olives and season with pepper.
- Bake in preheated oven for 20 minutes. Transfer chicken to a plate. Stir the vegetables and roast for 15 minutes more. Serve and enjoy.

Nutritional Information:

- Calories: 397
- Fat: 13g
- Protein: 38.3g
- Carbs: 31.4g

Recipe 189. Citrus Pork

Serving Size: 4

Preparation Time: 10 minutes

Cooking Time: 30 minutes

Ingredients:

- Zest of 2 limes, grated
- Zest of 1 orange, grated
- Juice of 1 orange
- Juice of 2 limes
- 4 teaspoons garlic, minced
- ¾ cup olive oil
- 1 cup cilantro, chopped
- 1 cup mint, chopped
- Black pepper to the taste
- 4 pork loin steaks

Directions:

- In your food processor, mix lime zest and juice with orange zest and juice, garlic, oil, cilantro, mint and pepper and blend well.
- Put the steaks in a bowl, add the citrus mix and toss really well.
- Heat up a large-sized pan over medium-high heat, add pork steaks and the marinade, cook for 4 minutes on each side, introduce the pan in the oven and bake at 350 degrees F for 20 minutes.
- Divide the steaks between plates, drizzle some of the cooking juices all over and serve with a side salad.
- Enjoy!

Nutritional Information:

- Calories 270
- Fat 7
- Carbs 8
- Protein 20

Recipe 190. Coconut Chicken and Mushrooms

Serving Size: 4

Preparation Time: 10 minutes

Cooking Time: 40 minutes

Ingredients:

- 2 tablespoons olive oil

- 1 yellow onion, chopped
- ½ pounds Bella mushrooms, sliced
- 2 pounds chicken thighs, boneless and skinless
- 3 carrots, sliced
- 2 celery stalks, chopped
- ½ cup coconut cream
- 1 tablespoon thyme, chopped
- 1 tablespoon cilantro, chopped

Directions:

- Heat up a pan with the oil over medium heat, add the onion, carrots and the celery and sauté for 5 minutes.
- Add the mushrooms and the meat and brown for 5 minutes more.
- Add the rest of the ingredients, toss, cook over medium heat for 30 minutes more, divide between plates and serve.

Nutritional Information:

- Calories 300
- Fat 6
- Carbs 15
- Protein 16

Recipe 191. Coconut Fried Shrimp with Cilantro Sauce

Serving Size: 2

Preparation Time: 10 minutes

Cooking Time: 20 minutes

Ingredients:

- 2 teaspoons coconut flour
- 2 tbsp grated Pecorino cheese
- 1 egg, beat in the bowl of
- 1/4 tsp curry powder
- 1/2 lb shrimp, shelled
- 2 tablespoons coconut oil
- Add salt to the sauce
- 2 Tbsp Ghee
- 2 tbsp cilantro leaves, chopped
- 1/2 onion, diced
- 1 cup of coconut cream
- 1/2 1 oz Paneer cheese grated

Directions:

- Mix the flour, Pecorino and curry, and salt into an ice-cold bowl. The coconut oil is melted in an oven over medium-high high heat. Dip the shrimp into the egg that has been beat, then coat them in this cheese mix. Grill until crispy and golden, around 5 minutes.
- In a separate skillet, melt the Ghee. Cook the onion for three minutes. Mix in coconut milk and Paneer cheese. Cook until the sauce becomes thicker, approximately 3-4 minutes. Add the shrimp and toss thoroughly. Serve warm with cilantro.

Nutritional Information:

- Cal 341
- Net Carbs 7.3g
- Fat 54g
- Protein 31g

Recipe 192. Cod Salad with Mustard

Serving Size: 4

Preparation Time: 12 minutes

Cooking Time: 12 minutes

Ingredients:

- 4 medium cod fillets, skinless and boneless
- 2 tablespoons mustard
- 1 tablespoon tarragon, chopped
- 1 tablespoon capers, drained
- 4 tablespoons olive oil+ 1 teaspoon
- Black pepper to the taste
- 2 cups baby arugula
- 1 small red onion, sliced
- 1 small cucumber, sliced
- 2 tablespoons lemon juice

Directions:

- In a bowl, mix mustard with 2 tablespoons olive oil, tarragon and capers and whisk.
- Heat up a pan with 1 teaspoon oil over medium-high heat, add fish, season with black pepper to the taste, cook for 6 minutes on each side and cut into medium cubes.
- In a salad bowl, combine the arugula with onion, cucumber, lemon juice, cod and mustard mix, toss and serve.
- Enjoy!

Nutritional Information:

- Calories 258
- Fat 12
- Carbs 12
- Protein 18

Recipe 193. Creamy Chicken Fried Rice

Serving Size: 4

Preparation Time: 15 minutes

Cooking Time: 45 minutes

Ingredients:

- 2 pounds of chicken; white and dark meat (diced into cubes)
- 2 Tablespoons butter or margarine
- 1 ½ cups instant rice
- 1 cup mixed frozen vegetables
- 1 can condensed cream of chicken soup
- 1 cup of water
- 1 cube instant chicken bouillon
- Salt and pepper to taste

Directions:

- Take the vegetables out of the freezer. Set aside. Warm large, deep skillet over medium heat, add the butter or margarine. Place the chicken in the skillet, season with salt and pepper. Fry until both sides are brown.
- Remove the chicken, then adjust the heat and add the rice. Add the water and bouillon. Cook the rice, then add the chicken, the vegetables. Mix in the soup, then simmer until the vegetables are tender. Serve immediately.

Nutritional Information:

- Calories - 319
- Protein - 22g
- Carbohydrates - 63g
- Fat - 18g

Recipe 194. Cumin Pork and Beans

Serving Size: 4

Preparation Time: 10 minutes

Cooking Time: 1 hour

Ingredients:

- 2 pounds pork stew meat, roughly cubed
- 1 cup canned pinto beans
- 4 scallions, chopped
- 2 tablespoons olive oil
- 1 tablespoon chili powder
- 2 teaspoons cumin, ground
- A pinch of salt and black pepper
- 2 garlic cloves, minced
- 1 cup vegetable stock
- A handful parsley, chopped

Directions:

- Heat up a pan with the oil over medium-high heat, add the scallions and the garlic and sauté for 5 minutes.
- Add the meat and brown for approximately about 5 minutes more.
- Add the beans and the other ingredients, toss, introduce the pan in the oven and cook everything at 380 degrees F for 50 minutes.
- Divide the mix between plates and serve.

Nutritional Information:

- Calories 291
- Fat 4
- Carbs 15
- Protein 24

Recipe 195. Feta and Mozarella Chicken

Serving Size: 4

Preparation Time: 25 minutes

Cooking Time: 45 minutes

Ingredients:

- 1.25 lbs chicken breasts chopped
- 1/2 teaspoon mixed spice seasoning
- Black pepper and salt to taste
- 1 cup baby spinach
- 2 tsp olive oil
- 4 oz feta cheese, crumbled
- 1/2 cup mozzarella, shredded

Directions:

- The chicken should be rubbed with the spice mix, salt, and black pepper. Place it into a baking dish, then place the spinach on top. Blend the olive oil, mozzarella cheese, and feta, as well as 1 cup of water and black pepper. Stir.
- Sprinkle the mix over the chicken, and then put the casserole on aluminum foil. Bake to cook for about 20 minutes. 350 F, remove the foil, and cook for 15 minutes or until a nice golden-brown color has formed over the top. Serve.

Nutritional Information:

- Cal 343

- Net Carbs 3.2g
- Fat 20g
- Protein 32g

Recipe 196. Gingered Grilled Chicken

Serving Size: 4

Preparation Time: 15 minutes

Cooking Time: 30 minutes

Ingredients:

- 1 lb chicken drumsticks
- 3 tbsp soy sauce
- 1/4 tbsp apple cider vinegar
- A little bit of red pepper flake
- 1 tbsp grated ginger
- 2 tablespoons sesame oil
- 1 clove of garlic, chopped
- 1/4 tsp lime zest
- 2 scallions finely chopped
- 1 tbsp sesame seeds

Directions:

- Mix the sesame oil, ginger vinegar, and garlic in a large mixing bowl. Add lime zest and soy sauce along with pepper flakes. Mix thoroughly. Incorporate the chicken and mix in a coating. Let it sit for one hour before chilling. Grill to high temperature.
- Take the chicken out of the marinade, removing any leftover marinade. Set the chicken skin-side to the side on the barbecue, and cook for 15 to 18 minutes, turning frequently and basting the chicken with marinade. Serve with scallions and sesame seeds. Serve.

Nutritional Information:

- Cal 293
- Net Carbs 3g
- Fat 21g
- Protein 21g

Recipe 197. Grilled Beef on Skewers with Fresh Salad

Serving Size: 2

Preparation Time: 15 minutes

Cooking Time: 20 minutes

Ingredients:

- 1 lb sirloin boneless cubed
- 1/4 cup ranch dressing
- 1 onion red, cut into slices
- 1/2 1 tbsp white wine vinegar
- 1 tablespoon extra olive oil
- 2 ripe tomatoes, sliced
- 2 tablespoons fresh parsley chopped
- 1 cucumber, sliced
- Salt to taste

Directions:

- Thread beef cubes over the skewers, approximately 4 - 5 cubes each skewer. Sprinkle one-third of the dressing onto the skewers (all around). The grill should be heated too high. Put the skewers onto the grill for six minutes and then cook. Then turn the skewers around and cook for another six minutes.
- Sprinkle any remaining dressing from the Ranch over the meat, then cook them for another minute per side. In a bowl for salad, mix the red onion, tomatoes, and cucumber. Sprinkle with vinegar, salt, and olive oil from extra virgin Mix well to mix. Serve the salad with skewers and scatter parsley over.

Nutritional Information:

- Cal 400
- Net Carbs 2.4g
- Fat 24g
- Protein 45g

Recipe 198. Grilled Chicken

Serving Size: 4

Preparation Time: 15 minutes

Cooking Time: 15 minutes

Ingredients:

- 4 chicken breasts, skinless and boneless
- 1 ½ teaspoon dried oregano
- 1 teaspoon paprika
- 5 garlic cloves, minced
- ½ cup fresh parsley, minced
- ½ cup olive oil
- ½ cup fresh lemon juice
- Pepper
- Salt

Directions:

- Add lemon juice, oregano, paprika, garlic, parsley, and olive oil to a large zip-lock bag. Season chicken with pepper and salt and add to bag. Seal bag and shake

well to coat chicken with marinade. Let sit chicken in the marinade for 20 minutes.
- Remove chicken from marinade and grill over medium-high heat for 5-6 minutes on each side. Serve and enjoy.

Nutritional Information:
- Calories: 512
- Fat: 36.5g
- Protein: 43.1g
- Carbs: 3g

Recipe 199. Grilled Pork Skewers with Chili Dipping Sauce

Serving Size: 6

Preparation Time: 55 minutes

Cooking Time: 1 hour 35 minutes

Ingredients:
- ¼ cup low-sodium soy sauce
- ¼ cup low-sodium teriyaki sauce
- 3 tablespoons cilantro, chopped
- 2 tablespoons garlic, chopped
- 2 tablespoons Splenda
- 1 teaspoon black pepper
- 2 tablespoons lime juice
- 1½ pounds pork tenderloin, cut into
- 16 long strips
- 16 bamboo skewers, soaked in water
- 1 recipe Chili Sauce
- 2 cups cooked rice

Directions:
- Whisk all liquids together, then add garlic, cilantro, Splenda, and pepper; stir to combine. Pour over pork. Marinate for 2 hours.
- Put one piece of meat on each skewer, laying it flat.
- Heat large-sized griddle pan on high heat and cook pork for 3 minutes per side.
- Serve with Chili Sauce and rice.

Nutritional Information:
- Calories: 280
- Fat: 4g
- Protein: 26g
- Carbohydrates: 9g

Recipe 200. Grilled Steak with Green Beans

Serving Size: 2

Preparation Time: 10 minutes

Cooking Time: 20 minutes

Ingredients:
- 2 ribeye steaks
- 2 tbsps unsalted butter
- 1 tsp olive oil
- 1/2 cup green beans, sliced
- Black pepper and salt to taste
- 1 tablespoon fresh thyme chopped
- 1 tbsp rosemary chopped,
- 1 tbsp fresh parsley chopped

Directions:
- Grill pans are heated up over high temperatures. Rub the prepared steaks with olive oil, then season with black pepper and salt. The steaks are cooked for approximately 4 minutes on each side; save them for later.
- Green beans are cooked in the steamer for about 3-4 minutes until they are tender. Add salt and pepper to taste. In the pan, cook the herbs for one minute. Mix with the green beans. Serve over the steaks and serve. Enjoy!

Nutritional Information:
- Cal 378
- Net Carbs 2.3g
- Fat 39g
- Protein 65g

Recipe 201. Grilled Swordfish with Lemon, Capers, and Olives

Serving Size: 4

Preparation Time: 15 minutes

Cooking Time: 30 minutes

Ingredients:
- 1 tablespoon canola oil
- 2 tablespoons lemon juice
- ½ red Thai chili, seeded and chopped
- 4 (6-ounce) swordfish fillets
- Zest of 1 lemon
- 1 clove garlic, chopped
- 2½ tablespoons capers, drained and rinsed
- 10 Kalamata olives, roughly chopped
- 2 tablespoons red onion, finely chopped
- 2 tablespoons low-fat Parmesan cheese, shredded

Directions:

- Preheat grill pan over high heat.
- In a bowl combine oil, lemon juice, and Thai chili and pour over swordfish.
- In another bowl, combine zest, garlic, capers, olives, red onion, and Parmesan cheese, and mix well.
- Place swordfish in hot pan and cook for 2 to 3 minutes per side.
- Place on fish plate and spoon prepared relish over fish. Garnish with parsley if desired.

Nutritional Information:

- Calories: 270
- Fat: 12g
- Protein: 35g
- Carbohydrates: 3g

Recipe 202. Hawaiian Chicken

Serving Size: 4

Preparation Time: 4 hours 10 minutes

Cooking Time: 12 minutes

Ingredients:

- 2 tablespoons tomato paste
- ¼ cup canned pineapple juice
- 2 tablespoons low sodium soy sauce
- 2 garlic cloves, minced
- 1 and ½ teaspoons ginger, grated
- 4 chicken breast halves, skinless and boneless
- Cooking spray
- Black pepper to the taste
- ¼ cup cilantro, chopped
- 2 cups brown rice, already cooked

Directions:

- In a bowl, mix pineapple juice with tomato paste, soy sauce, garlic and ginger and stir well.
- Reserve ¼ cup of mix, transfer the rest to a zip-top bag, add chicken, seal bag, shake and keep in the fridge for 4 hours.
- Heat up a pan after you've sprayed some cooking oil in it over medium high heat, add marinated chicken and season with black pepper to the taste.
- Add the reserved marinade, stir, and cook chicken for 6 minutes on each side.
- Add rice and cilantro, stir gently, take off heat and divide between plates.

Nutritional Information:

- Calories 340
- Fat 1
- Carbs 9
- Protein 12

Recipe 203. Kabobs with Peanut Curry Sauce

Serving Size: 4

Preparation Time: 9 minutes

Cooking Time: 9 minutes

Ingredients:

- 1 cup cream
- 4 teaspoon curry powder
- 1 1/2 teaspoon cumin
- 1 1/2 teaspoon salt
- 1 t minced garlic
- 1/3 cup peanut butter, sugar-free
- 2 t lime juice
- 3 t water
- 1/2 small onion, diced
- 2 t soy sauce
- 1 packet Splenda
- 8 oz. boneless, cooked chicken breast
- 8 oz. pork tenderloin

Directions:

- Blend together cream, onion, 2 teaspoons garlic, curry and cumin powder, and salt.
- Slice the meats into 1-inch pieces.
- Place the cream sauce into a bowl and put in the chicken and tenderloin to marinate. Let rest in sauce for 14 minutes.
- Blend peanut butter, water, 1 teaspoon. garlic, lime juice, soy sauce, and Splenda. This is your peanut dipping sauce.
- Remove the meats and thread on skewers. Broil or grill 4 minutes per side until meat is done.
- Serve with dipping sauce.

Nutritional Information:

- Calories: 530
- Total Fat: 29g
- Protein: 37g
- Total Carbs: 6g

Recipe 204. Lemon and Garlic Scallops

Serving Size: 4

Preparation Time: 10 minutes

Cooking Time: 5 minutes

Ingredients:

- 1 tablespoon olive oil
- 1 ¼ pounds dried scallops
- 2 tablespoons all-purpose flour
- ¼ teaspoon sunflower seeds
- 4-5 garlic cloves, minced
- 1 scallion, chopped
- 1 pinch of ground sage
- 1 lemon juice
- 2 tablespoons parsley, chopped

Directions:

- Take a nonstick skillet and place over medium-high heat.
- Add oil and allow the oil to heat up.
- Take a medium sized bowl and add scallops alongside sunflower seeds and flour.
- Place the scallops in the skillet and add scallions, garlic, and sage.
- Sauté for 3-4 minutes until they show an opaque texture.
- Stir in lemon juice and parsley.
- Remove heat and serve hot!

Nutritional Information:

- Calories: 351
- Fat: 4g
- Carbohydrates: 10g
- Protein: 18g

Recipe 205. Lemon-Parsley Chicken Breast

Serving Size: 2

Preparation Time: 15 minutes

Cooking Time: 15 minutes

Ingredients:

- 2 chicken breasts, skinless, boneless
- 1/3 cup white wine
- 1/3 cup lemon juice
- 2 garlic cloves, minced
- 3 Tablespoons breadcrumbs
- 2 Tablespoons flavorless oil (olive, canola, or sunflower)
- ¼ cup fresh parsley

Directions:

- Mix the wine, lemon juice, plus garlic in a measuring cup. Pound each chicken breast until they are ¼ inch thick. Coat the chicken with breadcrumbs, and heat the oil in a large skillet.
- Fry the chicken within 6 minutes on each side, until they turn brown. Stir in the wine mixture over the chicken. Simmer for 5 minutes. Pour any extra juices over the chicken. Garnish with parsley.

Nutritional Information:

- Calories - 317
- Protein - 14g
- Carbohydrates - 74 g
- Fat - 12g

Recipe 206. Mackerel and Orange Medley

Serving Size: 4

Preparation Time: 10 minutes

Cooking Time: 10 minutes

Ingredients:

- 4 mackerel fillets, skinless and boneless
- 4 spring onion, chopped
- 1 teaspoon olive oil
- 1-inch ginger piece, grated
- Black pepper as needed
- Juice and zest of 1 whole orange
- 1 cup low sodium fish stock

Directions:

- Season the fillets with black pepper and rub olive oil.
- Add stock, orange juice, ginger, orange zest and onion to Instant Pot.
- Place a steamer basket and add the fillets.
- Lock the lid and cook on HIGH pressure for 10 minutes.
- Release the pressure naturally over 10 minutes.
- Divide the fillets amongst plates and drizzle the orange sauce from the pot over the fish.
- Enjoy!

Nutritional Information:

- Calories: 300
- Fat: 4g
- Carbohydrates: 19g
- Protein: 14g

Recipe 207. Meatballs and Sauce

Serving Size: 6

Preparation Time: 10 minutes

Cooking Time: 32 minutes

Ingredients:

- 2 pounds pork, ground
- Black pepper to the taste
- ½ teaspoon garlic powder
- 1 tablespoon coconut aminos
- ¼ cup low sodium veggie
- ¾ cup almond flour
- 1 tablespoon parsley, chopped
- For the sauce:
- 1 cup yellow onion, chopped
- 2 cups mushrooms, sliced
- 2 tablespoons olive oil
- 1 teaspoon coconut aminos
- ½ cup coconut cream
- Black pepper to the taste

Directions:

- In a bowl, mix the pork with black pepper, garlic powder, 1 tablespoons coconut aminos, stock, almond flour, and parsley, stir well, shape medium meatballs out of this mix, arrange them on a baking sheet, introduce in the oven at 375 degrees F and bake for 20 minutes.
- Meanwhile, heat up a pan with the oil over medium heat, add mushrooms, stir, and cook for 4 minutes.
- Add onions, 1 teaspoon coconut aminos, cream and black pepper, stir and cook for 5 minutes more.
- Add the meatballs, toss gently, cook for 1-2 minutes more, divide everything into bowls and serve.
- Enjoy!

Nutritional Information:

- Calories 435
- Fat 23
- Carbs 6
- Protein 32

Recipe 208. Mushroom and Beef Stir-Fry

Serving Size: 4

Preparation Time: 15 minutes

Cooking Time: 30 minutes

Ingredients:

- 1 lb shiitake mushroom, cut in half
- 1 1 lb Chuck Steak
- 2 sprigs of rosemary chopped
- 1 bell pepper with a green color cut into pieces
- 4 slices prosciutto cut into slices, chopped
- 1 tablespoon coconut oil
- 1 tbsp of pureed garlic

Directions:

- Cut the chuck steak into thin slices against the grain, utilizing a sharp knife. Cut into smaller pieces. In a large skillet, heat it to medium-high heat. Cook the prosciutto until crispy and brown and set aside. In your skillet, cook the meat until golden brown, about 6-8 mins.
- Transfer to the prosciutto plate. Add the bell pepper and mushrooms to the skillet, and sauté until softened, about 5 minutes. Add beef, prosciutto rosemary, garlic, and prosciutto. Adjust seasoning to your taste, and cook in a slow cooker for four minutes. Serve with fried green beans.

Nutritional Information:

- Cal 249
- Net Carbs 7g
- Fat 17g
- Protein 32g

Recipe 209. Mussels Curry with Lime

Serving Size: 4

Preparation Time: 10 minutes

Cooking Time: 10 minutes

Ingredients:

- 2 and ½ pounds mussels, scrubbed
- 14 ounces canned coconut milk
- 3 tablespoons red curry paste
- 1 tablespoon olive oil
- Black pepper to the taste
- ½ cup low-sodium chicken stock
- Juice of 1 lime
- Zest of 1 lime, grated
- ¼ cup cilantro, chopped
- 3 tablespoons basil, chopped

Directions:

- Heat up a pan with the oil over medium-high heat, add curry paste, stir and cook for 2 minutes.

- Add stock, black pepper, coconut milk, lime juice, lime zest and mussels, toss, cover the pan and cook for 10 minutes.
- Divide this into bowls, sprinkle cilantro and basil on top and serve.
- Enjoy!

Nutritional Information:

- Calories 260
- Fat 12
- Carbs 10
- Protein 12

Recipe 210. Mustard Chicken with Rosemary

Serving Size: 4

Preparation Time: 20 minutes

Cooking Time: 20 minutes

Ingredients:

- 1 tbsp olive oil
- 1/2 cup chicken stock
- 1/2 cup onion chopped
- 1 lb of chicken thighs
- 1 cup of heavy cream
- 2 tbsp Dijon mustard
- 1 teaspoon rosemary Chop
- Black pepper and salt to taste

Directions:

- The olive oil is actually heated in a pan at medium-high temperature. Sprinkle the chicken with the black and salt. Let it cook for approximately 4 minutes on each side. Keep aside in this same skillet for three minutes.
- Add the stock, and let it simmer for about 5 minutes. Mix in heavy cream and mustard. Then pour the mixture over the chicken, then serve with rosemary sprinkled on top.

Nutritional Information:

- Cal 315
- Net Carbs 1.5g
- Fat 25g
- Protein 20g

Recipe 211. Nutmeg Salmon and Mushrooms

Serving Size: 4

Preparation Time: 10 minutes

Cooking Time: 20 minutes

Ingredients:

- 4 salmon fillets, boneless
- 2 tablespoons olive oil
- 1 cup mushrooms, sliced
- 3 green onions, chopped
- 1 tablespoon lime juice
- ¼ teaspoon nutmeg, ground
- ¼ cup almonds, toasted and chopped
- A pinch of salt and black pepper

Directions:

- Heat up a pan with the oil over medium-high heat, add the green onions and sauté for 5 minutes.
- Add the mushrooms and cook for 5 minutes more.
- Add the fish and the other ingredients, cook it for 5 minutes on each side, divide between plates and serve.

Nutritional Information:

- Calories 250
- Fat 10
- Carbs 7
- Protein 20

Recipe 212. Okra and Sausage Hot Pot

Serving Size: 4

Preparation Time: 20 minutes

Cooking Time: 30 minutes

Ingredients:

- 1 lb pork sausage, sliced
- 1 cup of mushrooms, cut into slices
- 1 onion chopped
- 1 tsp cayenne pepper
- Black pepper and salt to taste
- 1 tbsp fresh parsley chopped
- 2 tbsp of canola oil
- 1/4 cup beef soup
- 1 clove of garlic, chopped
- 2 cups tomatoes chopped
- 1 lb of okra, cut and cut
- 1/2 tbsp hot sauce
- 1 tablespoon coconut aminos

Directions:

- In the oil, heat it and sauté the onion, garlic, and mushroom for about 5 mins, until they are tender. Then add the hot sauce and stock, tomatoes, and coconut aminos.
- Add in cayenne peppers, okra, and sausage. Bring to a boil and cook for about 15 minutes. Check the seasoning and adjust by adding Salt and Pepper. Sprinkle fresh parsley on top to serve. Enjoy!

Nutritional Information:

- Cal 311
- Net Carbs 9g
- Fat 37g
- Protein 24g

Recipe 213. Oven-Baked Salami and Cheddar Chicken

Serving Size: 4

Preparation Time: 20 minutes

Cooking Time: 40 minutes

Ingredients:

- 1 tbsp olive oil
- 1 1/2 cups tomato paste canned
- 1-lb breasts of chicken
- Half-cut Salt and black pepper according to your taste
- 1 teaspoon dried oregano
- 4-ounce cheddar cheese slice
- 1 teaspoon garlic powder
- 2 oz salami, sliced

Directions:

- Preheat the oven up to 380 F. In a bowl, mix oregano, garlic and salt, and pepper. Apply the rub to your chicken using the mix. Cook a pan in the olive oil at moderate heat.
- Add the chicken and cook each side for two minutes. Transfer to an oven dish. Then, top with the cheddar cheese. Pour the tomato sauce over, and then arrange the salami slices over. Then bake for about 30 minutes. Serve warm and take your time!

Nutritional Information:

- Cal 317
- Net Carbs 3.5g
- Fat 28g
- Protein 35g

Recipe 214. Paella with Chicken, Leeks, and Tarragon

Serving Size: 2

Preparation Time: 10 minutes

Cooking Time: 20 minutes

Ingredients:

- 1 teaspoon extra-virgin olive oil
- 1 small onion, sliced
- 2 leeks (whites only), thinly sliced
- 3 garlic cloves, minced
- 1-pound boneless, skinless chicken breast, cut into strips 1/2-inch-wide and 2 inches long
- 2 large tomatoes, chopped
- 1 red pepper, sliced
- 2/3 cup long-grain brown rice
- 1 teaspoon tarragon, or to taste
- 2 cups fat-free, unsalted chicken broth
- 1 cup frozen peas
- 1/4 cup chopped fresh parsley
- 1 lemon, cut into 4 wedges

Directions:

- Preheat a nonstick pan with olive oil over medium heat. Toss in leeks, onions, chicken strips, and garlic. Sauté for 5 minutes. Stir in red pepper slices and tomatoes. Stir and cook for 5 minutes.
- Add tarragon, broth, and rice. Let it boil, then reduce the heat to a simmer. Continue cooking for 10 minutes, then add peas and continue cooking until the liquid is thoroughly cooked. Garnish with parsley and lemon. Serve.

Nutritional Information:

- Calories 388
- Fat 15.2 g
- Carbs 5.4 g
- Protein 27 g

Recipe 215. Pan-Seared Squids and Sausage

Serving Size: 4

Preparation Time: 15 minutes

Cooking Time: 20 minutes

Ingredients:

- 2 Tbsp butter

- Fresh 12 scallops cleaned
- 8 oz sausage, chopped
- One red bell pepper chopped
- 1 red onion finely chopped
- 1 Cup Grana Padano, grated
- Black pepper and salt to taste

Directions:

- Melt butter in a prepared medium-sized pan on medium heat. Stir-fry the bell pepper and onion for 5 minutes until they're tender. Add the sausage, and stir-fry for 5 minutes, then set aside.
- Dry the scallops with a towel, and then season with salt and black pepper. Place them in the skillet and sear for two minutes on each side until they are golden brown. The sausage mixture is returned to the skillet and heated to the desired temperature. Sprinkle the dish with Grana Padano cheese and serve.

Nutritional Information:

- Cal 334
- Net Carbs 9.5g
- Fat 62g
- Protein 56g

Recipe 216. Pancetta, Beef and Broccoli Bake

Serving Size: 4

Preparation Time: 30 minutes

Cooking Time: 55 minutes

Ingredients:

- 1 large broccoli head, cut into florets
- 1 lb ground beef
- 6 slices pancetta, chopped
- 2 tbsp olive oil
- 2 Tbsp butter
- 1 cup coconut cream
- 2 oz cream cheese, softened
- 1 1/4 cups cheddar grated
- 1 cup chopped up scallions
- Black pepper and salt to taste

Directions:

- The oven should be preheated to 325 F. Fill an empty pot with water, then bring to a simmer. Add broccoli and cook for two minutes. Remove and put aside. Put pancetta into the pot and cook for 5 minutes. Transfer to the plate. Heat oil and cook the steak until golden brown for 5-6 minutes in the pot.
- Add the coconut cream and cream cheese, two-thirds cheddar cheese, salt, and pepper, and mix for 7 minutes. Place the broccoli florets in a baking dish, pour the beef mixture on top and sprinkle the top with scallions and pancetta. In the oven, bake until cheese has become golden and bubbly after 20 minutes. Sprinkle with the remaining cheddar and bake for 10 minutes more. Serve.

Nutritional Information:

- Cal 361
- Net Carbs 5.3g
- Fat 71g
- Protein 49g

Recipe 217. Paprika Pork and Scallions

Serving Size: 4

Preparation Time: 10 minutes

Cooking Time: 30 minutes

Ingredients:

- 4 scallions, chopped
- 2 garlic cloves, minced
- 2 tablespoons olive oil
- 2 pounds pork stew meat, cubed
- 1 teaspoon sweet paprika
- A pinch of salt and black pepper
- ½ cup mustard
- 1 tablespoon chives, chopped

Directions:

- Heat up a pan with the oil over medium heat, add the scallions and the garlic and sauté for 5 minutes.
- Add the meat and brown it for 5 minutes.
- Add the rest of the ingredients, toss, cook over medium heat for 20 minutes more, divide into bowls and serve.

Nutritional Information:

- Calories 271
- Fat 5
- Carbs 15
- Protein 20

Recipe 218. Parmesan Beef Stuffed Mushrooms

Serving Size: 4

Preparation Time: 25 minutes

Cooking Time: 55 minutes

Ingredients:

- 1 2 lb ground beef
- 1/2 cup Romano cheese, grated
- 2 tbsp olive oil
- 1/2 celery stalk cut into pieces
- 1 shallot finely chopped
- 2 tbsp mayonnaise
- 1 teaspoon Old Bay seasoning
- 1/2 1 teaspoon garlic powder
- 2 large eggs
- 4 Portobello mushroom caps
- 1 tablespoon flaxseed meal
- 2 tbsp of shredded Parmesan
- 1 Tbsp chopped parsley

Directions:

- Preheat the oven to a heat of 360 F. In a pan and sauté celery and shallot for 3 minutes. Set aside. Add the beef to the pan and let it cook for 10 mins. Add the mixture to the shallots. Add mayonnaise Old Bay seasoning, garlic powder, Pecorino cheese, and crack eggs. Mix the ingredients equally.
- Then, arrange them on a baking sheet that has been greased and then fill them with the meat mixture. Mix flaxseed meal and Parmesan cheese into a large bowl. Sprinkle over the filling of the mushrooms. Bake until the cheese is melted in about 30 minutes. Sprinkle with parsley before serving.

Nutritional Information:

- Cal 352
- Net Carbs 3.5g
- Fat 28g
- Protein 42g

Recipe 219. Peach-Mustard Pork Shoulder

Serving Size: 8

Preparation Time: 2 minutes

Cooking Time: 55 minutes

Ingredients:

- 4 pounds pork shoulder
- 1 cup peach preserving:
- 1 cup white wine
- 1/3 cup salt
- 1 tablespoon grainy mustard

Directions:

- Season the pork well with salt.
- Mix mustard and peach and rub on the pork.
- Pour wine into cooker and add pork.
- Seal the lid.
- Hit "chicken/meat" and adjust time to 55 minutes.
- When time is up, hit "cancel" and wait 10 minutes before quick releasing.
- Pork should be cooked to at least 145-degrees.
- Move pork to a plate and tent with foil for 15 minutes before slicing and serving.

Nutritional Information:

- Total calories: 583
- Protein: 44
- Carbs: 26
- Fat: 32

Recipe 220. Pesto Chicken Breasts with Summer Squash

Serving Size: 4

Preparation Time: 15 minutes

Cooking Time: 10 minutes

Ingredients:

- 4 medium boneless, skinless chicken breast halves
- 1 tablespoon olive oil
- 2 tablespoons Homemade pesto
- 2 cups finely chopped zucchini
- 2 tablespoons Finely shredded Asiago

Directions:

- Cook your chicken in hot oil on medium heat within 4 minutes in a large nonstick skillet. Flip the chicken then put the zucchini.
- Cook for 10 minutes. Serve

Nutritional Information:

- Calories: 230
- Fat: 9 g
- Carbs: 8 g
- Protein: 30 g

Recipe 221. Pineapple Glazed Chicken

Serving Size: 4

Preparation Time: 10 minutes

Cooking Time: 1 hour 10 minutes

Ingredients:

- ½ cup apricot preserves
- ½ cup pineapple preserves
- 1 tablespoon low sodium soy sauce
- 1 onion, chopped
- ¼ teaspoon red pepper flakes
- 1 tablespoon vegetable oil
- Black pepper to the taste
- 6 chicken legs

Directions:

- In a bowl, mix soy sauce, pepper flakes, apricot and pineapple preserves and whisk really well.
- Heat up a large-sized pan with the oil over medium high heat, add chicken pieces, cook them for 5 minutes on each side and transfer to a bowl.
- Spread onion on the bottom of a baking dish and add chicken pieces on top.
- Season with black pepper, drizzle the tea glaze on top, cover dish, introduce in the oven at 350 degrees F and bake for 30 minutes.
- Uncover dish and bake for 20 minutes more.
- Divide chicken on plates and keep warm.
- Pour cooking juices into a pan, heat up over medium high heat, cook until sauce is reduced and drizzle it over chicken pieces.

Nutritional Information:

- Calories 198
- Fat 1
- Carbs 4
- Protein 19

Recipe 222. Pizzaiola Steaks

Serving Size: 4

Preparation Time: 10 minutes

Cooking Time: 25 minutes

Ingredients:

- 4 (4-ounce) sliced rump or chuck steaks
- Salt and pepper, to taste
- 3 tablespoons flour
- 3 tablespoons canola oil
- 3 cloves garlic, smashed
- 1 can plum tomatoes with juice, chopped
- 2 tablespoons fresh basil, chopped
- 2 cups packed baby spinach

Directions:

- Dredge steaks in flour to coat and tap to remove excess. Lightly season with salt and pepper.
- Heat nonstick pan over medium heat and add oil and garlic. Cook for 1 minute.
- Raise heat to high and add steaks to pan. Brown steaks quickly on both sides.
- Add in tomatoes, basil, and spinach. Reduce heat to low and simmer 12 to 15 minutes covered.

Nutritional Information:

- Calories: 320
- Fat: 19g
- Protein: 25g
- Carbohydrates: 11g

Recipe 223. Pork and Salsa

Serving Size: 4

Preparation Time: 10 minutes

Cooking Time: 15 minutes

Ingredients:

- 8 ounces canned pineapple, crushed
- 1 tablespoon olive oil
- 1 pound pork, ground
- 1 teaspoon chili powder
- 1 teaspoon garlic powder
- 1 teaspoon cumin, ground
- Black pepper to the taste
- 1 mango, chopped
- Juice of 1 lime
- 2 avocados, pitted, peeled, and chopped
- ¼ cup cilantro, chopped

Directions:

- Heat up a large-sized pan with the oil over medium heat, add pork meat stir and brown for 5 minutes.
- Add garlic, cumin, chili powder, pineapple, and pepper, stir and cook for 10 minutes.
- In a bowl, mix mango with avocados, lime juice, cilantro and pepper and stir.
- Divide the pork and pineapple mix between plates, top with the mango salsa and serve.
- Enjoy!

Nutritional Information:

- Calories 270
- Fat 6
- Carbs 12
- Protein 22

Recipe 224. Pork and Zucchini Stew

Serving Size: 4

Preparation Time: 10 minutes

Cooking Time: 50 minutes

Ingredients:

- 1 pound round pork, cubed
- Black pepper to the taste
- ¼ teaspoon sweet paprika
- 1 tablespoon olive oil
- 1 and ½ cups low-sodium veggie stock
- 3 cups zucchinis, cubed
- 1 yellow onion, chopped
- ½ cup low-sodium tomato sauce
- 1 tablespoon parsley, chopped

Directions:

- Heat up a large-sized pot with the oil over medium-high heat, add the pork, black pepper and paprika, stir and brown for 5 minutes.
- Add stock, onion and tomato sauce, toss, bring to a simmer, reduce heat to medium and cook for 40 minutes.
- Add the zucchinis and the parsley, toss, cook for 15 minutes more, divide into bowls and serve.
- Enjoy!

Nutritional Information:

- Calories 370
- Fat 7
- Carbs 12
- Protein 17

Recipe 225. Pork Chops with Green Beans and Avocado

Serving Size: 4

Preparation Time: 20 minutes

Cooking Time: 30 minutes

Ingredients:

- 4 - Pork shoulder chops
- 4 tbsp avocado oil
- 1 1/2 cups green beans
- 2 large avocados, chopped
- 6 green onions cut into pieces
- 1 Tbsp chopped parsley
- Black pepper and salt to taste

Directions:

- Heat the prepared avocado oil in a large skillet at medium-high temperature. Sprinkle your pork in salt and black pepper, cook until golden for 12 minutes, and then set aside. In the same pan, add green beans and sauté until they sweat and soften for 10 minutes.
- Add avocados and half of the green onions, cooking for about 2 minutes. Divide the saute among plates, decorate with the rest of the green onions, and sprinkle with parsley. Serve those pork chops.

Nutritional Information:

- Cal 321
- Net Carbs 3.9g
- Fat 36g
- Protein 43g

Recipe 226. Pork Meatballs

Serving Size: 4

Preparation Time: 10 minutes

Cooking Time: 10 minutes

Ingredients:

- 1 pound pork, ground
- 1/3 cup cilantro, chopped
- 1 cup red onion, chopped
- 4 garlic cloves, minced
- 1 tablespoon ginger, grated
- 1 Thai chili, chopped
- 2 tablespoons olive oil

Directions:

- In a bowl, combine the meat with cilantro, onion, garlic, ginger, and chili, stir well and shape medium meatballs out of this mix.
- Heat up a large-sized pan with the oil over medium-high heat, add the meatballs, cook them for 5 minutes on each side, divide them between plates and serve with a side salad.
- Enjoy!

Nutritional Information:

- Calories 220
- Fat 4
- Carbs 8
- Protein 14

Recipe 227. Pork Roast with Cranberry

Serving Size: 4

Preparation Time: 10 minutes

Cooking Time: 1 hour 30 minutes

Ingredients:

- 1 tablespoon coconut flour
- Black pepper to the taste
- 1 and ½ pounds pork loin roast
- ½ teaspoon ginger, grated
- ½ cup cranberries
- 2 garlic cloves, minced
- Juice of ½ lemon
- ½ cup low-sodium veggie stock

Directions:

- Put the stock in a small pan, heat it up over medium-high heat, add black pepper, ginger, garlic, cranberries, lemon juice and the flour, whisk well and cook for 10 minutes.
- Put the roast in a pan, add the cranberry sauce on top, introduce in the oven and bake at 375 degrees F for 1 hour and 20 minutes.
- Slice the roast, divide it and the sauce between plates and serve.
- Enjoy!

Nutritional Information:

- Calories 330
- Fat 13
- Carbs 13
- Protein 25

Recipe 228. Pork Sausage Sauerkraut

Serving Size: 4

Preparation Time: 30 minutes

Cooking Time: 1 hour 10 minutes

Ingredients:

- 2 tbsp olive oil
- 1 lb pork sausages, sliced
- 2 cups sauerkraut, drained
- Black pepper and salt to taste
- 1/2 cup Ham chopped
- 1 cup chicken broth
- 1 tbsp tomato paste
- 1 onion cut into pieces
- 2 cloves of garlic, minced
- 1 Tbsp butter
- 1/4 cup Parmesan cheese grated
- 1/2 teaspoon cumin
- 1/2 tsp nutmeg

Directions:

- Prepare a pot using butter and olive oil at medium-high temperature. Add the garlic and onion to cook for 3 mins. Add the pork sausages and ham and cook until lightly browned, approximately 5 to 4-5 minutes.
- Add the sauerkraut to the broth and cook for about 30 minutes. Add the tomato paste and cumin, black pepper, nutmeg, and salt. Serve with Parmesan cheese. Bake in the oven for about 20 mins at 350 F. Serve and have a blast!

Nutritional Information:

- Cal 355
- Net Carbs 6.6g
- Fat 22g
- Protein 25g

Recipe 229. Pork Stew with Shallots

Serving Size: 4

Preparation Time: 10 minutes

Cooking Time: 15 minutes

Ingredients:

- 2 shallots, chopped
- 2 tablespoons olive oil
- 4 garlic cloves, minced
- 1 pound pork, ground
- 1 eggplant, cubed
- 14 ounces canned tomatoes, no-salt-added and chopped
- Black pepper to the taste
- ½ cup basil, chopped
- 2 tablespoons low-sodium tomato paste
- ¾ cup coconut cream

Directions:

- Heat up a pan with half of the oil over medium heat, add garlic and shallots, stir, and cook for 5 minutes.
- Add pork, stir, and brown for 4 minutes.

- Heat up another pan with the rest of the oil over medium heat, add eggplant, stir, cook for 5 minutes, and add over the meat.
- Also add tomatoes, pepper, basil, tomato paste and coconut cream, stir, cook for 1 more minute, divide into bowls and serve.
- Enjoy!

Nutritional Information:

- Calories 261
- Fat 11
- Carbs 8
- Protein 22

Recipe 230. Pork with Dates Sauce

Serving Size: 6

Preparation Time: 10 minutes

Cooking Time: 40 minutes

Ingredients:

- 1 and ½ pounds pork tenderloin
- 2 tablespoons water
- 1/3 cup dates, pitted
- ¼ teaspoon onion powder
- ¼ teaspoon smoked paprika
- 2 tablespoons mustard
- ¼ cup coconut aminos
- Black pepper to the taste

Directions:

- In your prepared food processor, mix dates with water, coconut aminos, mustard, paprika, pepper and onion powder and blend well.
- Put pork tenderloin in a roasting pan, add the dates sauce, toss to coat very well, introduce everything in the oven at 400 degrees F, bake for 40 minutes, slice the meat, divide it and the sauce between plates and serve.
- Enjoy!

Nutritional Information:

- Calories 240
- Fat 8
- Carbs 13
- Protein 24

Recipe 231. Pork with Mushrooms Bowls

Serving Size: 6

Preparation Time: 10 minutes

Cooking Time: 23 minutes

Ingredients:

- Juice of 1 lime
- 1 and ½ pounds pork steak, cut into strips
- ½ teaspoon chili powder
- Black pepper to the taste
- 1 teaspoon sweet paprika
- ½ teaspoon oregano, dried
- 2 tablespoons olive oil
- 2 red bell peppers, chopped
- 1 yellow onion, sliced
- 5 ounces mushrooms, chopped
- 1 garlic clove, minced
- 2 green onions, chopped
- 1 jalapeno, chopped
- 1 cup low-sodium veggie stock
- ¼ cup parsley, chopped

Directions:

- In a bowl, mix lime juice with black pepper, chili powder, paprika, oregano and meat strips and toss well.
- Heat up a large-sized pan with the oil over medium-high heat, add the meat, cook for 4 minutes on each side and transfer to a plate.
- Heat up the same pan over medium heat, add bell peppers, mushrooms, garlic and onions, stir and cook for 5 minutes.
- Add stock, green onion, lime juice, jalapeno, return the meat, stir and cook for 10 minutes more.
- Divide everything between plates and serve with parsley on top.
- Enjoy!

Nutritional Information:

- Calories 250
- Fat 12
- Carbs 7
- Protein 14

Recipe 232. Pumpkin and Black Beans Chicken

Serving Size: 4

Preparation Time: 15 minutes

Cooking Time: 25 minutes

Ingredients:

- 1 tbsp. essential olive oil
- 1 tbsp. Chopped cilantro
- 1 c. coconut milk
- 15 oz canned black beans, drained
- 1 lb. skinless and boneless chicken breasts
- 2 c. water
- ½ c. pumpkin flesh

Directions:

- Heat a pan when using oil over medium-high heat, add the chicken and cook for 5 minutes.
- Add the river, milk, pumpkin, and black beans toss, cover the pan, reduce heat to medium and cook for 20 mins. Add the prepared cilantro, toss, divide between plates and serve. Enjoy!

Nutritional Information:

- Calories: 354
- Fat:6 g
- Carbs:16 g
- Protein:22 g

Recipe 233. Red Wine Beef Roast and Vegetables

Serving Size: 2

Preparation Time: 45 minutes

Cooking Time: 2 hours 20 minutes

Ingredients:

- 1 tbsp olive oil
- 1 lb of brisket
- 1/2 cup carrots peeled, 1 cup
- 1 onion red, cut in quarters
- 2 stalks of celery, cut into chunks
- 1 clove of garlic, chopped
- Black pepper and salt to taste
- 1 leaf from a bay
- 1 tablespoon fresh thyme chopped
- 1 cup red wine 1 cup red

Directions:

- Sprinkle the brisket using salt and black pepper. Cook the meat on both sides in hot olive oil at medium-high temperature for about 6-8 minutes. Transfer to a deep casserole dish. Arrange the onions, carrots, garlic, thyme bay leaf, and celery around the brisket.
- Pour into the red wine along with half a cup of water. Place the pot in a lid and place it in the preheated 350 F oven. Cook for two hours. When the dish is ready, you can remove the casserole. Transfer the beef onto a chopping board and slice it into long slices. Serve the beef with vegetables to serve.

Nutritional Information:

- Cal 300
- Net Carbs 8.6g
- Fat 22g
- Protein 52g

Recipe 234. Roasted Chicken

Serving Size: 8

Preparation Time: 45 minutes

Cooking Time: 1 hour 35 minutes

Ingredients:

- 1 medium yellow onion, peeled and chopped
- 2 stalks celery, chopped roughly
- 1 medium carrot, peeled and chopped
- 1 head garlic, cut in half
- 1 sprig fresh thyme
- 1 sprig fresh rosemary
- 1 teaspoon kosher salt
- ½ teaspoon black pepper
- 1 teaspoon garlic powder
- 1 teaspoon onion powder
- 2 tablespoons canola oil
- 1 (3½-pound) chicken, skin removed, rinsed, and dried

Directions:

- Preheat oven to 350°F.
- Place chopped vegetables and herbs in bottom of roasting pan.
- In a small bowl, combine oil and spices. Rub mixture on all surfaces of chicken.
- Place chicken on top of vegetables breast side down and cover. Cook for 35 minutes.
- Flip over chicken in pan. Cook uncovered for another 45 minutes.
- When internal temperature is 155°F, or chicken is fully cooked at the joints, remove from oven, and allow to rest. Carve and serve.

Nutritional Information:

- Calories: 240
- Fat: 8g
- Protein: 35g
- Carbohydrates: 5g

Recipe 235. Roasted Chicken Thighs

Serving Size: 4

Preparation Time: 15 minutes

Cooking Time: 55 minutes

Ingredients:

- 8 chicken thighs
- 3 tablespoons fresh parsley, chopped
- 1 tsp dried oregano
- 6 garlic cloves, crushed
- ¼ cup capers, drained
- 10 oz roasted red peppers, sliced
- 2 cups grape tomatoes
- 1 ½ lbs. potatoes, cut into small chunks
- 4 tablespoons olive oil
- Pepper
- Salt

Directions:

- Warm oven to 200 400 F. Season chicken with pepper and salt. Heat-up 2 tablespoons of olive oil in a pan over medium heat. Add chicken to the pan and sear until lightly golden brown from all the sides.
- Transfer chicken onto a baking tray. Add tomato, potatoes, capers, oregano, garlic, and red peppers around the chicken. Season with pepper and salt and drizzle with remaining olive oil. Bake in preheated oven for 45-55 minutes. Garnish with parsley and serve.

Nutritional Information:

- Calories: 448
- Fat: 29.1g
- Protein: 91.3g
- Carbs: 45.2g

Recipe 236. Roasted Lemon Swordfish

Serving Size: 4

Preparation Time: 10 minutes

Cooking Time: 1 hour 20 minutes

Ingredients:

- ¼ cup parsley, chopped
- ½ teaspoon garlic, chopped
- ½ teaspoon canola oil
- 4 swordfish fillets, 6 ounces each
- ¼ teaspoon sunflower seeds
- 1 tablespoon sugar
- 2 lemons, quartered and seeds removed

Directions:

- Preheat your oven to 375 degrees F.
- Take a small-sized bowl and add sugar, sunflower seeds, lemon wedges.
- Toss well to coat them.
- Take a shallow baking dish and add lemons, cover with aluminum foil.
- Roast for about 60 minutes until lemons are tender and browned (Slightly).
- Heat your grill and place the rack about 4 inches away from the source of heat.
- Take a baking pan and coat it with cooking spray.
- Transfer fish fillets to the pan and brush with oil on top spread garlic on top.
- Grill for about 5 minutes each side until fillet turns opaque.
- Transfer fish to a serving platter, squeeze roasted lemon on top.
- Sprinkle parsley serve with a lemon wedge on the side.
- Enjoy!

Nutritional Information:

- Calories: 280
- Fat: 12g
- Net Carbohydrates: 4g
- Protein: 34g

Recipe 237. Rosemary Chicken with Avocado Sauce

Serving Size: 2

Preparation Time: 15 minutes

Cooking Time: 35 minutes

Ingredients:

- Sauce
- 1/4 cup mayonnaise
- 1 avocado, pitted
- 1 2 tbsp lemon juice
- Salt to taste
- Chicken
- 2 tbsp olive oil
- 2 chicken breasts
- Black pepper and salt to taste
- 1/2 cup rosemary chopped

Directions:

- Mash the avocado using the help of a fork in the bowl. Mix in the mayonnaise mixture, juice of a lemon, and

salt. Stir to mix. The olive oil should be heated in the pan at a medium-low temperature. Sprinkle your chicken's meat with salt and pepper and cook for four minutes for each side until it is golden. Transfer the chicken to an apron. Place the 1 cup of hot liquid into the pan and put it in the rosemary.
- Bring the water to a boil, reduce the heat, and let it simmer for 3 minutes. Then add the chicken. Cover and cook for 10 to 15 minutes or until the liquid is reduced and the chicken is cooked. Divide the chicken between plates, and then spoon the avocado sauce on top. Serve and take a bite.

Nutritional Information:

- Cal 306
- Net Carbs 3.9g
- Fat 34g
- Protein 22g

Recipe 238. Rosemary Pork Medallions

Serving Size: 4

Preparation Time: 20 minutes

Cooking Time: 40 minutes

Ingredients:

- 1 lb tenderloin of pork, cut into medallions
- 2 onions cut into pieces
- 4 oz bacon, chopped
- 1/2 cup vegetable stock
- Black pepper and salt to taste
- 2 tbsp rosemary chopped

Directions:

- Cook the bacon on a skillet at medium-high heat until crisp for 5 minutes, then remove. Add onion, peppers, and salt. Cook for 5 minutes before transferring to the plate with bacon.
- Add the pork back into the pan. Cook for 3-4 mins, then flip and cook for another 3-4 minutes or until it is browned. Mix in the stock, then cook for another 10 minutes. Add bacon and onions back to the skillet and let them cook for one minute. Sprinkle with rosemary.

Nutritional Information:

- Cal 325
- Net Carbs 5.5g
- Fat 17g
- Protein 35g

Recipe 239. Salmon and Brussels Sprouts

Serving Size: 6

Preparation Time: 10 minutes

Cooking Time: 20 minutes

Ingredients:

- 2 tablespoons brown sugar
- 1 teaspoon onion powder
- 1 teaspoon garlic powder
- 1 teaspoon smoked paprika
- 3 tablespoons olive oil
- 1 and ¼ pounds Brussels sprouts, halved
- 6 medium salmon fillets, boneless

Directions:

- In a bowl, mix sugar with onion powder, garlic powder, smoked paprika and 2 tablespoon olive oil and whisk well.
- Spread Brussels sprouts on a prepared lined baking sheet, drizzle the rest of the olive oil, toss to coat, introduce in the oven at 450 degrees F and bake for 5 minutes.
- Add salmon fillets brush with sugar mix you've prepared, introduce in the oven, and bake for 15 minutes more.
- Divide everything between plates and serve.
- Enjoy!

Nutritional Information:

- Calories 212
- Fat 5
- Carbs 12
- Protein 8

Recipe 240. Saucy Chicken Legs with Vegetables

Serving Size: 4

Preparation Time: 25 minutes

Cooking Time: 50 minutes

Ingredients:

- 2 tbsp olive oil
- 1 parsnip, cut into pieces
- 2 celery stalks cut into pieces
- 2 cups chicken stock
- 1 onion chopped

- Red wine 1/4 cup
- 1 lb chicken legs
- 1 cup chopped tomatoes
- 1 cup spinach
- 1/4 teaspoon dried thyme
- Black pepper and salt to taste
- 1 tbsp chopped parsley, chopped

Directions:

- Set a large pan in medium-high heat and heat the olive oil within. Add celery, parsnips, and onions, season with salt and pepper, and cook for 5-6 minutes until the vegetables are tender.
- Add the chicken, stir in the meantime, and let it cook for five minutes. Add the red wine, stock tomatoes, thyme, and red wine to cook for 20 mins. Incorporate the spinach, and simmer for 4 minutes or until the spinach is wilted. Sprinkle with chopped parsley and serve.

Nutritional Information:

- Cal 264
- Net Carbs 7.5g
- Fat 15g
- Protein 22g

Recipe 241. Scallion and Egg Beef Bowls

Serving Size: 4

Preparation Time: 20 minutes

Cooking Time: 30 minutes

Ingredients:

- 2 tbsp olive oil
- 4 large eggs
- 1.25 lb. beef sirloin cut into strips
- 1/4 cup tamari sauce
- 2 1 tbsp lemon juice
- 3 teaspoons garlic powder
- 1 tablespoon served sugar
- 2 tablespoons coconut oil
- 6 cloves of garlic, chopped
- 1 lb cauliflower rice
- 2 TBSP chopped onions

Directions:

- In a bowl, make a mixture of tamari sauce, garlic powder, lemon juice, and the sugar you serve. Place the beef in a zip lock bag, and then add the mix. Massage the meat to coat thoroughly. Refrigerate overnight. The next day cooks coconut oil on a stove and cooks the beef until the liquid has evaporated and the meat has cooked for 12 minutes. Then, set aside.
- Sauté garlic for one min in that same pan. Mix in cauli rice until softened, 5 minutes. Serve in 4 bowls and put aside. Wipe the wok clean, then cook 1 tablespoon of olive oil. Crack two eggs into the wok and fry sunshine-style for one minute. Put an egg in each rice bowl of cauliflower and fry the remaining 2 eggs in the olive oil. Serve with scallions.

Nutritional Information:

- Cal 364
- Net Carbs 8g
- Fat 32g
- Protein 34g

Recipe 242. Scallops and Rosemary Potatoes

Serving Size: 4

Preparation Time: 5 minutes

Cooking Time: 22 minutes

Ingredients:

- 1-pound scallops
- ½ teaspoon rosemary, dried
- ½ teaspoon oregano, dried
- 2 tablespoons avocado oil
- 1 yellow onion, chopped
- 2 sweet potatoes, peeled and cubed
- ½ cup chicken stock
- 1 tablespoon cilantro, chopped
- A pinch of salt and black pepper

Directions:

- Heat up a pan with the oil over medium heat, add the onion and sauté for 2 minutes.
- Add the sweet potatoes and the stock, toss, and cook for 10 minutes more.
- Add the scallops and the remaining ingredients, toss, cook for another 10 minutes, divide everything into bowls and serve.

Nutritional Information:

- Calories 211
- Fat 2
- Carbs 26.9
- Protein 20.7

Recipe 243. Sesame Pork Bites

Serving Size: 4

Preparation Time: 20 minutes

Cooking Time: 45 minutes

Ingredients:

- 1 pork tenderloin, cubed
- 1 tablespoon sesame oil
- 1/2 cup plus
- 1 tbsp red wine
- 1 tbsp + 1/3 cup tamari sauce
- 1/2 cup maple syrup without sugar
- 1/2 cup sesame seeds
- 1 teaspoon pureed garlic
- 1/2 1 tsp freshly grated ginger
- 1 Tbsp chopped scallions, diced

Directions:

- Place 1 glass of wine and 1 tbsp of tamari in a zip-lock bag. Incorporate pork cubes, then seal the bag and let the meat marinate in the refrigerator for a night. Preheat the oven up to 350 F. Remove the meat from the refrigerator and wash it. Put the maple syrup, sesame seeds, and a little in two bowls.
- Roll your pork around in the maple syrup, and then roll it in sesame seeds. Put the pork on a baking tray and bake at 350 degrees for 35 minutes. A bowl is used to mix together the rest of the red wine with the remaining Tamari Sauce, Sesame Oil ginger, garlic, and garlic. Put the mix into the bowl. Transfer the pork onto a plate and decorate with scallions. Pour the sauce on top and serve.

Nutritional Information:

- Cal 289
- Net Carbs 6.4g
- Fat 18g
- Protein 30g

Recipe 244. Shrimp with Cilantro Sauce

Serving Size: 2

Preparation Time: 10 minutes

Cooking Time: 4 minutes

Ingredients:

- 1 pound shrimp, peeled and deveined
- 3 tablespoons cilantro, chopped
- 3 tablespoons olive oil
- 1 tablespoon pine nuts
- Zest of 1 lemon, grated
- Juice of ½ lemon

Directions:

- In your blender, combine the cilantro with 2 tablespoons oil, pine nuts, lemon zest and lemon juice and pulse well.
- Heat up a pan with the rest of the oil over medium-high heat, add the shrimp and cook for 3 minutes.
- Add the cilantro mix, toss, cook for 1 more minute, divide between plates and serve with a side salad.
- Enjoy!

Nutritional Information:

- Calories 210
- Fat 5
- Carbs 8
- Protein 12

Recipe 245. Smoked Sausage Casserole

Serving Size: 4

Preparation Time: 15 minutes

Cooking Time: 40 minutes

Ingredients:

- 1 lb smoked sausages, sliced
- 2 tbsp Lard
- 1 chili pepper finely chopped
- 1 onion chopped
- 1 lb green beans, chopped
- 1 cup of mushrooms, sliced
- 1/2 lb turnips, cut into wedges
- 1 teaspoon dried thyme
- Black pepper and salt to taste
- 1 clove of garlic finely minced
- 1 cup of cheddar cheese grated

Directions:

- Heat the lard in the saucepan on medium-high heat. Add the sausages, chili peppers, onions, garlic, and chili pepper. Stir fry for approximately about 5 minutes or until the onions are tender. Add the mushrooms, green beans, and turnips. Cook for 3-5 mins.
- Sprinkle with salt, pepper, thyme, and salt. Transfer the dish to the baking dish, then bake it in the heated 380 F oven for 12 to 15 minutes. Sprinkle with cheese

and bake for approximately another 5-8 minutes until the cheese is melted. Serve.

Nutritional Information:

- Cal 326
- Net Carbs 5.6g
- Fat 48g
- Protein 33g

Recipe 246. Spiced Winter Pork Roast

Serving Size: 6

Preparation Time: 10 minutes

Cooking Time: 3 hours 20 minutes

Ingredients:

- 2 and ½ pounds pork roast
- Black pepper to the taste
- 1 teaspoon chili powder
- ½ teaspoon onion powder
- ¼ teaspoon cumin, ground
- 1 teaspoon cocoa powder

Directions:

- In a large-sized roasting pan, combine the roast with black pepper, chili powder, onion powder, cumin and cocoa, rub, cover the pan, introduce in the oven, and bake at 325 degrees F for 3 hours and 20 minutes.
- Slice, divide between plates and serve with a side salad.
- Enjoy!

Nutritional Information:

- Calories 288
- Fat 5
- Carbs 12
- Protein 23

Recipe 247. Sriracha Tuna Kabobs

Serving Size: 4

Preparation Time: 9 minutes

Cooking Time: 4 minutes

Ingredients:

- 4 T Huy Fong chili garlic sauce
- 1 T sesame oil infused with garlic
- 1 T ginger, fresh, grated
- 1 T garlic, minced
- 1 red onion, quarters and separated by petals
- 2 cups bell peppers, red, green, yellow
- 1 can whole water chestnuts, halved
- ½ pound fresh mushrooms, halved
- 32 oz. boneless tuna, chunks, or steaks
- 1 Splenda packet
- 2 zucchinis, sliced 1 inch thick, keep skins on

Directions:

- Layer the tuna and the vegetable pieces evenly onto 8 skewers.
- Combine the spices and the oil and chili sauce, add the Splenda
- Quickly blend, either in blender or by quickly whipping.
- Brush onto the kabob pieces, make sure every piece is coated
- Grill 4 minutes on each side, check to ensure the tuna is cooked to taste.
- Serving size is two skewers.

Nutritional Information:

- Calories: 467
- Total Fat: 18g
- Protein: 56g
- Total Carbs: 21g

Recipe 248. Stuffed Chicken Breasts

Serving Size: 2

Preparation Time: 25 minutes

Cooking Time: 55 minutes

Ingredients:

- 2 tbsp butter
- 2 chicken breasts
- 1 cup baby spinach
- 1 carrot and chopped
- 1 tomato cut into pieces
- 1/4 cup goat cheese
- Black pepper and salt to taste
- 1 teaspoon dried oregano
- 2 cucumbers spiralized
- 2 tbsp olive oil
- 1 tbsp rice vinegar
- 1 tbsp fresh dill chopped

Directions:

- The oven should be heated up to 390 F. Lightly coat the baking dish using cooking spray. Place a skillet over moderate temperature. The butter should be melted to half the size, and sauté the carrots, spinach, and tomato until soft in approximately 5 minutes. Add salt and pepper to taste. Transfer the ingredients to an ice-cold bowl and let cool for about 10 minutes. Add either goat cheese or dried herbs, mix and put aside. Slice the breasts of chicken in length and stuff them with this cheese mix.

- Put the chicken in the dish for baking. Sprinkle with salt and pepper, then brush with the rest of the butter. Bake until the cucumbers are cooked for 20 to 30 minutes. Arrange the cucumbers on the platter, then toss them with salt, dill, olive oil, black pepper, and vinegar to coat. Serve the chicken stuffed.

Nutritional Information:

- Cal 361
- Net Carbs 9.5g
- Fat 38g
- Protein 37g

Recipe 249. Sweet Pork Chops with Spaghetti Squash

Serving Size: 4

Preparation Time: 35 minutes

Cooking Time: 1 hour 15 minutes

Ingredients:

- 1 tbsp olive oil
- 3 tablespoons peanut oil
- Pork chops with boneless bones
- 1 lb chopped kale
- 1 (3-lb) spaghetti squash
- 2 tablespoons lemongrass minced
- 3 tbsp fresh ginger paste
- 2 tablespoons sugar-free maple syrup
- 2 tablespoons coconut aminos
- 1 tbsp fish sauce
- 1/2 cup coconut milk
- 1 cup of peanut butter
- Black pepper and salt to taste

Directions:

- Cut longways the spaghetti squash, from the stem to the tail. Scoop the seeds in a bowl, blend lemongrass and 2 tablespoons of ginger paste aminos and fish sauce. The pork is coated with the liquid. Refrigerate for 45 minutes. Warm 2 tablespoons of peanut oil into a pan and remove the pork from the marinade. Sear in both Directions for 10 to 15 minutes. Transfer the spaghetti squash to a plate and protect it with aluminum foil to stay warm.
- Preheat the oven to 350 F. Put spaghetti squashes on baking sheets, rub with olive oil and sprinkle with pepper and salt. Cook for about 45 mins. Take the squash out and shred with forks into spaghetti-like strands. Place aside. The remaining peanut oil is heated in the same pan and sauté the remaining ginger paste. Then add kale and cook for two minutes. Set aside. Within a bowl, stir coconut milk and peanut butter until thoroughly combined. Divide the pork among four plates, then add spaghetti squash to one side, followed by the kale. Drizzle the peanut sauce over. Serve.

Nutritional Information:

- Cal 302 calories
- net carbs of 7g
- fats 34g
- Protein 49g

Recipe 250. Tandoori Chicken

Serving Size: 4

Preparation Time: 30 minutes

Cooking Time: 55 minutes

Ingredients:

- 4 chicken thigh/leg quarters
- 4 tablespoons vegetable oil
- 2 teaspoons salt
- 1 teaspoon curry powder
- 1 teaspoon paprika
- 1 teaspoon turmeric
- 1 teaspoon ground coriander
- 1 teaspoon chili powder
- 1 teaspoon allspice
- 1 teaspoon ground ginger
- 1 teaspoon fresh chopped parsley
- 1 teaspoon garlic powder
- 2 tablespoons plain yogurt
- 1 fresh lime

Directions:

- Preheat oven to 375°F. Line a prepared sheet pan with foil and place baking rack over foil.
- Pull skin from chicken to bottom of leg (do not remove).
- Combine all ingredients (except lime) and rub a thin coating onto chicken, then replace skin and place chicken on baking rack.

- Cook 50–60 minutes until done, then squeeze fresh lime juice over chicken before serving.

Nutritional Information:

- Calories: 290
- Fat: 24g
- Protein: 16g
- Carbohydrates: 4g

Recipe 251. Thyme Beef and Bacon Casserole

Serving Size: 4

Preparation Time: 25 minutes

Cooking Time: 40 minutes

Ingredients:

- 2 tbsp olive oil
- 2 tbsp of ghee
- 1 cup Pumpkin and chopped
- 1/2 cup celery Chopped
- 3 bacon slices, chopped
- 1 lb beef for stew Cubed
- 1 clove of garlic, minced
- 1 onion chopped
- 1 tbsp red vinegar
- Two cups of beef stock
- 1 tbsp tomato puree
- 1 cinnamon stick
- 1 lemon peel strip
- 3 thyme sprigs of thyme, chopped
- Black pepper and salt to taste

Directions:

- Place a pan on medium-high heat. Warm oil and add the garlic, celery, and onions to cook for 3 mins. Add bacon and beef and cook until lightly brown.
- Pour in the vinegar, ghee, lemon peel strip, tomato puree, stock, cinnamon stick, and pumpkin. Then cover and simmer for about 25 minutes. Take out the cinnamon and lemon peel stick. Adjust the seasoning and garnish with thyme before serving.

Nutritional Information:

- Cal 382
- Net Carbs 5.5g
- Fat 40g
- Protein 32g

Recipe 252. Turmeric Chicken Wings with Ginger Sauce

Serving Size: 4

Preparation Time: 15 minutes

Cooking Time: 35 minutes

Ingredients:

- 2 tbsp olive oil
- 1 lb chicken wings cut in half
- 1 tbsp of turmeric
- 1 2 tablespoons cumin
- 3 tablespoons fresh ginger, grated
- Black pepper and salt to taste
- A half lime and 1/2 lemon juice
- 1 cup of thyme leaves
- 3/4 cup chopped cilantro
- 1 jalapeno pepper, seeded

Directions:

- A bowl is used to mix 1 tbsp of ginger with cumin, salt, half olive oil, turmeric, pepper, and cilantro. In the chicken wings, mix to coat and then refrigerate for 20 mins. The grill should be heated to high temperatures.
- Take the wings out of the refrigerator and grill for 20-25 minutes, rotating at intervals, and then put them aside. Blend thyme with remaining ginger salt, jalapeno, salt, black pepper, and lime juice. Add the remainder of olive oil as well as 1 tablespoon of water. Blend thoroughly. Serve the wings of chicken alongside the sauce.

Nutritional Information:

- Cal 253
- Net Carbs 5.5g
- Fat 16g
- Protein 22g

Recipe 253. Turnip Greens and Artichoke Chicken

Serving Size: 4

Preparation Time: 15 minutes

Cooking Time: 40 minutes

Ingredients:

- 4 oz canned artichoke heart chopped
- 4 oz cream cheese

- 2 chicken breasts cut
- 1 cup turnip greens
- 1/4 cup Pecorino cheese, grated
- 1/2 tbsp onion powder
- 1/2 tbsp garlic powder
- Black pepper and salt to taste
- 2 oz Monterrey Jack Shredded

Directions:

- Prepare a large-sized baking dish by covering it with parchment paper and placing the chicken pieces in the bottom. Sprinkle salt and pepper on top. Bake to 350 F and bake for 20 to 25 minutes.
- In a mixing bowl, mix the other ingredients and mix thoroughly. Take the cooked chicken out of the oven and place it on top of the artichokes. Sprinkle the dish with Monterrey cheese and cook for five more minutes. Serve warm.

Nutritional Information:

- Cal 373
- Net Carbs 6.2g
- Fat 29g
- Protein 31g

Recipe 254. Vegetable Bake and Sausage

Serving Size: 6

Preparation Time: 15 minutes

Cooking Time: 35 minutes

Ingredients:

- 1 butternut squash that has been cut into pieces
- 1 cup mushrooms, quartered
- 1/4 lb smoked sausages, sliced
- 1 onion, cut into slices
- 1/4 1 lb Brussels sprouts
- 1 tbsp rosemary chopped,
- 1 tbsp chopped thyme
- 4 cloves of garlic peeled and only
- 3 tbsp olive oil
- Black pepper and salt to taste

Directions:

- Preheat the oven until the temperature of 450 F. Place the butternut squash and onion and garlic cloves, mushrooms, sausages, and Brussels sprouts on baking sheets.
- Sprinkle with salt and pepper, drizzle olive oil and toss to coat. Roast for 20 to 25 minutes. Sprinkle with rosemary and thyme to serve.

Nutritional Information:

- Cal 215
- Net Carbs 14.5g
- Fat 13g
- Protein 6g

Recipe 255. Winter Chicken and Vegetables

Serving Size: 4

Preparation Time: 15 minutes

Cooking Time: 40 minutes

Ingredients:

- 2 tbsp olive oil
- 2 cups of whipping cream
- 1-lb breasts of chicken chopped
- 1 onion cut into pieces
- 1 carrot chopped
- 2 cups chicken stock
- Black pepper and salt to taste
- 1 leaf from a bay
- 1 turnip and chopped
- 1 parsnip chopped
- 1 cup green beans, chopped
- 2 teaspoons fresh thyme chopped

Directions:

- Place a skillet on moderate heat. Warm your olive oil. Sauté the onion for 3 minutes before adding the stock, carrots and turnip, parsnip, chicken, and bay leaves. Bring the mixture to a boil and simmer for about 20 minutes.
- Add the green beans, and simmer for seven minutes. The bay leaf should be removed and stirred into the whipping cream, alter the flavor, and sprinkled with thyme before serving.

Nutritional Information:

- Cal 313
- Net Carbs 10g
- Fat 32g
- Protein 33g

CHAPTER 5. SIDES & SOUPS RECIPES

Recipe 256. Baby Spinach Salad

Serving Size: 2

Preparation Time: 10 minutes

Cooking Time: 5 minutes

Ingredients:

- 1 bag baby spinach, washed and dried
- 1 red bell pepper, cut in slices
- 1 cup cherry tomatoes, cut in halves
- 1 small red onion, finely chopped
- 1 cup black olives, pitted
- For dressing:
- 1 teaspoon dried oregano
- 1 large garlic clove
- 3 tablespoons red wine vinegar
- 4 tablespoons olive oil
- Sunflower seeds and pepper to taste

Directions:

- Prepare the dressing by blending in garlic, olive oil, vinegar in a food processor.
- Take a large-sized salad bowl and add spinach leaves, toss well with the dressing.
- Add remaining ingredients and toss again, season with sunflower seeds and pepper and enjoy!

Nutritional Information:

- Calories: 126
- Fat: 10g
- Carbohydrates: 10g
- Protein: 2g

Recipe 257. Bacon and Gorgonzola Salad

Serving Size: 4

Preparation Time: 15 minutes

Cooking Time: 15 minutes

Ingredients:

- 1 1/2 cups gorgonzola cheese, crumbled
- 1 head of lettuce, divided into leaves
- 4 oz bacon
- 1 tbsp white vinegar
- 3 tablespoons extra-virgin olive oil
- Black pepper and salt to taste
- 2 tablespoons pumpkin seeds

Directions:

- Chop the bacon into smaller pieces and fry them in an oven over moderate heat for about 6 minutes until it is brown and crispy. Mix white wine vinegar and olive oil, salt, and pepper within a bowl to ensure that the dressing is well blended.
- To put the salad together, lay the lettuce out on a platter for serving, then top with the gorgonzola and bacon. Sprinkle the dressing on the salad, lightly mix, then top with pumpkin seeds and serve.

Nutritional Information:

- Cal 239
- Net Carbs 3g
- Fat 32g
- Protein 16g

Recipe 258. Baked Potato with Thyme

Serving Size: 8

Preparation Time: 10 minutes

Cooking Time: 1 hour 15 minutes

Ingredients:

- 6 potatoes, peeled and sliced
- 2 garlic cloves, minced
- 2 tablespoons olive oil
- 1 and ½ cups coconut cream
- ¼ cup coconut milk
- 1 tablespoon thyme, chopped
- ¼ teaspoon nutmeg, ground
- A pinch of red pepper flakes
- 1 and ½ cups low-fat cheddar, shredded
- ½ cup low-fat parmesan, grated

Directions:

- Heat up a pan with the oil over medium heat, add garlic, stir, and cook for 1 minute.
- Add coconut cream, coconut milk, thyme, nutmeg, and pepper flakes, stir, bring to a simmer, reduce heat to low and cook for 10 minutes.
- Arrange 1/3 of the potatoes in a baking dish, add 1/3 of the cream, repeat with the rest of the potatoes and the cream, sprinkle the cheddar on top, cover with tin

foil, introduce in the oven and cook at 375 degrees F for 45 minutes.
- Uncover the dish, sprinkle the parmesan, bake everything for 20 minutes, divide between plates and serve as a side dish.
- Enjoy!

Nutritional Information:

- Calories 224
- Fat 8
- Carbs 16
- Protein 15

Recipe 259. Bean and Barley Soup

Serving Size: 6

Preparation Time: 30 minutes

Cooking Time: 1 hour 15 minutes

Ingredients:

- ¾ cup dried navy or great northern beans, soaked
- 1 medium potato, peeled and diced
- 1 medium onion, peeled and diced
- 1 celery stalk, diced
- 1 small carrot, diced
- 1 bay leaf
- 2 sage leaves
- 1 sprig fresh rosemary
- 4 sprigs parsley
- 1 clove garlic, minced
- ½ cup pearl barley
- ¼ pound turkey bacon

Directions:

- In a large stock pot combine beans, potatoes, onions, celery, carrots, bay leaf, sage, rosemary, parsley, garlic, and 1 quart of water. Bring to a boil and simmer covered over low heat for 1 hour.
- Rinse barley and place in sauté pan with bacon; cover with 1 quart of water and bring to a boil. Allow to boil for 5 minutes.
- Add barley and any remaining water to soup mixture, and simmer 1 more hour, then adjust seasoning to taste and serve.

Nutritional Information:

- Calories: 200
- Fat: 6g
- Protein: 10g
- Carbohydrates: 27g

Recipe 260. Bean Soup

Serving Size: 4

Preparation Time: 15 minutes

Cooking Time: 5 hours

Ingredients:

- ½ cup Pinto Beans (dried)
- ½ Bay Leaf
- 1 clove Garlic
- ½ onion (white)
- 2 cups Water
- 2 tablespoons. Cilantro (chopped)
- 1 cubed Avocado
- 1/8 cup White Onion (chopped)
- ¼ cup Roma Tomatoes (chopped)
- 2 tablespoons. Pepper Sauce (chipotle)
- ¼ teaspoon Kosher Salt
- 2 tablespoons. chopped Cilantro
- 2 tablespoons. Low Fat Monterrey Jack Cheese, shredded

Directions:

- Place water, salt, onion, pepper, garlic, bay leaf, and beans in the slow cooker.
- Cook on high for 5-6 hours. Discard the Bay leaf.
- Serve in heated bowls.

Nutritional Information:

- Calories 258
- Fats 19 g
- Cholesterol 2 mg
- Carbohydrates 25 mg
- Protein 8 g

Recipe 261. Bell Peppers Cakes

Serving Size: 6

Preparation Time: 10 minutes

Cooking Time: 10 minutes

Ingredients:

- 1 tablespoon olive oil
- ½ cup cilantro, chopped
- 2 spring onions, chopped
- 1 red bell pepper, chopped
- 1 green bell pepper, chopped
- 1 egg
- ½ cup almond flour
- A pinch of salt and black pepper
- 2 garlic cloves, minced

- 3 zucchinis, grated

Directions:

- In a bowl, combine the zucchinis with the bell peppers and the other ingredients except the oil, stir well and shape medium cakes out of this mix.
- Heat up a pan with the oil over medium heat, add the cakes, cook for 5 minutes on each side, arrange on a platter, and serve.

Nutritional Information:

- Calories 120
- Fat 4
- Carbs 6
- Protein 6

Recipe 262. Black Bean Soup

Serving Size: 6

Preparation Time: 15 minutes

Cooking Time: 8 hours

Ingredients:

- 1-pound dried black beans, soaked overnight and rinsed
- 1 onion, chopped
- 1 carrot, peeled and chopped
- 2 jalapeño peppers, seeded and diced
- 6 cups Vegetable Broth or store-bought
- 1 teaspoon ground cumin
- 1 teaspoon ground coriander
- 1 teaspoon chili powder
- ½ teaspoon ground chipotle pepper
- ½ teaspoon of sea salt
- ¼ teaspoon freshly ground black pepper
- Pinch cayenne pepper
- ¼ cup fat-free sour cream, for garnish (optional)
- ¼ cup grated low-fat Cheddar cheese, for garnish (optional)

Directions:

- In your slow cooker, combine all the fixing listed, then cook on low for 8 hours.
- If you'd like, mash the beans with a potato masher, or purée using an immersion blender, blender, or food processor.
- Serve topped with the optional garnishes, if desired.

Nutritional Information:

- Calories: 320
- Fat: 3g
- Carbohydrates: 57g
- Protein: 18g

Recipe 263. Butternut Squash Soup

Serving Size: 6

Preparation Time: 15 minutes

Cooking Time: 8 hours

Ingredients:

- 1 butternut squash, peeled, seeded, and diced
- 1 onion, chopped
- 1 sweet-tart apple (such as Braeburn), peeled, cored, and chopped
- 3 cups Vegetable Broth or store-bought
- 1 teaspoon garlic powder
- ½ teaspoon ground sage
- ¼ teaspoon of sea salt
- ¼ teaspoon freshly ground black pepper
- Pinch cayenne pepper
- Pinch nutmeg
- ½ cup fat-free half-and-half

Directions:

- In your slow cooker, combine the squash, onion, apple, broth, garlic powder, sage, salt, black pepper, cayenne, and nutmeg. Cook on low within 8 hours.
- Using an immersion blender, counter-top blender, or food processor, purée the soup, adding the half-and-half as you do. Stir to combine and serve.

Nutritional Information:

- Calories: 106
- Fat: 0g
- Carbohydrates: 26g
- Protein: 3g

Recipe 264. Caprese Salad Stacks Anchovies

Serving Size: 4

Preparation Time: 10 minutes

Cooking Time: 10 minutes

Ingredients:

- 4 fillets of anchovy in oil
- 12 fresh mozzarella slices
- 4 slices of red tomatoes
- 4 tomato slices of yellow
- 1 cup basil pesto

Directions:

- Use a serving plate and alternately place slices of tomato and a mozzarella slice, an orange tomato slice, another slice of mozzarella and the red tomato slice, and finally a slice of mozzarella on top.
- Repeat this process for three more stacks using the same method. Sprinkle pesto on top. Place anchovies on top and serve.

Nutritional Information:

- Cal 292
- Net Carbs 5g
- Fat 20g
- Protein 22g

Recipe 265. Cauliflower Butternut Soup

Serving Size: 6

Preparation Time: 5 minutes

Cooking Time: 25 minutes

Ingredients:

- 1 diced onion
- 2-3 cloves minced garlic
- 1-pound frozen butternut squash
- 1 teaspoon paprika
- ½ teaspoon red pepper flakes
- ½ cup cream
- 1-pound frozen cauliflower
- 2 cups vegetable broth
- 1 teaspoon diced thyme
- ¼ teaspoon sea salt
- 2 teaspoons oil for sautéing
- topping such as cheddar cheese, crumbled bacon, sour cream, chives, cheddar, and crumbled bacon

Directions:

- Heat oil up in pressure cooker, and sauté onion, adding garlic to mixture. Add the cauliflower, broth, spices, and butternut, and from there, mix it together.
- Cook on manual high for approximately about 5 minutes, and natural pressure release, and from there, blend it through an immersion blender, and then serve!

Nutritional Information:

- Calories: 100
- Fat: 3g
- Carbs: 16g
- Protein: 5g

Recipe 266. Cauliflower Cheese Soup

Serving Size: 4

Preparation Time: 15 minutes

Cooking Time: 25 minutes

Ingredients:

- 1/2 head of cauliflower, into pieces
- 2 tablespoons coconut oil
- 1/2 cup chopped leeks, chopped
- 1 celery stalk cut into pieces
- 1 serrano pepper, chopped
- 1 teaspoon garlic puree
- 1 1/2 1 tbsp flaxseed meal
- 1 1/2 cups coconut milk
- 6 Oz Monterey Jack, shredded
- Black pepper and salt to taste
- Fresh parsley chopped and fresh

Directions:

- In a deep large-sized skillet over medium-high heat, melt the coconut oil, then sauté the serrano pepper, celery, and leeks until soft for approximately 5 minutes. Incorporate the coconut milk and garlic purée cauliflower in two cups of water and a flaxseed meal.
- After covering, let it simmer for over 10 minutes or for as long as it takes until cooked. Blend with the aid of an immersion blender till it is smooth. Incorporate the shredded cheese and stir until the cheese has melted completely and is a homogeneous mixture. Sprinkle with salt and pepper according to your preference. Decorate with chopped parsley to serve hot.

Nutritional Information:

- Cal 372
- Net Carbs 7g
- Fat 43g
- Protein 13g

Recipe 267. Cauliflower Soup with Crispy Bacon

Serving Size: 4

Preparation Time: 20 minutes

Cooking Time: 25 minutes

Ingredients:

- 2 tbsp olive oil
- 1 onion chopped
- 1/4 celery root and grated
- 10 oz cauliflower florets
- Black pepper and salt to taste
- 1 cup almond milk.
- 1 cup almond
- 1 cup of white cheddar shred
- 2 oz bacon, cut into strips

Directions:

- A large pan is heated to medium heat. Fry the bacon for 5 minutes or until crisp. Remove to a plate lined with paper towels. In the same skillet, warm olive oil and sauté onions for three minutes until it becomes fragrant. Include the cauliflower florets and the celery root and cook for 3 minutes until soft. Include 3 cups of boiling water, and season by adding salt and pepper.
- Bring the water to a boil and lower the heat to a simmer. The soup will be covered and cooked for about 10 minutes. Puree the soup using the aid of an immersion blender until all the ingredients are evenly mixed, and then add almond milk and cheese, stirring until the cheese melts. Taste the soup and adjust with the black and salt. Add crispy bacon to the top, then serve it hot.

Nutritional Information:

- Cal 333
- Net Carbs 7.6g
- Fat 27g
- Protein 13g

Recipe 268. Cauliflower-Watercress Salad

Serving Size: 4

Preparation Time: 10 minutes

Cooking Time: 15 minutes

Ingredients:

- 2 tablespoons sesame oil
- 1 lemon, juiced and zested
- 10 oz cauliflower florets
- 12 olives of green chopped
- 8 sun-dried tomatoes that have been a drain
- 3 tablespoons chopped scallions
- a handful of toasted peanuts
- 3 tbsp chopped parsley
- 1/2 cup watercress
- Black pepper and salt to taste

Directions:

- In a pot at medium-low temperature, bring the water to the boiling point. Place a steamer basket in the large-sized pot and add the cauliflower. It will soften for about 8 minutes. Transfer the cauliflower into a salad bowl.
- Include tomatoes, olives, and scallions. Add lemon juice and zest Sesame oil, peanuts, watercress, parsley, and parsley. Sprinkle with salt and pepper. Mix with the spoon. Serve.

Nutritional Information:

- Cal 198
- Net Carbs 8.4g
- Fat 10g
- Protein 6g

Recipe 269. Cheddar and Turkey Meatball Salad

Serving Size: 4

Preparation Time: 10 minutes

Cooking Time: 30 minutes

Ingredients:

- 3 tbsp olive oil
- 1 2 tbsp lemon juice
- 1 Lb ground turkey
- Black pepper and salt to taste
- 1 head romaine lettuce, torn
- 2 tomatoes, sliced
- 1 red onion 1/4, cut into slices
- 3 Oz yellow cheddar shred

Directions:

- Mix ground turkey in a bowl with black pepper and salt, then form meatballs. Refrigerate for 10 minutes. The olive oil inside a skillet at medium temperature. Cook the meatballs on both sides for 10 minutes or until cooked and brown inside. Transfer the meatballs to a wire rack to drain the oil.
- Mix the tomatoes, lettuce, and red onion in a bowl for salad. Add the olive oil remaining and lemon juice, salt, and pepper. Mix and place the meatballs. Sprinkle the cheese on top of the salad and serve.

Nutritional Information:

- Cal 382
- Net Carbs 3.5g

- Fat 27g
- Protein 30g

Recipe 270. Cheesy Beef Salad

Serving Size: 4

Preparation Time: 10 minutes

Cooking Time: 15 minutes

Ingredients:

- 1/2 lb of beef Rump steak, cut into strips
- 1 teaspoon cumin
- 3 tbsp olive oil
- Black pepper and salt to taste
- 1 tbsp of thyme
- 1 clove of garlic, chopped
- 1/2 cup ricotta, crumbled
- 1/2 cup pecans, toasted
- 2 cups baby spinach
- 1 1/2 Tbsp lemon juice
- 1 cup mint fresh cut into pieces

Directions:

- The grill should be preheated to medium-high. The beef should be rubbed with salt. Add 1 tablespoon of olive oil, garlic, black pepper, thyme, and cumin. Grill the beef on the barbecue and grill to cook 10 minutes, turning often.
- Sprinkle the pecans in a dry pan on moderate heat and cook for a couple of minutes, shaking it frequently. Transfer the cooked beef to a cutting table, allow it to cool, and cut into strips. In a bowl for salad, mix baby spinach with mint, olive oil, salt, citrus juice, ricotta, and pecans. Toss thoroughly to cover. Serve with slices of beef.

Nutritional Information:

- Cal 237
- Net Carbs 4.2g
- Fat 42g
- Protein 16g

Recipe 271. Cheesy Chicken Soup with Spinach

Serving Size: 4

Preparation Time: 25 minutes

Cooking Time: 45 minutes

Ingredients:

- 2 tbsp olive oil
- 1 onion chopped
- 2 cloves of garlic, chopped
- One carrot chopped
- 1 celery stalk chopped
- 1 chicken breast cubed
- 1 cup Spinach
- 4 cups chicken broth
- 1 cup cheddar, shredded
- 1/2 tsp chili powder
- 1/2 teaspoon ground cumin
- Black pepper and salt to taste

Directions:

- Heat the olive oil inside a pan at medium-high heat and cook the chicken for a couple of minutes. Stir fry the onion, garlic, carrot, and celery for 5 minutes until vegetables become soft. Sprinkle with chili powder along with cumin, salt, and pepper.
- Incorporate the broth of chicken and bring it to the point of boiling. Simmer for 15-20 minutes. Add spinach, stir, then cook another 5-6 mins until the spinach has softened. Serve with cheddar cheese.

Nutritional Information:

- Cal 381
- Net Carbs 5.3g
- Fat 28g
- Protein 22g

Recipe 272. Chicken, Avocado and Egg Bowls

Serving Size: 2

Preparation Time: 20 minutes

Cooking Time: 25 minutes

Ingredients:

- 1 chicken breast cubed
- 1 tbsp avocado oil
- 2 eggs
- 2 cups green beans
- 1 avocado, sliced
- 2 tbsp olive oil
- 2 1 tbsp lemon juice
- 1 tsp Dijon mustard
- 1 2 tbsp mint and chopped
- Black pepper and salt to taste

Directions:

- Blanch the beans in salted, boiling water over medium-low heat for 4-5 mins to ensure that the beans remain crisp and bright green. Rinse with cold water and take them out to drain. In the same boiling water, add the eggs and cook for about 10 minutes. Move them to an Ice tub to let them cool. Peel and cut the avocados. The avocado oil is heated in a skillet over medium-high temperatures.

- In the pan, cook chicken until around 4 minutes. Split the beans into 2 salad bowls. Serve with eggs, chicken as well as avocado pieces. In a separate bowl, mix the juice of the lemon and olive oil with salt, mustard, and pepper. Drizzle it over the salad. Add fresh mint and serve.

Nutritional Information:

- Cal 292
- Net Carbs 6.9g
- Fat 33g
- Protein 30g

Recipe 273. Chicken Salad with Parmesan

Serving Size: 2

Preparation Time: 15 minutes

Cooking Time: 30 minutes

Ingredients:

- 1 lb breast of chicken chopped
- 1 cup juice of a lemon
- 2 cloves of garlic, minced
- 2 tablespoons olive oil
- 1 Romaine lettuce, chopped
- 3 Parmesan crisps
- 2 tbsp Parmesan Grated Dressing
- 2 tbsps extra olive oil
- 1 tbsp lemon juice
- Black pepper and salt to taste

Directions:

- Add the chicken with lemon juice, oil, and garlic to the Ziploc bag. Close in the bag, shake it to blend, and chill for one hour. The grill should be heated to medium and grill the chicken for approximately 3-4 minutes on each side.
- Mix the dressing ingredients in one bowl, and mix thoroughly on a serving plate layout, with salad leaves and Parmesan crisps. Sprinkle the dressing over them and then toss in a coating. Add Chicken and Parmesan cheese. Serve.

Nutritional Information:

- Cal 329
- Net Carbs 5g
- Fat 32g
- Protein 34g

Recipe 274. Chickpea and Kale Soup

Serving Size: 6

Preparation Time: 15 minutes

Cooking Time: 9 hours

Ingredients:

- 1 summer squash, quartered lengthwise and sliced crosswise
- 1 zucchini, quartered lengthwise and sliced crosswise
- 2 cups cooked chickpeas, rinsed
- 1 cup uncooked quinoa
- 2 cans diced tomatoes, with their juice
- 5 cups Vegetable Broth, Poultry Broth, or store-bought
- 1 teaspoon garlic powder
- 1 teaspoon onion powder
- 1 teaspoon dried thyme
- ½ teaspoon of sea salt
- 2 cups chopped kale leaves

Directions:

- In your slow cooker, combine the summer squash, zucchini, chickpeas, quinoa, tomatoes (with their juice), broth, garlic powder, onion powder, thyme, and salt.
- Cover and cook on low within 8 hours. Stir in the kale.
- Cover and cook on low for 1 more hour.

Nutritional Information:

- Calories: 221
- Fat: 3g
- Carbohydrates: 40g
- Protein: 10g

Recipe 275. Chorizo and Tomato Salad with Olives

Serving Size: 4

Preparation Time: 10 minutes

Cooking Time: 10 minutes

Ingredients:

- 2 tbsp olive oil

- 4 chorizo sausages, chopped
- 2 1/2 cups cherry tomatoes
- 2 teaspoons red wine vinegar
- Small, red onion chopped
- 2 tbsp chopped cilantro
- 8 slices Kalamata olives
- One head of Boston lettuce with a shred
- Black pepper and salt to taste

Directions:

- Warm 1 tbsp olive oil on a large skillet and cook chorizo until golden. Cut cherry tomatoes in half. In a salad bowl, whisk the prepared olive oil, vinegar, salt, and pepper.
- Add the onion, lettuce, tomatoes, cilantro, and chorizo, and toss in a bowl to make sure they are coated. Add olives for garnish.

Nutritional Information:

- Cal 211
- Net Carbs 5.2g
- Fat 17g
- Protein 10g

Recipe 276. Clam Chowder

Serving Size: 6

Preparation Time: 15 minutes

Cooking Time: 8 hours

Ingredients:

- 1 red onion, chopped
- 3 carrots, peeled and chopped
- 1 fennel bulb and fronds, chopped
- 1 (10-ounce) can chopped clams, with their juice
- 1-pound baby red potatoes, quartered
- 4 cups Poultry Broth or store-bought
- ½ teaspoon of sea salt
- 1/8 teaspoon freshly ground black pepper
- 2 cups skim milk
- ¼ pound turkey bacon, browned and crumbled, for garnish

Directions:

- In your slow cooker, combine the onion, carrots, fennel bulb and fronds, clams (with their juice), potatoes, broth, salt, and pepper.
- Cover and cook on low within 8 hours. Stir in the milk and serve garnished with the crumbled bacon.

Nutritional Information:

- Calories: 172
- Fat: 1g
- Carbohydrates: 29g
- Protein: 10g

Recipe 277. Coriander Seeds Cabbage

Serving Size: 6

Preparation Time: 10 minutes

Cooking Time: 4 hours

Ingredients:

- 2 yellow onions, chopped
- 10 cups red cabbage, shredded
- 1 cup plums, pitted and chopped
- 1 teaspoon cinnamon powder
- 1 garlic clove, minced
- 1 teaspoon cumin seeds
- 1 teaspoon coriander seeds
- ¼ teaspoon cloves, ground
- 2 tablespoons red wine vinegar
- ½ cup water

Directions:

- In your slow cooker, mix cabbage with onions, plums, garlic, cinnamon, cumin, cloves, vinegar, coriander, and water, stir, cover and cook on low for 4 hours.
- Divide between plates and serve as a side dish.

Nutritional Information:

- Calories 252
- Fat 0.3g
- Carbohydrate 12g
- Protein 2.1g

Recipe 278. Cream Soup with Avocado and Zucchini

Serving Size: 4

Preparation Time: 15 minutes

Cooking Time: 40 minutes

Ingredients:

- 3 tbsp of vegetable oil
- 1 leek cut into pieces
- 1/2 rutabaga, sliced
- 3 cups zucchinis, chopped
- 1 avocado, chopped
- Black pepper and salt to taste
- 4 cups vegetable broth

- 2 tbsp fresh mints and chopped

Directions:

- The vegetable oil is heated in a pan at medium temperature. Cook the leeks and the zucchini and rutabaga for about 7-10 minutes. Add salt and pepper to taste. Pour the broth in and bring it to the point of boiling.
- Reduce the heat and let it simmer for 20 minutes. Remove from the heat. In small portions, take the Avocado and soup to the blender. Blend until smooth and creamy. Serve with mint.

Nutritional Information:

- Cal 278
- Net Carbs 9.3g
- Fat 20g
- Protein 8g

Recipe 279. Creamy White Chicken Chili

Serving Size: 10

Preparation Time: 30 minutes

Cooking Time: 45 minutes

Ingredients:

- 1-pound boneless, skinless chicken breast, cubed
- 2 teaspoons garlic powder
- 1 large onion, chopped
- 2 tablespoons onion powder
- 1 tablespoon vegetable oil
- 3 (15-ounce) cans great northern beans
- 32 ounces low-fat chicken broth
- ½ cup chopped green chilies
- 1 teaspoon salt
- 1 teaspoon cumin
- 1 teaspoon oregano
- ¼ teaspoon cayenne pepper
- ½ teaspoon black pepper
- 16 ounces sour cream

Directions:

- In a large saucepan, sauté the chicken, garlic, onion, and onion powder in oil until chicken is just cooked through, approximately 7 minutes.
- Add beans, broth, chilies, salt, cumin, oregano, cayenne, and pepper. Reduce heat, simmer uncovered for 30 minutes.
- Remove from heat, stir in sour cream. Serve while hot.

Nutritional Information:

- Calories: 350
- Fat: 12g
- Protein: 27g
- Carbohydrates: 32g

Recipe 280. Crispy Garlic Baked Potato Wedges

Serving Size: 3

Preparation Time: 5 minutes

Cooking Time: 10 minutes

Ingredients:

- 3 teaspoon salt
- 1 teaspoon minced garlic & 6 large russet
- ¼ cup olive oil & 1 teaspoon paprika
- 2/3 finely grated parmesan cheese
- 2 teaspoons freshly chopped parsley

Directions:

- Preheat the oven into 350 degrees Fahrenheit and line the baking sheet with a parchment pepper.
- Cut the potatoes into halfway length and cut each half in half lengthways again. Make 8 wedges.
- In a small jug combine garlic, oil, paprika and salt and place your wedges in the baking sheets. Pour the oil combo on top of the potatoes and toss them to ensure that they are evenly coated.
- Position the potato chunks in a single layer on the baking tray and sprinkle salt and parmesan cheese if needed. Bake for 35 minutes turning the wedges once half side is cooked.
- Flip the other side until they are both golden brown.
- Sprinkle parsley and the remaining parmesan before serving.

Nutritional Information:

- Calories: 324
- Fat: 6 Gram
- Carbs: 8 Gram
- Protein: 2g

Recipe 281. Cumin Black Beans and Peppers

Serving Size: 4

Preparation Time: 10 minutes

Cooking Time: 20 minutes

Ingredients:

- 1 tablespoon olive oil
- 2 cups canned black beans
- 1 green bell pepper, chopped
- 1 yellow onion, chopped
- 4 garlic cloves, minced
- 1 teaspoon cumin, ground
- ½ cup chicken stock
- 1 tablespoon coriander, chopped
- A pinch of salt and black pepper

Directions:

- Heat up a pan with the oil over medium heat, add the onion and the garlic and sauté for 5 minutes.
- Add the black beans and the other ingredients, toss, cook over medium heat for 15 minutes more, divide between plates and serve.

Nutritional Information:

- Calories 221
- Fat 5
- Carbs 9
- Protein 11

Recipe 282. Curry Eggplant

Serving Size: 4

Preparation Time: 10 minutes

Cooking Time: 3 hours

Ingredients:

- 2 cups cherry tomatoes, halved
- 1 eggplant, sliced
- ½ teaspoon cumin, ground
- 1 teaspoon mustard seed
- ½ teaspoon coriander, ground
- ½ teaspoon curry powder
- A pinch of nutmeg, ground
- ½ yellow onion, chopped
- 1 tablespoon cilantro, chopped
- 1 teaspoon red wine vinegar
- 1 tablespoon olive oil
- 1 garlic clove, minced
- Black pepper to the taste

Directions:

- Grease the slow cooker with the oil and add eggplant slices inside.
- Add cumin, mustard seeds, coriander, curry powder, nutmeg, tomatoes, onion, garlic, vinegar, black pepper and cilantro, cover and cook on High for 3 hours.
- Divide between plates and serve as a side dish.

Nutritional Information:

- Calories 94
- Fat 4.6g
- Carbohydrate 13.2g
- Protein 2.5g

Recipe 283. Fiery Shrimp Cocktail Salad

Serving Size: 4

Preparation Time: 10 minutes

Cooking Time: 15 minutes

Ingredients:

- 2 tbsp olive oil 1/2 head Romaine lettuce, torn
- 1 cucumber, cut into ribbons
- 1/2 lb shrimp, deveined
- 1 cup of arugula
- 1/2 cup mayonnaise
- 2 tbsp Cholula hot sauce
- 1/2 tsp Worcestershire sauce
- Chili pepper and salt to taste
- 1 2 tbsp lemon juice
- 1 lemon Cut into wedges
- 4 Dill Weed

Directions:

- Sprinkle the shrimp with salt and pepper. Heat the prepared olive oil on moderate heat, and fry for three minutes per side until opaque and pink. Place the shrimp aside to cool.
- Mix your mayonnaise mix, juice of a hot lemon sauce, and Worcestershire sauce in a bowl, mixing until it is smooth and creamy in the bowl. Divide the cucumber and lettuce into four glass bowls. Serve with shrimp, then pour the hot dressing on top. Sprinkle arugula all over and garnish using lemon wedges and dill. Serve.

Nutritional Information:

- Cal 241
- Net Carbs 3.9g
- Fat 18g
- Protein 14g

Recipe 284. Green Lentil and Olive Salad

Serving Size: 6

Preparation Time: 10 minutes

Cooking Time: 30 minutes

Ingredients:

- Juice of 1 lemon
- 1 teaspoon Dijon mustard
- 1 tablespoon olive oil
- 1 cup green lentils, soaked and cooked until tender
- 2 tomatoes, diced
- 1 small red onion, diced
- 1 small serrano chili, seeded and diced
- Salt and pepper, to taste
- 1 bunch fresh parsley, chopped
- 4 mint leaves, chopped
- 2 romaine lettuce crowns

Directions:

- In a small-sized bowl, combine lemon juice, mustard, and olive oil to make dressing. Set aside.
- Combine lentils, tomatoes, onion, chili, salt and pepper, parsley, and mint. Serve on the romaine lettuce and top with prepared dressing.

Nutritional Information:

- Calories: 150
- Fat: 3g
- Protein: 9g
- Carbohydrates: 24g

Recipe 285. Green Salad with Feta and Blueberries

Serving Size: 4

Preparation Time: 10 minutes

Cooking Time: 10 minutes

Ingredients:

- 2 cups of broccoli 2 cups slaw
- 2 cups baby spinach
- 2 tablespoons poppy seeds
- 1/3 cup sunflower seeds
- 1/3 cup blueberries
- 2/3 cup chopped cheese
- 1/3 cup walnuts chopped
- 2 tbsp olive oil
- 1 tbsp white vinegar
- Black pepper and salt to taste

Directions:

- A bowl mixes vinegar, olive oil, poppy seeds, salt, and pepper. Keep aside.
- Mix the broccoli slaw with spinach, walnuts, sunflower seeds, blueberries, and feta cheese in a salad bowl. Sprinkle the dressing over and toss. Serve.

Nutritional Information:

- Cal 201
- Net Carbs 7.5g
- Fat 24g
- Protein 9g

Recipe 286. Grilled Avocado Caprese Crostini

Serving Size: 2

Preparation Time: 10 minutes

Cooking Time: 20 minutes

Ingredients:

- 1 avocado thinly sliced
- 9 ounces ripened cherry tomatoes
- ounces fresh bocconcini in water
- 2 teaspoon balsamic glaze
- 8 pieces Italian baguette
- ½ a cup basil leaves

Directions:

- Preheat your oven to 375 degrees Fahrenheit
- Arrange your baking sheet properly before spraying them on top with olive oil.
- Bake your item of choice until they are well done or golden brown. Rub your crostini with the cut side of garlic while they are still warm, and you can season them with pepper and salt.
- Divide the basil leaves on each side of bread and top up with tomato halves, avocado slices and bocconcini. Season it with pepper and salt.
- Broil it for 4 minutes and when the cheese starts to melt through remove and sprinkle balsamic glaze before serving.

Nutritional Information:

- Calories: 278
- Fat: 10 Gram
- Carbs: 37 Gram
- Protein: 10g

Recipe 287. Kale-Poppy Seed Salad

Serving Size: 6

Preparation Time: 10 minutes

Cooking Time: 5 minutes

Ingredients:

- ½ cup nonfat plain Greek yogurt
- 2 tablespoons apple cider vinegar
- ½ tablespoon extra-virgin olive oil
- 1 teaspoon poppy seeds
- 1 teaspoon sugar
- 4 cups firmly packed finely chopped kale
- 2 cups broccoli slaw
- 2 cups thinly sliced Brussels sprouts
- 6 tablespoons dried cranberries
- 6 tablespoons hulled pumpkin seeds

Directions:

- Mix the yogurt, vinegar, oil, poppy seeds, sugar in a small bowl. Store the dressing in 6 condiment cups.
- In a large bowl, mix the kale, broccoli slaw, and Brussels sprout. Divide the greens into 6 large storage containers and top each salad with cranberries and pumpkin seeds. To serve, toss the greens with the poppy seed dressing to coat.

Nutritional Information:

- Calories: 129
- Fat: 6g
- Carbohydrates: 13g
- Protein: 8g

Recipe 288. Lettuce, Beet and Tofu Salad

Serving Size: 4

Preparation Time: 20 minutes

Cooking Time: 55 minutes

Ingredients:

- 2 tbsp butter
- 2 oz tofu, cubed
- 8 Oz of red beets washed
- 1 red onion cut in half
- 1 cup mayonnaise
- 1 small romaine salad Torn
- 2 Tbsp fresh chopped chives
- Black pepper and salt to taste

Directions:

- Place the beets into a pot at medium heat, cover them with salted water, and simmer for about 40 minutes or until they are soft. Let them cool and drain. Take off the skin and cut the beets.
- Make butter by melting it in a pan on medium heat. Fry tofu until it is browned, about 3-4 minutes. Transfer to an ice-cold plate. Mix tofu, beets, red onion, and lettuce in a salad bowl. Add salt, pepper, mayonnaise, and salt. Sprinkle with chives and serve.

Nutritional Information:

- Cal 215
- Net Carbs 6g
- Fat 30g
- Protein 7g

Recipe 289. Minestrone Soup

Serving Size: 6

Preparation Time: 20 minutes

Cooking Time: 30 minutes

Ingredients:

- 3½ cups whole peeled tomatoes with juice
- 1½ cups chopped onion
- 1 clove garlic, minced
- 1½ cups low-sodium chicken stock
- 1 cup celery, chopped
- 1 cup frozen corn
- 1 cup chopped zucchini
- 1 cup canned red kidney beans
- 1 cup cabbage, chopped
- 1 teaspoon Italian seasoning

Directions:

- Chop tomatoes, then combine all ingredients in a large soup pot.
- Bring to a steady simmer, then allow to simmer for 30 minutes or until vegetables are tender.
- Adjust seasoning as desired and serve.

Nutritional Information:

- Calories: 120
- Fat: 1g
- Protein: 6g
- Carbohydrates: 25g

Recipe 290. Moroccan Sweet Potato Soup

Serving Size: 6

Preparation Time: 15 minutes

Cooking Time: 25 minutes

Ingredients:

- 1 tablespoon olive oil
- 2 diced carrots
- 1 zested lemon
- 2 teaspoons cumin
- 2 diced yellow onions
- 1 can drained chickpeas
- 2 diced yellow onions
- 1 tablespoon turmeric
- ½ teaspoon coriander
- 2 tablespoons harissa
- 6 cups vegetable stock
- Parsley, mint, harissa, labneh, and lemon wedges to garnish

Directions:

- Turn the pot on to sauté and put oil in there, then dice the onion and sauté till golden.
- Add in the carrots, sweet potatoes, zest, spices, stock, and chickpeas, and then seal the vent, manually cooking for 20 minutes.
- Get garnish ready while it cooks.
- Once finished, let it depressurize naturally, then pop off lid.
- Take the soup and use a stick blender to puree it, or blend it in blender
- Season to taste.
- Serve it with garnishees, or even a swirl of coconut cream.

Nutritional Information:

- Calories: 260
- Fat: 2g
- Carbs: 15g
- Protein: 1g

Recipe 291. Mushroom Cream Soup with Herbs

Serving Size: 4

Preparation Time: 15   minutes

Cooking Time: 25 minutes

Ingredients:

- 12 oz white mushroom and chopped
- 1 onion chopped
- 1 cup of heavy cream
- 1/4 cup butter
- 1 tsp thyme leaf, chopped
- 1 tsp parsley leaves chopped
- 1 teaspoon cilantro leaves chopped
- 2 cloves of garlic, minced
- 4 cups vegetable broth
- Black pepper and salt to taste

Directions:

- In a big pan at high heat. Cook the garlic and onion for approximately about 3 minutes until they are tender. Add the mushrooms, salt, and pepper, and cook until the mushrooms are tender for five minutes.
- Add the broth and bring it to a boil. Reduce the heat, and let it simmer for 10 minutes. Puree soup using the aid of a hand blender until it is smooth. Mix in heavy cream. Sprinkle with herbs.

Nutritional Information:

- Cal 232
- Net Carbs 6.4g
- Fat 20g
- Protein 8g

Recipe 292. Mushroom Sausages

Serving Size: 12

Preparation Time: 10 minutes

Cooking Time: 2 hours

Ingredients:

- 6 celery ribs, chopped
- 1 pound no-sugar, beef sausage, chopped
- 2 tablespoons olive oil
- 1/2-pound mushrooms, chopped
- 1/2 cup sunflower seeds, peeled
- 1 cup low-sodium veggie stock
- 1 cup cranberries, dried
- 2 yellow onions, chopped
- 2 garlic cloves, minced
- 1 tablespoon sage, dried
- 1 whole wheat bread loaf, cubed

Directions:

- Heat up a pan with the oil over medium-high heat, add beef, stir and brown for a few minutes.
- Add mushrooms, onion, celery, garlic, and sage, stir, cook for a few more minutes and transfer to your slow cooker.
- Add stock, cranberries, sunflower seeds and the bread cubes, cover and cook on High for 2 hours. Stir the whole mix, divide between plates, and serve as a side dish.

Nutritional Information:

- Calories 188
- Fat 13.8g
- Carbohydrate 8.2g
- Protein 7.6g

Recipe 293. Parmesan Artichokes

Serving Size: 8

Preparation Time: 10 minutes

Cooking Time: 5 hours

Ingredients:

- 4 artichokes, trimmed and halved
- 2 cups whole wheat breadcrumbs
- 1 cup low-sodium vegetable stock
- Juice of 1 lemon
- 3 garlic cloves, minced
- 1 tablespoon lemon zest, grated
- 2 tablespoons parsley, chopped
- 1/3 cup low-fat parmesan, grated
- Black pepper to the taste
- 1 tablespoon olive oil
- 1 tablespoon shallot, minced
- 1 teaspoon oregano, chopped

Directions:

- Rub artichokes with the lemon juice and the oil and put them in your slow cooker.
- Add breadcrumbs, garlic, parsley, parmesan, lemon zest, black pepper, shallot, oregano and stock, cover and cook on Low for 5 hours.
- Divide the whole mix between plates, sprinkle parsley on top and serve as a side dish.

Nutritional Information:

- Calories 149
- Fat 2.8g
- Carbohydrate 26g
- Protein 7.7g

Recipe 294. Parsley Red Potatoes

Serving Size: 8

Preparation Time: 10 minutes

Cooking Time: 6 hours

Ingredients:

- 16 baby red potatoes, halved
- 2 cups low-sodium chicken stock
- 1 carrot, sliced
- 1 celery rib, chopped
- 1/4 cup yellow onion, chopped
- 1 tablespoon parsley, chopped
- 2 tablespoons olive oil
- A pinch of black pepper
- 1 garlic clove minced

Directions:

- In your slow cooker, mix the potatoes with the carrot, celery, onion, stock, parsley, garlic, oil and black pepper, toss, cover and cook on Low for 6 hours.
- Divide between plates and serve as a side dish.

Nutritional Information:

- Calories 257
- Fat 9.5g
- Carbohydrate 43.4g
- Protein 4.4g

Recipe 295. Peach and Carrots

Serving Size: 6

Preparation Time: 10 minutes

Cooking Time: 6 hours

Ingredients:

- 2 pounds small carrots, peeled
- 1/2 cup low-fat butter, melted
- 1/2 cup canned peach, unsweetened
- 2 tablespoons cornstarch
- 3 tablespoons stevia
- 2 tablespoons water
- 1/2 teaspoon cinnamon powder
- 1 teaspoon vanilla extract
- A pinch of nutmeg, ground

Directions:

- In your slow cooker, mix the carrots with the butter, peach, stevia, cinnamon, vanilla, nutmeg, and cornstarch mixed with water, toss, cover and cook on low for 6 hours.
- Toss the carrots one more time, divide between plates and serve as a side dish.

Nutritional Information:

- Calories 139
- Fat 10.7g
- Carbohydrate 35.4g
- Protein 3.8g

Recipe 296. Plantain and Corn Soup

Serving Size: 4

Preparation Time: 15 minutes

Cooking Time: 20 minutes

Ingredients:

- 1 tablespoon vegetable oil
- 1 medium onion, diced
- 1 clove garlic, smashed
- 1 medium plantain, sliced
- 1½ cups peeled diced tomatoes
- ½ cup frozen corn
- ½ teaspoon tarragon
- 1 quart low-sodium chicken stock
- 1 mild serrano chili pepper, seeded
- 1 pinch nutmeg
- Salt and freshly ground black pepper
- Fresh chopped parsley, for garnish

Directions:

- Heat large sauté pan over medium heat. When hot, add oil, onion, and garlic; cook until onions become translucent, approximately 8 minutes.
- Add plantain, tomatoes, corn, and tarragon and cook for 5 minutes.
- Add stock, chili pepper, nutmeg, salt, and pepper and simmer for 10 minutes.
- Garnish with parsley and serve.

Nutritional Information:

- Calories: 170
- Fat: 5g
- Protein: 7g
- Carbohydrates: 29g

Recipe 297. Potato Soup

Serving Size: 6

Preparation Time: 10 minutes

Cooking Time: 12 minutes

Ingredients:

- 6 cups cubed gold potatoes
- ½ chopped yellow onion
- black pepper for taste
- a pinch of crushed red pepper flakes
- 2 cups coconut cream
- 1 cup corn
- 1 cup fat-free shredded cheddar cheese
- 3 oz. Cream cheese, cubed
- 2 tablespoons avocado oil
- 28 oz. Chicken stock, low sodium
- 2 tablespoons dried parsley

Directions:

- Turn IP to sauté mode, then add oil, onion, and then cook for 5 minutes.
- Put the pepper, pepper flakes, parsley, and half the stock in, and then stir.
- Put potatoes in steamer basket, and cook on high for 5 minutes, and then put them in bowl Add cream cheese and cheese and sauté in instant pot, and then add the rest of the ingredients, stirring it, and then ladle it to bowls to serve this!

Nutritional Information:

- Calories: 200
- Fat: 7g
- Carbs: 20g
- Protein: 8g

Recipe 298. Quinoa and Scallops Salad

Serving Size: 6

Preparation Time: 10 minutes

Cooking Time: 20 minutes

Ingredients:

- 12 ounces sea scallops
- 4 tablespoons olive oil+ 2 teaspoons
- 4 teaspoons coconut aminos
- 1 and ½ cup quinoa, already cooked
- 2 teaspoons garlic, minced
- 1 cup snow peas, sliced
- 1/3 cup balsamic vinegar
- 1 cup scallions, sliced
- 1/3 cup red bell pepper, chopped
- ¼ cup cilantro, chopped

Directions:

- In a bowl, mix scallops with half of the aminos and toss.
- Heat up a pan with 1 tablespoon olive oil over medium heat, add quinoa, stir, and cook for 8 minutes.
- Add garlic and snow peas, stir, cook for 5 more minutes, and take off heat.
- Meanwhile, in a bowl, mix 3 tablespoons olive oil with the rest of the coconut aminos and vinegar, whisk well, add the quinoa mix, scallions and bell pepper and toss.

- Heat up another pan with 2 teaspoons olive oil over medium-high heat, add scallops, cook for 1 minute on each side, add over the quinoa mix, toss a bit, sprinkle cilantro on top and serve.
- Enjoy!

Nutritional Information:

- Calories 221
- Fat 5
- Carbs 7
- Protein 8

Recipe 299. Refried Beans with Baked Tortilla or Pita Chips

Serving Size: 6

Preparation Time: 15 minutes

Cooking Time: 2 hours 10 minutes

Ingredients:

- 1 tablespoon canola oil
- 1 yellow onion, diced fine
- 2 cloves garlic, smashed
- 1 pound pinto beans
- 2 bay leaves
- 2 tablespoons cumin
- ½ teaspoon cayenne
- 1 tablespoon coriander
- 4 cups vegetable stock or water
- 6 slices turkey bacon, diced 1 bunch cilantro

Directions:

- Heat oil in large-sized saucepan and cook onions and garlic until tender, approximately 4 minutes.
- Add remaining ingredients and cover with stock by 2 inches.
- Bring to a very hot boil and then reduce to a covered simmer.
- Cook for about 2 hours — checking and adding additional stock if needed until beans are tender.
- Drain and remove bay leaves and bacon.
- Add beans to food processor and blend, adding liquid to form consistency of mashed potatoes.
- Adjust seasoning and serve with low-fat sour cream and baked tortilla/pita chips.

Nutritional Information:

- Calories: 310
- Fat: 4.5g
- Protein: 19g
- Carbohydrates: 50g

Recipe 300. Roasted Corn Salad

Serving Size: 6

Preparation Time: 15 minutes

Cooking Time: 20 minutes

Ingredients:

- 2 cups fresh or frozen shelled edamame
- ½ cup fresh corn kernels
- ½ cup red peppers, diced
- ¼ cup red onions, diced
- ¼ cup green onions, diced
- 1 clove garlic, minced
- ¾ teaspoon salt
- ¼ teaspoon fresh ground black pepper
- 1 tablespoon olive oil
- 1 cup fresh tomatoes, chopped
- ¼ cup fresh basil leaves, chopped
- 1 tablespoon red wine vinegar
- Juice of 1 lime

Directions:

- Preheat oven to 400°F.
- Toss edamame, corn, peppers, onion, green onion, garlic, salt, and pepper in bowl to coat.
- Place on a prepared medium-sized sheet pan in a single layer on middle oven rack and roast until beans start to turn brown (approximately 10–12 minutes).
- Place in the refrigerator to cool completely, then toss with remaining ingredients and serve chilled.

Nutritional Information:

- Calories: 120
- Fat: 4.5g
- Protein: 6g
- Carbohydrates: 13g

Recipe 301. Roasted Garlic Soup

Serving Size: 10

Preparation Time: 15 minutes

Cooking Time: 60 minutes

Ingredients:

- 1 tablespoon olive oil
- 2 bulbs garlic, peeled
- 3 shallots, chopped
- 1 large head cauliflower, chopped
- 6 cups vegetable broth
- Sunflower seeds and pepper to taste

Directions:

- Warm your oven to 400 degrees F. Slice ¼ inch top of the garlic bulb and place it in aluminum foil. Oiled it using olive oil and roast in the oven for 35 minutes. Squeeze flesh out of the roasted garlic.
- Heat-up oil in a saucepan and add shallots, sauté for 6 minutes. Add garlic and remaining ingredients. Adjust heat to low. Let it cook for 15-20 minutes.
- Puree the mixture using an immersion blender. Season soup with sunflower seeds and pepper. Serve and enjoy!

Nutritional Information:

- Calories: 142
- Fat: 8g
- Carbohydrates: 3.4g
- Protein: 4g

Recipe 302. Roasted Vegetables

Serving Size: 4

Preparation Time: 15 minutes

Cooking Time: 25 minutes

Ingredients:

- 1 carrot, peeled and cut in thin diagonal cuts
- 1 medium red onion, peeled and cut into quarters
- 1 large zucchini, cut in 1-inch cubes
- 1 large yellow squash, cut into 1-inch cubes
- ½ small eggplant, cut in 1-inch cubes
- 1 red bell pepper, cut into cubes and seeded
- ¼ cup low-fat balsamic vinaigrette dressing
- ½ teaspoon ground black pepper
- 1 teaspoon dried Italian seasoning

Directions:

- Preheat oven to 375°F.
- Toss vegetables in dressing, pepper, and Italian seasonings to coat.
- Coat a prepared sheet pan with nonstick cooking spray. Place vegetables in a single layer and roast for 12 to 15 minutes. Stir every 5 minutes while cooking.

Nutritional Information:

- Calories: 90
- Fat: 1g
- Protein: 4g
- Carbohydrates: 21g

Recipe 303. Rosemary Carrots

Serving Size: 4

Preparation Time: 5 minutes

Cooking Time: 25 minutes

Ingredients:

- 1-pound carrots, peeled and roughly sliced
- 1 yellow onion, chopped
- 1 tablespoon olive oil
- Zest of 1 orange, grated
- Juice of 1 orange
- 1 orange, peeled and cut into segments
- 1 tablespoon rosemary, chopped
- A pinch of salt and black pepper

Directions:

- Heat up a pan with the oil over medium-high heat, add the onion and sauté for 5 minutes.
- Add the carrots, the orange zest and the other ingredients, toss, cook over medium heat for 20 minutes more, divide between plates and serve.

Nutritional Information:

- Calories 140
- Fat 3.9
- Carbs 26.1
- Protein 2.1

Recipe 304. Sausage and Pesto Salad with Cheese

Serving Size: 2

Preparation Time: 10 minutes

Cooking Time: 10 minutes

Ingredients:

- 1/4 cup cherry tomatoes mixed cut in half
- 1/2 lb pork sausage links, sliced
- 1 cup mixed lettuce greens
- 1/4 cup radicchio, sliced
- 1 tbsp olive oil
- 1/4 lb feta cheese, cubed
- 1/2 1 tbsp lemon juice
- 1/4 cup basil pesto
- 6 black olives, pitted, halved
- Black pepper and salt to taste
- 1 tbsp Parmesan shavings

Directions:

- Sauté the sausages in olive oil on medium heat for 5 to 6 minutes, turning them frequently. Mix the mixed greens of lettuce and radicchio, pesto, feta cheese,

black olives, cherry tomatoes, and lemon juice within a bowl of salad.
- Mix thoroughly to make sure that everything is covered. Sprinkle with salt and black pepper, and then include the sausages. Sprinkle the sausages with Parmesan shavings, and then serve.

Nutritional Information:

- Cal 311
- Net Carbs 7.5g
- Fat 38g
- Protein 31g

Recipe 305. Smoked Mackerel Lettuce Cups

Serving Size: 2

Preparation Time: 10 minutes

Cooking Time: 20 minutes

Ingredients:

- 1 Head Iceberg lettuce, leaves firm removed to make cups
- 4 oz smoked mackerel, flaked
- Black pepper and salt to taste
- 2 eggs
- 1 tomato, seed, and chopped
- 2 tbsp mayonnaise
- 1 red onion 1/4, cut into slices
- 1 teaspoon lemon juice
- 1 tbsp chopped chives, chopped

Directions:

- Boil eggs in the small saucepan using salted and boiled water for about 10 minutes. After that, wash the eggs under cold water, peel them and chop them into pieces. Transfer them into a salad bowl. Include the smoked mackerel and tomatoes and red onion, and mix them all together using the help of a spoon.
- Blend the mayonnaise mixture, the juice of a lemon, salt, and black pepper together in small bowls, and stir until well-mixed. Place two lettuce leaves as cups and divide the salad ingredients among the leaves. Sprinkle with chives and serve.

Nutritional Information:

- Cal 234
- Net Carbs 8g
- Fat 25g
- Protein 26g

Recipe 306. Smoked Salmon, Bacon and Egg Salad

Serving Size: 4

Preparation Time: 10 minutes

Cooking Time: 20 minutes

Ingredients:

- 2 eggs
- 1 head romaine lettuce, torn
- 4 oz smoked salmon, chopped
- 3 slices bacon
- 4 cherry tomatoes, halved
- Black pepper and salt to taste
- Dressing: 1/2 cup mayonnaise
- 1/2 1 tsp garlic puree
- 1 tbsp lemon juice
- 1 tsp tabasco sauce

Directions:

- In a large-sized bowl, mix the dressing ingredients thoroughly, then put them aside. Make the salted water in a pot to a simmer. Break each egg in a bowl, then gently drop it into the boiling water. Poach for about 2 minutes. Remove with a spoon perforated and transfer to the towel to dry, then place on a plate.
- Place bacon in a pan at medium-high heat, and cook until crispy and browned, approximately 6 minutes. Turn once. Remove, let cool to cool, then cut into small pieces. Mix the salad with bacon, smoked salmon, bacon, and the dressing into a bowl. Divide the salad among plates, top with the eggs, and serve right away or cool.

Nutritional Information:

- Cal 321
- Net Carbs 5.4g
- Fat 24g
- Protein 15g

Recipe 307. Spicy Brussels Sprouts

Serving Size: 6

Preparation Time: 10 minutes

Cooking Time: 20 minutes

Ingredients:

- 2 pounds Brussels sprouts, halved
- 2 tablespoons olive oil
- A pinch of black pepper

- 1 tablespoon sesame oil
- 2 garlic cloves, minced
- ½ cup coconut aminos
- 2 teaspoons apple cider vinegar
- 1 tablespoon coconut sugar
- 2 teaspoons chili sauce
- A pinch of red pepper flakes
- Sesame seeds for serving

Directions:

- Spread the sprouts on a lined baking dish, add the olive oil, the sesame oil, black pepper, garlic, aminos, vinegar, coconut sugar, chili sauce and pepper flakes, toss well, introduce in the oven, and bake at 425 degrees F for 20 minutes.
- Divide the sprouts between plates, sprinkle sesame seeds on top and serve as a side dish.
- Enjoy!

Nutritional Information:

- Calories 176
- Fat 3
- Carbs 14
- Protein 9

Recipe 308. Spinach and Brussels Sprout Salad

Serving Size: 2

Preparation Time: 15 minutes

Cooking Time: 35 minutes

Ingredients:

- 1 lb Brussels sprouts, halved
- 2 tablespoons olive oil
- Black pepper and salt to taste
- 1 tablespoon balsamic vinegar
- 2 tablespoons extra-virgin olive oil
- 1 cup baby spinach
- 1 tbsp Dijon mustard
- 1/2 cup hazelnuts

Directions:

- The oven should be heated at 400 F. Drizzle the Brussels sprouts with olive oil, then sprinkle with salt and black pepper and place them on a baking tray. Bake until they are tender, about 20 minutes, turning them frequently.
- In a dry skillet over moderate temperature, toast the hazelnuts for 2 minutes, let them cool, and then cut them into smaller pieces. Move the Brussels sprouts into a salad bowl, including baby spinach. Mix until well-combined. In the bowl of a small serving dish, mix vinegar along with mustard and olive oil. Pour the dressing over the salad, and then top it with hazelnuts and serve.

Nutritional Information:

- Cal 311
- Net Carbs 10g
- Fat 43g
- Protein 14g

Recipe 309. Spinach and Lentil Soup

Serving Size: 6

Preparation Time: 20 minutes

Cooking Time: 55 minutes

Ingredients:

- 1 cup dried lentils
- 5 cups low-sodium chicken or vegetable stock
- 1 teaspoon salt
- 2 tablespoons olive oil
- 2 cups onions, chopped
- 3 cloves garlic, smashed
- ¼ teaspoon cayenne
- ½ cup raw bulgur wheat
- 2 bay leaves
- ¼ cup parsley, chopped
- 2 cups tomatoes, chopped
- ¼ cup tomato paste
- 1 pinch dried rosemary
- 2 cups frozen spinach, chopped and drained
- Salt and pepper, to taste

Directions:

- Rinse lentils in cold water. In a large pot, bring lentils, stock, and salt to a boil. Cover and reduce heat to a simmer for 40 minutes.
- Heat large sauté pan over medium heat, then add oil, onions, garlic, cayenne, and wheat until lightly brown, then add in the bay leaves, parsley, tomatoes, tomato paste, and rosemary, and simmer for 15 minutes.
- Combine stock and sautéed mixture (add more stock if needed) and add in the spinach right before serving. Season as desired with salt and pepper.

Nutritional Information:

- Calories: 290
- Fat: 7g

- Protein: 19g
- Carbohydrates: 45g

Recipe 310. Spinach Salad with Goat Cheese and Nuts

Serving Size: 2

Preparation Time: 15 minutes

Cooking Time: 20 minutes

Ingredients:

- 2 cups spinach
- 1/4 cup pine nuts
- 1 cup goat's hard cheese grated
- 2 1 tbsp white vinegar
- 2 tablespoons extra-virgin olive oil
- Black pepper and salt to taste

Directions:

- Preheat the oven to 390 F. Spread goat cheese that has been grated into 2 circles on top of two pieces. Put them in the oven and wait for 10 mins to bake. Take two bowls of the same size, place them upside-down, and carefully put the parchment paper over to create an appearance of a bowl.
- Allow cooling for about 15 minutes. Divide the spinach between the bowls. Sprinkle with salt and pepper and drizzle it with olive oil. Sprinkle with pine nuts and serve.

Nutritional Information:

- Cal 240
- Net Carbs 4.4g
- Fat 52g
- Protein 19g

Recipe 311. Spinach Salad with Pancetta and Mustard

Serving Size: 2

Preparation Time: 15 minutes

Cooking Time: 20 minutes

Ingredients:

- 1 cup spinach
- 1 large avocado, sliced
- One spring onion chopped
- 2 pancetta slices
- 1/2 head of lettuce, chopped
- 1 hard-boiled egg with a little chopped Vinaigrette
- Salt to taste
- 1/4 teaspoon garlic powder
- 3 tbsp olive oil
- 1 tsp Dijon mustard
- 1 tbsp white vinegar

Directions:

- Chop the pancetta into pieces and fry in a skillet on medium-high heat for about 5 minutes or until crisp. Place the pancetta aside and let it cool.
- Mix the lettuce, spinach egg, and spring onion in one bowl. Mix all the vinaigrette components in a separate bowl. Pour the prepared dressing on top and mix to combine. Serve with pancetta and Avocado. Serve immediately.

Nutritional Information:

- Cal 267
- Net Carbs 7g
- Fat 42g
- Protein 12g

Recipe 312. Split Pea Cream Soup

Serving Size: 6

Preparation Time: 10 minutes

Cooking Time: 15 minutes

Ingredients:

- 2 tablespoons olive oil
- 1 chopped yellow onion
- ½ cup chopped celery
- 18 oz, low-salt chicken stock
- 2 cups water
- ½ cup coconut cream
- 1 pound chicken sausage, ground
- ½ cup chopped carrots
- 2 minced garlic cloves
- black pepper for taste
- 16 oz, split peas, rinsed
- ¼ teaspoon dried pepper flakes

Directions:

- Press sauté mode and add sausage, browning for 2-3 minutes then transferring to plate.
- Add oil to IP, then add celery, onions, carrots, water, garlic, stock, pepper flakes, and peas, stirring, and cooking on manual for 10 minutes.
- Blend with an immersion blender and then sauté once more, and add the pepper, sausage, and corn, simmering and mix it all together.

Nutritional Information:

- Calories: 281
- Fat: 7g
- Carbs: 19g
- Protein: 16g

Recipe 313. Sweet Butternut

Serving Size: 8

Preparation Time: 10 minutes

Cooking Time: 4 hours

Ingredients:

- 1 cup carrots, chopped
- 1 tablespoon olive oil
- 1 yellow onion, chopped
- 1/2 teaspoon stevia
- 1 garlic clove, minced
- 1/2 teaspoon curry powder
- 1 butternut squash, cubed
- 2 and 1/2 cups low-sodium veggie stock
- 1/2 cup basmati rice
- ¾ cup coconut milk
- 1/2 teaspoon cinnamon powder
- 1/4 teaspoon ginger, grated

Directions:

- Heat up a pan with the oil over medium-high heat, add the oil, onion, garlic, stevia, carrots, curry powder, cinnamon, and ginger, stir, cook for 5 minutes and transfer to your slow cooker.
- Add squash, stock and coconut milk, stir, cover and cook on Low for 4 hours.
- Divide the butternut mix between plates and serve as a side dish.

Nutritional Information:

- Calories 134
- Fat 7.2g
- Carbohydrate 16.5g
- Protein 1.8g

Recipe 314. Sweet Corn Soup

Serving Size: 4

Preparation Time: 20 minutes

Cooking Time: 1 hour 15 minutes

Ingredients:

- 10 ears fresh corn
- 1 tablespoon canola oil
- 1 yellow onion, chopped
- ½ cup smoked chicken meat or ½ cup diced turkey bacon (optional)
- 2 tablespoons cumin
- 1 teaspoon dry thyme
- 1 teaspoon dry mustard
- 2 tablespoons Worcestershire sauce
- 1 chipotle chili
- 2½ quarts vegetable stock Juice of 1 lime

Directions:

- Brush corn with oil and grill. Roast until most of the kernels are brown, approximately 10 minutes. Cut kernels from ear and set aside.
- In a large pan, sauté onion and chicken (or bacon) until tender, approximately 10 minutes.
- Add cumin, thyme, mustard, and Worcestershire.
- Add corn and chili with stock and simmer for 1 hour.
- Using a blender, puree until smooth and strain into bowls. Season with lime juice. Garnish with fresh cilantro sprig.

Nutritional Information:

- Calories: 310
- Fat: 8g
- Protein: 13g
- Carbohydrates: 56g

Recipe 315. Tahini Beans

Serving Size: 4

Preparation Time: 10 minutes

Cooking Time: 10 minutes

Ingredients:

- 1 and ½ tablespoons tahini paste
- Juice of 1 lemon
- Zest of 1 lemon, grated
- 2 tablespoons olive oil
- 1 garlic clove, minced
- 1 red onion, sliced
- 1 yellow bell pepper, sliced
- 10 ounces green beans, halved
- A pinch of black pepper

Directions:

- In a bowl, mix lemon zest, lemon juice, tahini and black pepper and whisk well.
- Heat up a pan with the oil over medium-high heat, add onion, stir and cook for 5 minutes.

- Add the bell pepper, garlic and green beans, toss and cook for 10 minutes.
- Add tahini dressing, toss, cook for 2 minutes more, divide between plates and serve as a side dish.
- Enjoy!

Nutritional Information:

- Calories 180
- Fat 10
- Carbs 13
- Protein 8

Recipe 316. Thyme Sweet Potatoes

Serving Size: 10

Preparation Time: 10 minutes

Cooking Time: 3 hours

Ingredients:

- 4 pounds sweet potatoes, sliced
- 3 tablespoons stevia
- 2 tablespoons olive oil
- ½ teaspoon sage, dried
- ½ cup orange juice
- ½ teaspoon thyme, dried
- A pinch of black pepper

Directions:

- In a bowl, mix orange juice with salt, pepper, stevia, thyme, sage and oil and whisk well.
- Add the prepared potatoes to your slow cooker, drizzle the sage and orange mix all over, cover, cook on High for 3 hours, divide between plates and serve as a side dish.

Nutritional Information:

- Calories 244
- Fat 0.3g
- Carbohydrate 56.4g
- Protein 2.9g

Recipe 317. Toasted Orzo Pasta

Serving Size: 6

Preparation Time: 10 minutes

Cooking Time: 15 minutes

Ingredients:

- ½ pound orzo pasta
- 3 cups low-sodium chicken stock
- ¼ cup dry-packed sun-dried tomatoes, chopped
- Salt and pepper, to taste
- 1 tablespoon dried thyme

Directions:

- Preheat oven to 350°F.
- Place orzo on sheet pan in single layer and bake for 10 minutes until lightly browned.
- In a large-sized pot, bring stock to a boil. Add orzo, cook until tender.
- Place sun-dried tomatoes in strainer and drain pasta into it.
- Add salt and pepper and thyme and serve.

Nutritional Information:

- Calories: 160
- Fat: 1.5g
- Protein: 8g
- Carbohydrates: 31g

Recipe 318. Tuna Bites

Serving Size: 4

Preparation Time: 10 minutes

Cooking Time: 10 minutes

Ingredients:

- 1 pound tuna fillets, boneless, skinless, and cubed
- 1 pound shrimp, peeled and deveined
- 2 tablespoons olive oil
- 4 scallions, chopped
- Juice of 1 lime
- 1 teaspoon sweet paprika
- 1 teaspoon turmeric powder
- 2 tablespoons coconut aminos
- A pinch of salt and black pepper

Directions:

- Heat up a pan with the oil over medium heat, add the scallions and sauté for 2 minutes.
- Add the tuna bites and cook them for 2 minutes on each side.
- Add the shrimp and the remaining ingredients, toss gently, cook everything for 4 minutes more, arrange everything on a platter and serve.

Nutritional Information:

- Calories 210
- Fat 7
- Carbs 6
- Protein 7

Recipe 319. Turkey Bacon and Turnip Salad

Serving Size: 4

Preparation Time: 15 minutes

Cooking Time: 40 minutes

Ingredients:

- 2 turnips, cut into wedges
- 2 tsp olive oil
- 1/3 cup black olives, sliced
- 1 cup baby spinach
- 6 radishes, cut
- 3 oz turkey bacon, sliced
- 4 tbsp buttermilk
- 2 teaspoon mustard seeds
- 1 tsp Dijon mustard1
- 2 tbsp red wine vinegar
- Black pepper and salt to taste
- 1 tbsp chopped chives

Directions:

- Cook the turkey bacon in a large-sized skillet on moderate heat until crispy for approximately 5 minutes. Put aside and then break it up. Cover a baking tray with parchment paper and sprinkle the turnips with black pepper. Then drizzle with olive oil and bake in a 25-minute timer at 390 F, Turning halfway through. Allow cooling.
- Spread the baby spinach on the base of the salad plate and cover it with bacon, radishes, and turnips. Combine the mustard seeds, buttermilk vinegar, mustard, and salt. Sprinkle the salad dressing on top, mix thoroughly, and sprinkle with olives and chives. Serve.

Nutritional Information:

- Cal 135
- Net Carbs 6g
- Fat 10g
- Protein 6g

Recipe 320. Turkey Ginger Soup

Serving Size: 6

Preparation Time: 15 minutes

Cooking Time: 8 hours

Ingredients:

- 1-pound boneless, skinless turkey thighs, cut into 1-inch pieces
- 1-pound fresh shiitake mushrooms halved
- 3 carrots, peeled and sliced
- 2 cups frozen peas
- 1 tablespoon grated fresh ginger
- 6 cups Poultry Broth or store-bought
- 1 tablespoon low-sodium soy sauce
- 1 teaspoon toasted sesame oil
- 2 teaspoons garlic powder
- 1½ cups cooked Brown Rice

Directions:

- In your slow cooker, combine the turkey, mushrooms, carrots, peas, ginger, broth, soy sauce, sesame oil, and garlic powder.
- Cover and cook on low within 8 hours. About 30 minutes before serving, stir in the rice to warm it through.

Nutritional Information:

- Calories: 318
- Fat: 7g
- Carbohydrates: 42g
- Protein: 24g

Recipe 321. Vegetable Beef Stew

Serving Size: 6

Preparation Time: 20 minutes

Cooking Time: 1 hour

Ingredients:

- 2 pounds cubed beef chuck and 1 tablespoon olive oil
- ½ cup peeled turnip, diced
- ¼ cup rolled carrots
- ¼ cup sliced celery
- ¼ cup cut string beans
- 2 cloves sliced garlic
- ½ cup red wine
- ¾ cup diced red onions
- 4 cups low-sodium beef broth
- 2 tablespoons red tomato paste
- 2 tablespoons beef base
- 1 tablespoon porcini mushroom powder
- 2 cloves
- 2 teaspoons gelatin powder
- 2 bay leaves
- ½ teaspoon dried marjoram
- Salt and pepper for taste
- 1 teaspoon rubbed thyme

- 4 tablespoons cooking butter

Directions:

- Trim beef chuck of silver skin and fat and cube it, prepare veggies as well.
- Turn on sauté mode and brown beef in batches, and from there, you add the rest of the ingredients and then stir together.
- Press soup button, and let it natural pressure release, when finished, you can adjust with seasonings.

Nutritional Information:

- Calories: 321
- Fat: 15g
- Carbs: 10g
- Protein: 33g

Recipe 322. Vegetarian Chili Mac

Serving Size: 6

Preparation Time: 10 minutes

Cooking Time: 25 minutes

Ingredients:

- 1 tablespoon olive oil
- 1 diced red bell pepper
- 2 tablespoons chili powder
- 1 teaspoon of chipotle powder
- 1 clove minced garlic
- 1 can tomato sauce
- 1 can drained and rinsed kidney beans
- 1 diced yellow onion
- 1 minced jalapeno pepper
- 2 teaspoons cumin
- 2 teaspoons salt
- 1 can diced tomatoes
- 1 can black beans, drained and rinsed
- 8 oz. Elbow pasta, whole wheat
- 1 cup cheddar cheese
- 2 cups vegetable broth
- 1 cup Monterey jack cheese
- Cilantro and Greek yogurt to top

Directions:

- Put olive oil in instant pot, sautéing for 5 minutes.
- Add the onions, peppers, cumin, powders, salt, and pepper and then combine, and then put garlic in, sautéing for a minute.
- Put the rest of the ingredients besides the cheese into there and combine it.
- Let it pressurize and cook for 5 minutes.

- Quick release the valve, then add cheese till combined.

Nutritional Information:

- Calories: 230
- Fat: 10g
- Carbs: 5g
- Protein: 7g

Recipe 323. Veggie Fritters

Serving Size: 4

Preparation Time: 10 minutes

Cooking Time: 10 minutes

Ingredients:

- 2 garlic cloves, minced
- 2 yellow onions, chopped
- 4 scallions, chopped
- 2 carrots, grated
- 2 teaspoons cumin, ground
- ½ teaspoon turmeric powder
- Salt and black pepper to the taste
- ¼ teaspoon coriander, ground
- 2 tablespoons parsley, chopped
- ¼ teaspoon lemon juice
- ½ cup almond flour
- 2 beets, peeled and grated
- 2 eggs, whisked
- ¼ cup tapioca flour
- 3 tablespoons olive oil

Directions:

- In a container, combine the garlic with the onions, scallions, and the rest of the ingredients except the oil, stir well and shape medium fritters out of this mix.
- Heat up a skillet with the oil over medium-high heat, add the fritters, cook for 5 minutes on each side, arrange on a platter, and serve.

Nutritional Information:

- Calories: 209
- Fat: 11.2 Gram
- Carbs: 4.4 Gram
- Protein: 4.8g

Recipe 324. Wonton Soup

Serving Size: 8

Preparation Time: 20 minutes

Cooking Time: 25 minutes

Ingredients:

- 1 recipe of Asian Broth
- 2½ cups Napa cabbage leaves, core removed and chopped
- 1-pound lean ground pork
- 1/3 cup green onions, chopped
- ¼ teaspoon garlic powder
- ¼ teaspoon onion powder
- ½ teaspoon low-sodium soy sauce
- ½ cup water chestnuts, chopped
- 1 package wonton wrappers
- 3 tablespoons egg substitute

Directions:

- Preheat oven to 400°F.
- Place broth and cabbage in a deep pan and bring to a simmer.
- Combine pork, green onions, garlic powder, onion powder, soy sauce, egg substitute, water chestnuts, and 2 cups of cooked cabbage.
- Mix well to combine and form into teaspoon-size balls.
- Place balls on parchment-lined sheet pan and bake in oven for 5 minutes. Remove from oven and allow to cool.
- Once cooled, place meatball in wonton wrapper; fold into a triangle and seal edges of the wrappers by moistening with water and pressing the edges together firmly.
- Place in simmering broth and cook 3 to 4 minutes until they float. Serve immediately.

Nutritional Information:

- Calories: 320
- Fat: 13g
- Protein: 16g
- Carbohydrates: 34g

Recipe 325. Zucchini and Leek Turkey Soup

Serving Size: 4

Preparation Time: 20 minutes

Cooking Time: 40 minutes

Ingredients:

- 2 cups turkey, cooked and chopped
- 1 onion chopped
- 1 clove of garlic, minced
- 3 celery stalks and chopped
- 2 leeks 2 leeks, chopped
- 2 Tbsp butter
- 4 cups chicken stock
- Black pepper and salt to taste
- 1 cup of fresh parsley chopped
- 1 large zucchini, spiralized

Directions:

- In a pan on medium flame. Add the leeks, celery, onion, garlic, and other vegetables to the pot and let them cook for 5 mins.
- Add the turkey, meat and salt, black pepper, and stock. Cook over 20 minutes. Add the zucchini, stir in the meantime, and let it cool down for five minutes. Serve in bowls topped with parsley.

Nutritional Information:

- Cal 235
- Net Carbs 9.3g
- Fat 10g
- Protein 23g

CHAPTER 6. SNACKS RECIPES

Recipe 326. Apple Crisp

Serving Size: 12

Preparation Time: 30 minutes

Cooking Time: 45 minutes

Ingredients:

- Crust/Crumble
- 1 cup rolled oats
- 1 cup whole wheat flour
- ½ cup Grape Nuts cereal
- 1 teaspoon cinnamon
- 1 cup unsweetened apple juice
  - Filling
- 2 apples, sliced
- ½ cup raisins
- 1 cup unsweetened apple juice
- 2 teaspoons cinnamon
- 1 tablespoon lemon juice
- 2 teaspoons cornstarch

Directions:

- Preheat oven to 350°F.
- Combine all crust/crumble ingredients and press half of mixture into the bottom of a 9-inch nonstick pan and bake for 5 minutes. Remove from oven and set aside.
- Raise oven to 375°F.
- In saucepan combine apples, raisins, apple juice, cinnamon, lemon juice, and cornstarch, and boil for 10 minutes.
- Remove apples and raisins, placing them in the prepared crust, and reduce liquid until thick, approximately 5 minutes.
- Pour liquid into crust and top with the remaining crumble mixture.
- Bake for 30 minutes.

Nutritional Information:

- Calories: 100
- Fat: 1g
- Protein: 3g
- Carbohydrates: 20g

Recipe 327. Avocado Tuna Bites

Serving Size: 4

Preparation Time: 10 minutes

Cooking Time: 5 minutes

Ingredients:

- 1/3 cup coconut oil
- 1 avocado, cut into cubes
- 10 ounces canned tuna, drained
- ¼ cup parmesan cheese, grated
- ¼ teaspoon garlic powder
- 1/4 teaspoon onion powder
- 1/3 cup almond flour
- ¼ teaspoon pepper
- ¼ cup low fat mayonnaise
- Pepper as needed

Directions:

- Take a bowl and add tuna, mayo, flour, parmesan, spices and mix well.
- Fold in avocado and make 12 balls out of the mixture.
- Melt coconut oil in pan and cook over medium heat, until all sides are golden.
- Serve and enjoy!

Nutritional Information:

- Calories: 185
- Fat: 18g
- Carbohydrates: 1g
- Protein: 5g

Recipe 328. Baked Eggplant Chips with Salad and Aioli

Serving Size: 4

Preparation Time: 15 minutes

Cooking Time: 30 minutes

Ingredients:

- 2 eggplants, sliced
- 1 egg, beaten
- 3 1/2 oz of cooked beets shred
- 3 1/2 oz of red cabbage shred
- 2 cups almond meal
- 2 Tbsp butter, melt
- 2 egg yolks
- 2 cloves of garlic, chopped
- 1 cup olive oil
- 1/2 1 tsp red chili flakes
- 2 Tbsp lemon juice
- 3 tbsp yogurt

- 2 tablespoons fresh cilantro chopped
- Black pepper and salt to taste

Directions:

- Preheat the oven to 400 F. On a thick plate, make a mixture of flour, salt, and pepper. Dip the eggplants in the egg and then dip them in the flour. Place them on a baking sheet, and then brush with butter. Cook for about 15 mins.
- For aioli to make, whisk egg yolks and garlic. Gradually add 3 cups olive oil as you whisk. Add chili flakes, salt pepper, 1 tbsp lemon juice and yogurt. In a bowl for salad, mix cabbage, beets, cilantro, the rest of the oil, the remaining lemon juice, salt, and pepper. Toss in a dressing. The fries are served alongside Aioli and the beet salad.

Nutritional Information:

- Cal 377
- Net Carbs 10.5g
- Fat 65g
- Protein 8g

Recipe 329. Baked Scotch Eggs

Serving Size: 4

Preparation Time: 20 minutes

Cooking Time: 35 minutes

Ingredients:

- 4 eggs, hard-boiled
- 1 egg
- 1/2 cup pork rinds, crushed
- 1 lb pork sausages, skinless
- 2 Tbsp Grana Padano, grated
- 1 clove of garlic, chopped
- 1/2 teaspoon onion powder
- 1/2 tsp cayenne pepper
- 1 tsp fresh chopped parsley chopped
- Black pepper and salt to taste

Directions:

- Preheat the oven to 350 F. Within a mixing dish, mix all the ingredients, except for the egg and the pork rinds. Grab a few tablespoons from the sausage mixture and put it in each of the eggs.
- Utilizing your fingers, you can mold the mixture until it's sealed. Mix the egg using a fork in the bowl. Dip the sausage eggs into the egg, coat them with pork rinds, and put them in a baking dish. Bake for 25 minutes or until crisp and golden brown. Serve.

Nutritional Information:

- Cal 265
- Net Carbs 1.1g
- Fat 15g
- Protein 29g

Recipe 330. Cashew and Carrot Muffins

Serving Size: 4

Preparation Time: 10 minutes

Cooking Time: 3 hours

Ingredients:

- 4 tablespoons cashew butter, melted
- 4 eggs, whisked
- ½ cup coconut cream
- 1 cup carrots, peeled and grated
- 4 teaspoons maple syrup
- ¾ cup coconut flour
- ½ teaspoon baking soda

Directions:

- In a bowl, mix the cashew butter with the eggs, cream, and the other ingredients, whisk well and pour into a muffin pan that fits the slow cooker.
- Put the lid on, cook the muffins on High for 3 hours, cool down and serve.

Nutritional Information:

- Calories 245
- Fat 21.7g
- Carbohydrate 28.6g
- Protein 12.3g

Recipe 331. Cheese and Nut Zucchini Boats

Serving Size: 4

Preparation Time: 20 minutes

Cooking Time: 35 minutes

Ingredients:

- 2 medium zucchinis, halved
- 1 cup cauliflower rice
- 2 tbsp olive oil
- 1/4 cup vegetable broth
- 1 1/4 cups diced tomatoes
- 1 red onion chopped
- 1 cup of pine nuts

- 1/4 cup hazelnuts
- 1 tablespoon balsamic vinegar
- 1 tbsp smoked paprika
- 1 cup of grated Monterey Jack
- 4 TBSP chopped cilantro

Directions:

- Preheat the oven to 350 F. Put the cauli rice, broth and cauli in an oven-proof pot. Cook up to 5 mins. Then, you can fluff the rice and let it cool. Scoop the pulp out of the zucchini halves, then slice the flesh.
- The zucchini shells should be brushed with olive oil. In a bowl, mix together cauli rice, tomatoes, red onion, hazelnuts, pine nuts, cilantro, vinegar and paprika and the zucchini pulp. Pour the mix into the zucchini halves. Drizzle with the remaining prepared olive oil, then sprinkle the cheese over. Then bake for approximately around 20 minutes, or until the cheese is melted. Serve.

Nutritional Information:

- Cal 228
- Net Carbs 7g
- Fat 31g
- Protein 12g

Recipe 332. Cheese Chips

Serving Size: 8

Preparation Time: 15 minutes

Cooking Time: 15 minutes

Ingredients:

- 3 tablespoons. coconut flour
- ½ cup strong cheddar cheese, grated and divided
- ¼ cup Parmesan cheese, grated
- 2 tablespoons. butter, melted
- 1 organic egg
- 1 teaspoon. fresh thyme leaves, minced

Directions:

- Preheat the oven to 350o F. Line a large baking sheet with parchment paper.
- In a bowl, place the coconut flour, ¼ cup of grated cheddar, Parmesan, butter, and egg and mix until well combined.
- Set the mixture aside for about 3-5 minutes.
- Make 8 equal-sized balls from the mixture.
- Arrange the prepared balls onto the prepared baking sheet in a single layer about 2-inch apart.
- With your hands, press each ball into a little flat disc.
- Sprinkle each disc with the remaining cheddar, followed by thyme.
- Bake for about 13-15 minutes or until the edges become golden brown.
- Remove from the preheated oven and let them cool completely before serving.

Nutritional Information:

- Calories: 189 Cal
- Fat: 28 g
- Carbs: 4 g
- Protein: 14 g

Recipe 333. Cheesy Mashed Sweet Potato Cakes

Serving Size: 4

Preparation Time: 10 minutes

Cooking Time: 30 minutes

Ingredients:

- ¾ cup breadcrumbs
- 4 cups mashed potatoes
- ½ cup onions
- 2 cup of grated mozzarella cheese
- ¼ cup fresh grated parmesan cheese
- 2 large cloves finely chopped
- 1 egg
- 2 teaspoons finely chopped parsley
- Salt and pepper to taste

Directions:

- Line your baking sheet with foil. Wash, peel and cut the prepared sweet potatoes into 6 pieces. Arrange them inside the baking sheet and drizzle a small amount of oil on top before seasoning with salt and pepper.
- Cover with a baking sheet and bake it for 45 minutes. Once cooked transfer them into a mixing bowl and mash them well with a potato masher.
- To the sweet potatoes in a bowl add green onions, parmesan, mozzarella, garlic, egg, parsley, and breadcrumbs. Mash and combine the mixture together using the masher.
- Put the remaining ¼ cup of the breadcrumbs in a place. Scoop a teaspoon of mixture into your palm and form round patties around ½ and inch thick. Dredge your patties in the breadcrumbs to cover both sides and set them aside.
- Heat a tablespoon of oil in a medium nonstick pan. When the oil is hot, begin to cook the patties in

batches 4 or 5 per session and cook each side for 6 minutes until they turn golden brown. Using a spoon or spatula flip them. Add oil to prevent burning.

Nutritional Information:

- Calories 126
- Fat 6g
- Carbs 15g
- Proteins 3g

Recipe 334. Cherry Clafouti

Serving Size: 6

Preparation Time: 30 minutes

Cooking Time: 45 minutes

Ingredients:

- ¼ cup + 2 teaspoons flour
- ½ teaspoon baking powder
- ¼ cup egg substitute
- 2 egg whites
- 1/3 cup Splenda
- ½ cup cherry or pomegranate juice
- 2½ cups frozen cherries, thawed and chopped
- Zest of 1 orange

Directions:

- Preheat oven to 375°F.
- Spray 8-inch baking dish with cooking spray.
- In a medium-sized bowl, combine flour and baking powder.
- In a separate medium-sized bowl, combine egg substitute and egg whites; whip until frothy; add in Splenda, juice, and flour mixture; and mix until smooth and blended.
- Fold in cherries and zest and ladle into baking dish; bake for 35–45 minutes until golden brown.
- Allow to cool and serve with fat-free vanilla, frozen yogurt, or a dollop of low-fat whipped topping.

Nutritional Information:

- Calories: 140
- Fat: 0.5g
- Protein: 4g
- Carbohydrates: 30g

Recipe 335. Cinnamon Peach Cobbler

Serving Size: 4

Preparation Time: 10 minutes

Cooking Time: 4 hours

Ingredients:

- 4 cups peaches, peeled and sliced
- Cooking spray
- ¼ cup coconut sugar
- 1 and ½ cups whole wheat sweet crackers, crushed
- ½ cup almond milk
- ½ teaspoon cinnamon powder
- ¼ cup stevia
- 1 teaspoon vanilla extract
- ¼ teaspoon nutmeg, ground

Directions:

- In a bowl, mix peaches with sugar, cinnamon, and stir.
- In a separate bowl, mix crackers with stevia, nutmeg, almond milk, and vanilla extract and stir.
- Spray your slow cooker with cooking spray, spread peaches on the bottom, and add the crackers mix, spread, cover, and cook on Low for 4 hours.
- Divide into bowls and serve.

Nutritional Information:

- Calories 249
- Fat 11.4g
- Carbohydrate 42.7g
- Protein 3.5g

Recipe 336. Fat-Free Fries

Serving Size: 2

Preparation Time: 20 minutes

Cooking Time: 20 minutes

Ingredients:

- Butter-flavored nonfat cooking spray
- 2 large Yukon gold potatoes, cut thin into fries
- 2 egg whites, beaten
- Salt and pepper, to taste
- Toasted garlic powder
- Ground red chili flakes
- Fresh minced chives

Directions:

- Thoroughly spray nonstick baking sheet with butter flavored cooking spray.
- Coat potatoes in egg whites and lay out single layer on sheet pan.
- Sprinkle with salt and pepper, garlic powder, and chili flakes.
- Bake at 350°F for 20 minutes, adding chives when almost done.

Nutritional Information:
- Calories: 260
- Fat: 0g
- Protein: 11g
- Carbohydrates: 53g

Recipe 337. Ginger and Pumpkin Pie

Serving Size: 10

Preparation Time: 10 minutes

Cooking Time: 2 hours

Ingredients:
- 2 cups almond flour
- 1 egg, whisked
- 1 cup pumpkin puree
- 1 and ½ teaspoons baking powder
- Cooking spray
- 1 tablespoon coconut oil, melted
- 1 tablespoon vanilla extract
- ½ teaspoon baking soda
- 1 and ½ teaspoons cinnamon powder
- ¼ teaspoon ginger, ground
- 1/3 cup maple syrup
- 1 teaspoon lemon juice

Directions:
- In a bowl, flour with baking powder, baking soda, cinnamon, ginger, egg, oil, vanilla, pumpkin puree, maple syrup and lemon juice, stir and pour in your slow cooker greased with cooking spray and lined with parchment paper, cover the pot and cook on Low for 2 hours and 20 minutes.
- Leave the pie to cool down, slice and serve.

Nutritional Information:
- Calories 191
- Fat 4.8g
- Carbohydrate 10.8g
- Protein 2g

Recipe 338. Ginger Snaps

Serving Size: 18

Preparation Time: 15 minutes

Cooking Time: 10 minutes

Ingredients:
- 4 tablespoons unsalted butter
- 1/2 cup light brown sugar
- 2 tablespoons molasses
- 1 egg white
- 21/2 teaspoons ground ginger
- 1/4 teaspoon ground allspice
- 1 teaspoon sodium-free baking soda
- 1/2 cup unbleached all-purpose flour
- 12 cup white whole-wheat flour
- 1 tablespoon sugar

Directions:
- Warm oven to 375°F. Put aside a baking sheet with parchment paper. Put the butter, sugar, plus molasses into a mixing bowl and beat well.
- Mix the egg white, ginger, and allspice. Mix in the baking soda, then put the flours, then beat.
- Roll the dough into small balls. Put the balls on a prepared baking sheet and press down using a glass dipped in the tablespoon sugar.
- Once the glass presses on the dough, it will moisten sufficiently to coat with sugar. Bake within 10 minutes. Let it cool, then serve.

Nutritional Information:
- Calories: 81
- Fat: 2 g
- Protein: 1 g
- Carbohydrates: 14 g

Recipe 339. Goat Cheese and Rutabaga Puffs

Serving Size: 4

Preparation Time: 20 minutes

Cooking Time: 35 minutes

Ingredients:
- 1/2 oz goat cheese, crumbled
- 1 rutabaga, peeled, and cut into pieces
- 2 tablespoons of butter that is melted
- One cup of ground pork rinds

Directions:
- Preheat the oven to 350 F. Spread rutabaga on baking sheets and drizzle with butter. Roast until soft, about 15 minutes. Transfer the cooked vegetables to an ice cube. Let it cool before adding goat cheese.
- Utilizing a fork, mash to mix all the components. Put the pork rinds on the plate. Form 1-inch balls from the rutabaga and then wrap them around the rinds, pressing them lightly to adhere. Put them on the

baking pan and cook for about 10 minutes or until golden. Serve.

Nutritional Information:

- Cal 131
- Net Carbs 5.9g
- Fat 9g
- Protein 3g

Recipe 340. Grilled Fruit

Serving Size: 4

Preparation Time: 10 minutes

Cooking Time: 20 minutes

Ingredients:

- 2 tablespoons brown sugar
- ½ teaspoon chili powder
- ¼ teaspoon ground ginger
- ¼ teaspoon cinnamon Pinch salt
- 2 cups fruit of choice (pineapple, peach, pear, apricot, apple), cut into thick slices and seeded/cored

Directions:

- Combine brown sugar, chili powder, ginger, cinnamon, and salt. Place cut side of fruit onto mixture to coat.
- Place fruit on grill or nonstick pan at medium-high heat to allow sugars to caramelize, approximately 4 minutes.
- Flip and cook for 2 more minutes. Flip and cook for approximately an additional 2 minutes if fruit is not tender.
- Serve with fat-free vanilla frozen yogurt.

Nutritional Information:

- Calories: 260
- Fat: 5g
- Protein: 2g
- Carbohydrates: 67g

Recipe 341. Halloumi and Cheddar Sticks

Serving Size: 4

Preparation Time: 10 minutes

Cooking Time: 20 minutes

Ingredients:

- 1 lb halloumi cut into strips
- 1/2 cup cheddar, cut into strips
- 1/3 cup almond flour
- 2 tsp smoked paprika
- 2 Tbsp chopped parsley
- 1/2 tsp cayenne powder

Directions:

- Set your oven at 360 F. Blend the almond flour with the paprika in a large bowl. Lightly coat the cheddar cheese and halloumi strips in the mix.
- Place them on a baking tray that is greased. Sprinkle them with cayenne and parsley powder and spray the baking sheet with cooking spray. Cook for approximately about 10 minutes or until golden brown. Serve and have a blast!

Nutritional Information:

- Cal 361
- Net Carbs 8g
- Fat 35g
- Protein 22g

Recipe 342. Hoisin Meatballs

Serving Size: 12

Preparation Time: 20 minutes

Cooking Time: 10 minutes

Ingredients:

- 1 cup beef broth of choice
- 2 tablespoons soy sauce
- 4 chopped green onions
- ¼ cup minced cilantro
- ¼ cup chopped onion
- 1 lightly beaten egg
- 3 tablespoons hoisin sauce
- 2 minced garlic cloves
- ½ teaspoon salt and pepper each
- 1 pound ground beef
- 1 pound ground pork of choice
- sesame seeds for topping

Directions:

- In instant pot, put the wine, sauces, and boil them, then reduce heat.
- Combine next 7 ingredients in bowl, then mix it together with the meats, shaping into meatballs, and then put it in instant pot.
- Set it to manual high pressure for 10 minutes, quick release, and then top with sesame seeds.

Nutritional Information:

- Calories: 78

- Fat: 5g
- Carbs: 1g
- Protein: 6g

Recipe 343. Honey Granola

Serving Size: 8

Preparation Time: 20 minutes

Cooking Time: 30 minutes

Ingredients:

- 4 cups oatmeal
- 1 cup flaked or shredded unsweetened coconut
- 1 cup raw, hulled sunflower seeds
- 1 cup chopped walnuts
- ½ cup raw wheat germ
- ¼ cup flaxseed meal
- ¼ cup oil (canola or olive)
- ¼ cup pasteurized honey

Directions:

- Preheat oven to 350°F.
- In a large bowl, mix oatmeal, coconut, sunflower seeds, walnuts, wheat germ, and flaxseed meal.
- Combine oil and honey in microwaveable container and add a splash of water. Microwave for 15 seconds, then stir to combine thoroughly.
- Pour honey mixture over dry ingredients in bowl, stir thoroughly to coat granola.
- Spread mixture evenly on 2 cookie sheets and bake for 30 minutes or until granola reaches desired crunchiness. Use a spatula to stir granola every few minutes.
- Allow to actually cool on cookie sheet, then store in an airtight container.

Nutritional Information:

- Calories: 150
- Fat: 9g
- Protein: 4g
- Carbohydrates: 15g

Recipe 344. Hot Marinated Shrimp

Serving Size: 8

Preparation Time: 1 hour 10 minutes

Cooking Time: 2 minutes

Ingredients:

- 2 tablespoons capers
- ½ cup lime juice
- 1 red onion, chopped
- ½ teaspoon chili powder
- 1 tablespoon mustard
- ½ cup rice vinegar
- 1 cup water
- 1 bay leaf
- 3 cloves
- 1 pound shrimp, peeled and deveined

Directions:

- In a baking dish, mix capers with mustard, lime juice and chili and whisk well.
- Put the water in a pot and heat up over medium heat.
- Add cloves, bay leaf and vinegar, stir and bring to a boil.
- Add shrimp, cook for 1 minute, drain and transfer shrimp to the baking dish.
- Toss to coat well, cover and keep in the fridge for 1 hour.
- Divide into bowls and serve.

Nutritional Information:

- Calories 150
- Fat 0
- Carbs 3
- Protein 12

Recipe 345. Jalapeno Vegetable Frittata Cups

Serving Size: 2

Preparation Time: 20 minutes

Cooking Time: 35 minutes

Ingredients:

- 1 tbsp olive oil
- 2 green onions chopped
- 1 clove of garlic, minced
- 1/2 jalapeno pepper, chopped
- Half a carrot chopped
- 1 zucchini, shredded
- 2 tbsp mozzarella, shredded
- 4 eggs whisked
- Black pepper and salt to taste
- 1/2 1 tsp dried oregano

Directions:

- Sauté garlic and green onions in olive oil warm on moderate heat for three minutes. Add zucchini, carrots, and jalapeno pepper and cook for an

additional 4 minutes. Transfer the cooked mixture to an oven pan that has been lightly greased.
- Top with mozzarella cheese. Cover with whisked eggs, then sprinkle with black pepper, oregano, and salt. In the oven, bake for approximately around twenty minutes at a temperature of 360 F.

Nutritional Information:

- Cal 335
- Net Carbs 5.7g
- Fat 18g
- Protein 14g

Recipe 346. Leafy Greens and Cheddar Quesadillas

Serving Size: 4

Preparation Time: 15 minutes

Cooking Time: 25 minutes

Ingredients:

- 1 tbsp butter softened
- 1/2 cup cream cheese
- 3 eggs
- 1 1/2 1 tsp 1 1/2 tsp psyllium husk powder
- 1 tbsp of coconut flour
- 1/2 teaspoon salt
- 5 OZ grated cheddar cheese
- 1 oz of leafy greens

Directions:

- Preheat the oven to 400 F. In a bowl, mix the eggs together with cream cheese. In a different bowl, mix coconut flour, psyllium husk and salt. Mix in eggs and stir until completely integrated. Then let it rest for a few minutes. Prepare a baking sheet using parchment paper. Add half of the mix.
- The tortilla is baked for seven minutes until brown on the edges. Repeat the very same process with the rest of the batter. Prepare a skillet by greasing it with butter, then place it in the tortilla. Add cheddar cheese and green leaves and then the tortilla with another. Brown every side of the tortilla for one minute.

Nutritional Information:

- Cal 320
- Net Carbs 2.6g
- Fat 28g
- Protein 15g

Recipe 347. Lemon Zest Pudding

Serving Size: 4

Preparation Time: 10 minutes

Cooking Time: 5 hours

Ingredients:

- 1 cup pineapple juice, natural
- Cooking spray
- 1 teaspoon baking powder
- 1 cup coconut flour
- 3 tablespoons avocado oil
- 3 tablespoons stevia
- ½ cup pineapple, chopped
- ½ cup lemon zest, grated
- ½ cup coconut milk
- ½ cup pecans, chopped

Directions:

- Spray your slow cooker with cooking spray.
- In a bowl, mix flour with stevia, baking powder, oil, milk, pecans, pineapple, lemon zest and pineapple juice, stir well, pour into your slow cooker greased with cooking spray, cover and cook on Low for 5 hours.
- Divide into bowls and serve.

Nutritional Information:

- Calories 231
- Fat 29.7g
- Carbohydrate 47.1g
- Protein 8.1g

Recipe 348. Lentil Sweet Bars

Serving Size: 14

Preparation Time: 10 minutes

Cooking Time: 25 minutes

Ingredients:

- 1 cup lentils, cooked, drained and rinsed
- 1 teaspoon cinnamon powder
- 2 cups whole wheat flour
- 1 teaspoon baking powder
- ½ teaspoon nutmeg, ground
- 1 cup low-fat butter
- 1 cup coconut sugar
- 1 egg
- 2 teaspoons almond extract
- 1 cup raisins
- 2 cups coconut, unsweetened and shredded

Directions:

- Put the lentils in a bowl, mash them well using a fork, add cinnamon, flour, baking powder, nutmeg, butter, sugar, egg, almond extract, raisins, and coconut, stir, spread on a lined baking sheet, introduce in the oven, bake at 350 degrees F for 25 minutes, cut into bars and serve cold.
- Enjoy!

Nutritional Information:

- Calories 214
- Fat 4
- Carbs 5
- Protein 7

Recipe 349. Mini Teriyaki Turkey Sandwiches

Serving Size: 20

Preparation Time: 20 minutes

Cooking Time: 30 minutes

Ingredients:

- 2 chicken breast halves
- 1 cup soy sauce, low salt
- ¼ cup cider vinegar
- 3 minced garlic cloves
- 1 tablespoon fresh ginger root
- 2 tablespoons cornstarch
- 20 Hawaiian sweet rolls
- ½ teaspoon pepper
- 2 tablespoons melted butter

Directions:

- Put turkey in pressure cooker and combine the first six ingredients over it.
- Cook it on manual for 25 minutes, and when finished, natural pressure release.
- Push sauté after removing the turkey, then mix cornstarch and water, stirring into cooking juices, and cook until sauce is thickened. Shred meat and stir to heat.
- You can split the rolls, buttering each side, and bake till golden brown, adding the meat mixture to the top.

Nutritional Information:

- Calories: 252
- Fat: 5g
- Carbs: 25g
- Protein: 26g

Recipe 350. Pesto Veggie Pinwheels

Serving Size: 4

Preparation Time: 15 minutes

Cooking Time: 40 minutes

Ingredients:

- 3 whole eggs
- 1 egg, beaten for brushing
- 1 cup grated cheese
- 1 cup of almond flour
- 3 tablespoons coconut flour
- 1/2 tsp 1 tsp
- 4 tbsp cream cheese, softened
- 1/4 tsp yogurt
- One cup of cold butter
- 1 cup of mushrooms, chopped
- 1 cup basil pesto
- 2 cups baby spinach
- Salt to taste

Directions:

- Mix coconut and almond flour, Xanthan gum, and 1/2 teaspoon salt in a bowl. Add cream cheese, yogurt, and butter; mix until it is crumbly. Incorporate three eggs in succession and mix until the dough is formed into an oval. Make the dough flat on a flat, clean surface, wrap it in plastic wrap and chill for an hour.
- Dust a clean, flat area with almond flour. Cut off the dough and then roll out to 15x12 inches. Spread pesto over the top using a spatula, leaving a 2-inch border along one side. A bowl mixes baby mushrooms and spinach, season with salt and black pepper, and spreads the mixture on top of the pesto. Sprinkle with cheese, and wrap as tightly as possible, starting at the lower end. Refrigerate for 10 minutes. Preheat the oven to 350 F. Take the pastry from the fridge onto a flat surface, and then use the sharp edge of a knife, cut it into 24 small discs. Lay them out in a baking tray, brush with the remaining egg and bake for about 25 minutes until they are golden. Allow cooling.

Nutritional Information:

- Cal 241
- Net Carbs 3.4g
- Fat 39g
- Protein 20g

Recipe 351. Plum Cake

Serving Size: 8

Preparation Time: 1 hour 20 minutes

Cooking Time: 40 minutes

Ingredients:

- 7 ounces whole wheat flour
- 1 teaspoon baking powder
- 1-ounce low-fat butter, soft
- 1 egg, whisked
- 5 tablespoons coconut sugar
- 3 ounces warm almond milk
- 1 and ¾ pounds plums, pitted and cut into quarters
- Zest of 1 lemon, grated
- 1-ounce almond flakes

Directions:

- In a bowl, combine the flour with baking powder, butter, egg, sugar, milk, and lemon zest, stir well, transfer dough to a lined cake pan, spread plums and almond flakes all over, introduce in the oven and bake at 350 degrees F for 40 minutes.
- Slice and serve cold.
- Enjoy!

Nutritional Information:

- Calories 222
- Fat 4
- Carbs 7
- Protein 7

Recipe 352. Pork Beef Bean Nachos

Serving Size: 10

Preparation Time: 15 minutes

Cooking Time: 40 minutes

Ingredients:

- 1 package beef jerky
- 4 cans black beans, drained and rinsed
- 6 bacon strips, crumbled
- 3 pounds pork spareribs
- 1 cup chopped onion
- 4 teaspoons minced garlic
- 4 cups divided beef broth
- optional toppings such as cheddar, sour cream, green onions, jalapeno slices
- 1 teaspoon crushed red pepper flakes

Directions:

- Pulse jerky in processor till ground, working in batches, put the ribs in the instant pot, topping with half jerky, two beans, ½ cup onion, three pieces of bacon, 2 teaspoons garlic, 2 cups broth, and half teaspoon red pepper flakes. Cook on high for forty minutes.
- Let it natural pressure release for approximately about 10 minutes, then quick release what's next, and do the same with the second batch.
- Discard bones, and shred meat and then sauté it, and strain the mixture, and then discard juice and serve with chips and your desired toppings.

Nutritional Information:

- Calories: 269
- Fat: 24g
- Carbs: 27g
- Protein: 33g

Recipe 353. Pumpkin Pie

Serving Size: 8

Preparation Time: 15 minutes

Cooking Time: 45 minutes

Ingredients:

- 1 Cup ginger snaps
- ½ Cup egg white
- 16 Ounces canned pumpkin
- ½ Cup sugar
- 2 Teaspoons pumpkin pie spice
- 12 Ounces (can) skim milk, evaporated

Directions:

- Using a food processor, grind the cookies thoroughly.
- Set the oven to 350°F and preheat.
- Take a 10" glass pie pan and sprinkle little vegetable cooking oil.
- Spread the cookies crumbs evenly in the pan.
- In a medium mixing bowl, combine all the remaining Ingredients.
- Pour over the crust and bake.
- Continue baking about 45 minutes, until you can insert a knife and take out clean.
- Once it baked well, allow it cool and refrigerate.
- Slice it into eight wedges.

Nutritional Information:

- Calories: 184
- Total Carbs: 39.4 g
- Total Fat: 0.5 g

- Cholesterol: 2 mg

Recipe 354. Raspberry and Goat Cheese Focaccia Bites

Serving Size: 4

Preparation Time: 20 minutes

Cooking Time: 30 minutes

Ingredients:

- 6 zero carb buns, cut into
- Each square is 4 squares
- 1 cup of mushrooms, cut into slices
- 1 cup of fresh raspberries
- 2 cups of erythritol
- 1 lemon juiced
- 1 tbsp olive oil
- 1/2 1 tsp dried thyme
- 2 oz goat cheese, crumbled
- 1 green onion chopped

Directions:

- Put the raspberries in a saucepan and break them into a puree using a potato masher. Then mix in erythritol and lemon juice. Place the saucepan over the simmering point and cook it with constant stirring until sugar melts. Increase the heat to medium, and let the mixture simmer for 4 minutes, continuously stirring to stop it from burning. Allow cooling.
- Preheat the oven to 350 F. Lay the buns on a baking sheet and bake for six minutes. In an oven-proof skillet. Sauté mushrooms and thyme for 10 minutes. Remove the bread slices from the oven, cut each one in half horizontally, and then top with mushrooms. Sprinkle goat cheese and green onions as well as raspberry jam. Wrap with 6 focaccia pieces and serve.

Nutritional Information:

- Cal 171
- Net Carbs 5.7g
- Fat 9g
- Protein 7g

Recipe 355. Rosemary Feta Cheese Bombs

Serving Size: 4

Preparation Time: 25 minutes

Cooking Time: 50 minutes

Ingredients:

- 6 Tbsp butter
- 1/3 cup almond meal
- 3 eggs
- 1 cup of crumbled cheese feta
- Half cup whipping heavy cream inconsistency
- 1 tbsp olive oil
- 2 sprigs of rosemary
- Two onions of white, thinly cut
- 2 Tbsp of red wine vinegar
- 1 tsp Serve Brown Sugar

Directions:

- Preheat the oven up to 350 F. Line a baking tray with parchment paper. In a pan, warm 1 cup of butter and 1 cup of water. Bring to a simmer and add the almond flour. Beat with a bouncy beat until a ball is formed. Then turn off the heat and keep beating, adding eggs, one at each time, until the dough is soft and slightly more pliable. Scoop out mounds of the dough into the baking dish.
- Create a small hole in the middle of each of the mounds. Then bake for around 20 minutes until the buns are golden and risen. Take them out of the oven and puncture the buns' sides using the toothpick. Return to the oven to bake for two minutes until crisp. Allow cooling.
- Take the middle of the bun (keep the part that is torn out) to make an opening to place the filling of cream. Set aside. Place olive oil in an oven and cook rosemary and onions for 2 minutes. Mix in served vinegar and sugar, then simmer for 3 minutes or when the caramelization has occurred. In a bowl, mix whipping cream with feta. Pour the mixture into a piping bag and place a spoonful of the mixture into each bun. Place the buns on top of the torn portion of the pastry. Top with the relish of onions to serve.

Nutritional Information:

- Cal 279
- Net Carbs 3.5g
- Fat 37g
- Protein 10g

Recipe 356. Salmon Apple Salad Sandwich

Serving Size: 4

Preparation Time: 15 minutes

Cooking Time: 10 minutes

Ingredients:

- 4 ounces (125 g) canned pink salmon, drained, and flaked
- 1 medium (180 g) red apple, cored and diced
- 1 celery stalk (about 60 g), chopped
- 1 shallot (about 40 g), finely chopped
- 1/3 cup (85 g) light mayonnaise
- 8 slices whole grain bread (about 30 g each), toasted
- 8 (15 g) Romaine lettuce leaves
- Salt and freshly ground black pepper

Directions:

- Combine the salmon, apple, celery, shallot, and mayonnaise in a mixing bowl. Season with salt and pepper.
- Place 1 slices bread on a plate, top with lettuce and salmon salad, and then covers with another slice of bread. Repeat procedure for the remaining Ingredients.
- Serve and enjoy.

Nutritional Information:

- Calories: 315
- Fat - 11.3 g
- Carbohydrates - 40.4 g
- Protein - 15.1 g

Recipe 357. Salmon Spinach and Cottage Cheese Sandwich

Serving Size: 4

Preparation Time: 15 minutes

Cooking Time: 10 minutes

Ingredients:

- 4 ounces (125 g) cottage cheese
- 1/4 cup (15 g) chives, chopped
- 1 teaspoon (5 g) capers
- 1/2 teaspoon (2.5 g) grated lemon rind
- 4 (2 oz. or 60 g) smoked salmon
- 2 cups (60 g) loose baby spinach
- 1 medium (110 g) red onion, sliced thinly
- 8 slices rye bread (about 30 g each)
- Kosher salt and freshly ground black pepper

Directions:

- Preheat your griddle or Panini press.
- Mix together cottage cheese, chives, capers, and lemon rind in a small bowl.
- Spread and divide the cheese mixture on 4 bread slices. Top with spinach, onion slices, and smoked salmon.
- Cover with remaining bread slices.
- Grill the sandwiches until golden and grill marks form on both sides.
- Transfer to a serving dish.
- Serve and enjoy.

Nutritional Information:

- Calories: 261
- Fat 9.9 g
- Carbohydrates 22.9 g
- Protein 19.9 g

Recipe 358. Shrimps Ceviche

Serving Size: 8

Preparation Time: 3 hours 10 minutes

Cooking Time: 6 minutes

Ingredients:

- ¼ pound shrimp, peeled, deveined and chopped
- Zest and juice of 2 limes
- Zest and juice of 2 lemons
- 2 teaspoons cumin, ground
- 2 tablespoons olive oil
- 1 cup tomato, chopped
- ½ cup red onion, chopped
- 2 tablespoons garlic, minced
- 1 Serrano chili pepper, chopped
- 1 cup black beans, canned and drained
- 1 cup cucumber, chopped
- ¼ cup cilantro, chopped

Directions:

- In a bowl, mix lime juice and lemon juice with shrimp, toss well, cover and keep in the fridge for 3 hours.
- Heat up a pan with the oil over medium high heat, add shrimp and citrus juices, cook for 2 minutes on each side and transfer everything to a bowl.
- Add lime and lemon zest, cumin, tomato, onion, garlic, chili pepper, cucumber, black beans, and cilantro, toss well and serve with some tortilla chips on the side.

Nutritional Information:

- Calories 100
- Fat 3
- Carbs 10
- Protein 5

Recipe 359. Spinach Chips with Avocado Hummus

Serving Size: 4

Preparation Time: 20 minutes

Cooking Time: 25 minutes

Ingredients:

- 1 tbsp olive oil
- 1/2 cup baby spinach
- 1/2 tsp plain vinegar
- 3 avocados, chopped
- Half cup chopped parsley
- 1/2 cup butter
- 1 cup of pumpkin seeds
- 1/4 cup sesame paste
- Juice from half a lemon
- 1 clove of garlic, minced
- 1/2 teaspoon coriander powder
- Black pepper and salt to taste

Directions:

- Preheat the oven to 350 F. Place leaves in bowls and mix in simple vinegar, olive oil, and salt. Spread the spinach on a parchment-lined baking tray and bake till the leaves are crisp but not burnt, about 15 minutes.
- Place the avocados into the food processor. Add pumpkin seeds, butter, sesame paste, garlic, lemon juice, coriander, salt, and pepper. Puree until smooth. Serve in a large-sized bowl and garnish with chopped parsley. Serve with chips of spinach.

Nutritional Information:

- Cal 348
- Net Carbs 7g
- Fat 50g
- Protein 10g

Recipe 360. Vegan Rice Pudding

Serving Size: 8

Preparation Time: 15 minutes

Cooking Time: 20 minutes

Ingredients:

- 1-quart vanilla nondairy milk
- 1 cup basmati or jasmine rice, rinsed
- 1/4 cup sugar
- 1 teaspoon pure vanilla extract
- 1/8 teaspoon pure almond extract
- 1/2 teaspoon ground cinnamon
- 1/8 teaspoon ground cardamom

Directions:

- Mix all the fixings into a saucepan and stir well to combine. Bring to a boil over medium-high heat. Adjust heat to low and simmer, stirring very frequently, about 15–20 minutes. Remove from heat and cool. Serve sprinkled with additional ground cinnamon if desired.

Nutritional Information:

- Calories: 148
- Fat: 2 g
- Protein: 4 g
- Carbohydrates: 26 g

Recipe 361. Avocado Caprese Wrap

Serving Size: 2

Preparation Time: 20 minutes

Cooking Time: 15 minutes

Ingredients:

- 2 tortillas
- Balsamic vinegar, as needed
- 1 ball of mozzarella cheese, grated
- ½ cup of arugula
- 1 tomato, sliced
- 2 tablespoons of fresh basil leaves, chopped
- Kosher salt, to taste
- 1 avocado, sliced
- Olive oil, as required
- Black pepper, to taste

Directions:

- Divide the tomato slices and cheese evenly among the tortilla wraps. Then add the avocado and basil.
- Drizzle olive oil and also the vinegar over the top. Wrap the tortilla and season with pepper and salt and serve. Garnish with parsley.

Nutritional Information:

- Calories: 191
- Fat: 4.7g
- Protein: 2.3g
- Carbohydrates: 7.1g

Recipe 362. Brussels Sprouts with Pistachios

Serving Size: 4

Preparation Time: 20 minutes

Cooking Time: 40 minutes

Ingredients:

- 1-pound of Brussels sprouts, tough bottoms trimmed, halved lengthwise
- 4 shallots, peeled and quartered
- 1 tablespoon of extra-virgin olive oil
- Sea salt
- Freshly ground black pepper
- ½ cup of chopped roasted pistachios
- Zest of ½ lemon
- Juice of ½ lemon

Directions:

- Preheat the oven to 400°F. In a large-sized bowl, toss the Brussels sprouts and shallots with the olive oil until well coated.
- Bake for 15 minutes. Take away from the oven and transfer to a serving bowl. Toss with the pistachios, lemon zest, and lemon juice. Season with pepper and sea salt. Serve warm.

Nutritional Information:

- Calories: 126
- Fat: 7g
- Protein: 6g
- Carbohydrates: 14g

Recipe 363. Caramelized Onions

Serving Size: 5

Preparation Time: 20 minutes

Cooking Time: 40 minutes

Ingredients:

- 15.8 oz of golden onions
- 15.8 of red onions
- 0.7 oz of extra virgin olive oil
- 2 tablespoons water
- 2 pinches of salt

Directions:

- Peel the prepared onions and cut them into thin slices about 0.4 inch thick.
- In a large pan, heat the olive oil and add the onions and cook over low heat with a lid for 25 minutes, stirring often.
- Cook for 10 minutes and serve

Nutritional Information:

- Calories: 75.5
- Fat: 5.3g
- Protein: 1.2g
- Carbohydrates: 5.5g

Recipe 364. Creamy Panini

Serving Size: 6

Preparation Time: 15 minutes

Cooking Time: 20 minutes

Ingredients:

- 8 slices rustic whole grain bread
- 4 slices provolone cheese
- 2 tablespoons finely chopped oil-cured black olives
- ¼ cup chopped fresh basil leaves
- 1 small zucchini, thinly sliced
- ½ cup Mayonnaise dressing with olive oil
- 7 ounces roasted red peppers

Directions:

- In a small bowl, mix together olives, basil and mayonnaise dressing. Spread the dressing evenly on 4 slices of whole grain bread. Then top it with zucchini, peppers and provolone before covering with another slice of bread.
- Spread the remaining mayonnaise mixture around the bread and cook over medium heat on a nonstick skillet for about approximately 2 minutes on each side or until bread is golden brown on both sides and cheese is melted.

Nutritional Information:

- Calories: 250
- Fat: 21.8g
- Protein: 14.4g
- Carbohydrates: 24.2g

Recipe 365. Zingy Zucchini Bites

Serving Size: 5

Preparation Time: 5 minutes

Cooking Time: 15 minutes

Ingredients:

- 2 tablespoons vegetable oil
- 1 red chili pepper, chopped
- 1 pound zucchini, dig thick slices
- 1 teaspoon garlic powder
- 1 cup chicken stock
- salt and black pepper, to taste
- 1/2 teaspoon paprika
- 1/2 teaspoon ground coriander

Directions:

- Oil and heat the pan and cook chili pepper for 1 minute. Add the remaining ingredients.
- Cook for 5 minutes and serve

Nutritional Information:

- Calories: 70
- Fat: 5.1g
- Protein: 3.2g
- Carbohydrates: 4.4g

CHAPTER 7. 93+1 MEAL PLANS

Meal Plan 1

- Breakfast: Apple Quinoa Muffins ~ **200 Calories**
- Lunch: Beef and Cheese Avocado Boats ~ **400 Calories**
- Dinner: Citrus Pork ~ **270 Calories**
- Sides/Snacks: Cauliflower Soup with Crispy Bacon ~ **333 Calories**

Total Calorie Count: 1203 Calories

Meal Plan 2

- Breakfast: Eggs and Broccoli Casserole ~ **373 Calories**
- Lunch: Chicken and Brussels Sprout Bake ~ **318 Calories**
- Dinner: Okra and Sausage Hot Pot ~ **311 Calories**
- Sides/Snacks: Potato Soup ~ **200 Calories**

Total Calorie Count: 1202 Calories

Meal Plan 3

- Breakfast: Onion Frittata ~ **217 Calories**
- Lunch: Olive Capers Chicken ~ **433 Calories**
- Dinner: Smoked Sausage Casserole ~ **326 Calories**
- Sides/Snacks: Baked Potato with Thyme ~ **224 Calories**

Total Calorie Count: 1200 Calories

Meal Plan 4

- Breakfast: Sweet Chia Bowls ~ **321 Calories**
- Lunch: Buffalo Chicken Salad Wrap ~ **300 Calories**
- Dinner: Chicken with Potatoes Olives and Sprouts ~ **397 Calories**
- Sides/Snacks: Mushroom Sausages ~ **188 Calories**

Total Calorie Count: 1206 Calories

Meal Plan 5

- Breakfast: Morning Herbed Eggs ~ **273 Calories**
- Lunch: Eggplant Beef Lasagna ~ **399 Calories**
- Dinner: Sesame Pork Bites ~ **289 Calories**
- Sides/Snacks: Thyme Sweet Potatoes ~ **244 Calories**

Total Calorie Count: 1205 Calories

Meal Plan 6

- Breakfast: Roasted Root Vegetable Hash ~ **343 Calories**
- Lunch: Garlic Pork and Kale ~ **350 Calories**
- Dinner: Mussels Curry with Lime ~ **260 Calories**
- Sides/Snacks: Mini Teriyaki Turkey Sandwiches ~ **252 Calories**

Total Calorie Count: 1205 Calories

Meal Plan 7

- Breakfast: Apple Pancakes ~ **378 Calories**
- Lunch: Thyme Chicken with Mushrooms and Turnip ~ **394 Calories**
- Dinner: Chicken and Sausage Gumbo ~ **303 Calories**
- Sides/Snacks: Spicy Brussels Sprouts ~ **176 Calories**

Total Calorie Count: 1251 Calories

Meal Plan 8

- Breakfast: Roasted Red Pepper and Pesto Omelet ~ **314 Calories**
- Lunch: Ground Pork Stuffed Mushrooms ~ **382 Calories**
- Dinner: Roasted Lemon Swordfish ~ **280 Calories**
- Sides/Snacks: Bean Soup ~ **258 Calories**

Total Calorie Count: 1234 Calories

Meal Plan 9

- Breakfast: Scrambled Eggs with Tofu and Mushrooms ~ **385 Calories**
- Lunch: Pimiento Cheese Pork Meatballs ~ **393 Calories**
- Dinner: Paprika Pork and Scallions ~ **271 Calories**
- Sides/Snacks: Avocado Tuna Bites ~ **185 Calories**

Total Calorie Count: 1234 Calories

Meal Plan 10

- Breakfast: Zucchini and Pepper Caprese Gratin ~ **283 Calories**
- Lunch: Pesto Chicken Cacciatore ~ **371 Calories**
- Dinner: Mustard Chicken with Rosemary ~ **315 Calories**
- Sides/Snacks: Split Pea Cream Soup ~ **281 Calories**

Total Calorie Count: 1250 Calories

Meal Plan 11

- Breakfast: Egg Muffins with Quinoa ~ **221 Calories**
- Lunch: Chicken and Acorn Squash Bake ~ **391 Calories**
- Dinner: Grilled Chicken ~ **512 Calories**
- Sides/Snacks: Ginger and Pumpkin Pie ~ **91 Calories**

Total Calorie Count: 1215 Calories

Meal Plan 12

- Breakfast: Arugula Pesto Egg Scramble ~ **392 Calories**

- Lunch: Barbecued Pork Chops ~ **342 Calories**
- Dinner: Stuffed Chicken Breasts ~ **361 Calories**
- Sides/Snacks: Vegan Rice Pudding ~ **148 Calories**

Total Calorie Count: 1243 Calories

Meal Plan 13

- Breakfast: Chorizo and Cheese Frittata ~ **335 Calories**
- Lunch: Pork with Apple Sauce ~ **356 Calories**
- Dinner: Sesame Pork Bites ~ **289 Calories**
- Sides/Snacks: Plum Cake ~ **222 Calories**

Total Calorie Count: 1202 Calories

Meal Plan 14

- Breakfast: Goat Cheese Frittata with Asparagus ~ **345 Calories**
- Lunch: Tamari Chicken Thighs and Capers ~ **329 Calories**
- Dinner: Pork Roast with Cranberry ~ **330 Calories**
- Sides/Snacks: Potato Soup ~ **200 Calories**

Total Calorie Count: 1204 Calories

Meal Plan 15

- Breakfast: Hash Brown Vegetable Breakfast Casserole ~ **363 Calories**
- Lunch: Turkey and Vegetable Casserole ~ **364 Calories**
- Dinner: Cod Salad with Mustard ~ **258 Calories**
- Sides/Snacks: Cinnamon Peach Cobbler ~ **249 Calories**

Total Calorie Count: 1234 Calories

Meal Plan 16

- Breakfast: Crabmeat Frittata with Onion ~ **345 Calories**
- Lunch: Teriyaki Chicken Wings ~ **296 Calories**
- Dinner: Mushroom and Beef Stir-Fry ~ **259 Calories**
- Sides/Snacks: Vegetable Beef Stew ~ **321 Calories**

Total Calorie Count: 1221 Calories

Meal Plan 17

- Breakfast: Ham and Egg Casserole ~ **310 Calories**
- Lunch: Salmon with Mushroom ~ **220 Calories**
- Dinner: Chicken Tikka ~ **417 Calories**
- Sides/Snacks: Roasted Garlic Soup & Hot Marinated Shrimp ~ **292 Calories**

Total Calorie Count: 1239 Calories

Meal Plan 18

- Breakfast: Mexican Eggs ~ **395 Calories**
- Lunch: Chicken Sliders ~ **224 Calories**
- Dinner: Roasted Chicken Thighs ~ **448 Calories**
- Sides/Snacks: Lentil Sweet Bars ~ **214 Calories**

Total Calorie Count: 1281 Calories

Meal Plan 19

- Breakfast: Creamy Oatmeal ~ **368 Calories**
- Lunch: Chili Shrimp with Scallions Rice ~ **240 Calories**
- Dinner: Turnip Greens and Artichoke Chicken ~ **373 Calories**
- Sides/Snacks: Parsley Red Potatoes ~ **257 Calories**

Total Calorie Count: 1238 Calories

Meal Plan 20

- Breakfast: Bacon and Blue Cheese Cups ~ **380 Calories**
- Lunch: Saffron Shrimp ~ **210 Calories**
- Dinner: Asparagus and Lemon Salmon ~ **434 Calories**
- Sides/Snacks: Tahini Beans ~ **180 Calories**

Total Calorie Count: 1204 Calories

Meal Plan 21

- Breakfast: Pepper and Cheese Frittata ~ **201 Calories**
- Lunch: Fennel and Chicken Wrapped in Bacon ~ **357 Calories**
- Dinner: Bacon and Parsnip Chicken Bake ~ **351 Calories**
- Sides/Snacks: Turkey Ginger Soup ~ **318 Calories**

Total Calorie Count: 1227 Calories

Meal Plan 22

- Breakfast: Rolled Smoked Salmon with Avocado ~ **320 Calories**
- Lunch: Ground Pork Stuffed Mushrooms ~ **382 Calories**
- Dinner: Chicken with Garlic and Fennel ~ **200 Calories**
- Sides/Snacks: Spinach and Brussels Sprout Salad ~ **311 Calories**

Total Calorie Count: 1213 Calories

Meal Plan 23

- Breakfast: Hash Browns with Quinoa ~ **191 Calories**
- Lunch: Prosciutto Broccoli Chicken Stew ~ **399 Calories**
- Dinner: Meatballs and Sauce ~ **435 Calories**
- Sides/Snacks: Cumin Black Beans and Peppers ~ **221 Calories**

Total Calorie Count: 1246 Calories

Meal Plan 24

- Breakfast: Snazzy Baked Eggs ~ **175 Calories**
- Lunch: Honey Spiced Cajun Chicken ~ **312 Calories**
- Dinner: Paella with Chicken, Leeks, and Tarragon ~ **388 Calories**
- Sides/Snacks: Cheddar and Turkey Meatball Salad ~ **382 Calories**

Total Calorie Count: 1257 Calories

Meal Plan 25

- Breakfast: Broccoli, Egg and Pancetta Gratin ~ **399 Calories**
- Lunch: Juicy Beef Meatballs ~ **398 Calories**
- Dinner: Pork and Salsa ~ **270 Calories**
- Sides/Snacks: Clam Chowder ~ **172 Calories**

Total Calorie Count: 1239 Calories

Meal Plan 26

- Breakfast: Poached Eggs ~ **200 Calories**
- Lunch: Pimiento Chicken Pork Meatballs ~ **393 Calories**
- Dinner: Pan-Seared Squids and Sausage ~ **334 Calories**
- Sides/Snacks: Smoked Salmon, Bacon and Egg Salad ~ **321 Calories**

Total Calorie Count: 1248 Calories

Meal Plan 27

- Breakfast: Quinoa Patties with Parmesan ~ **201 Calories**
- Lunch: Braised Chicken with Tomato and Garlic ~ **353 Calories**
- Dinner: Oven-Baked Salami and Cheddar Chicken ~ **317 Calories**
- Sides/Snacks: Cheesy Chicken Soup with Spinach ~ **381 Calories**

Total Calorie Count: 1252 Calories

Meal Plan 28

- Breakfast: Amazing Quinoa Hash Browns ~ **191 Calories**
- Lunch: Baked Chicken Nuggets ~ **373 Calories**
- Dinner: Pork Roast with Cranberry ~ **330 Calories**
- Sides/Snacks: Chicken Salad with Parmesan ~ **329 Calories**

Total Calorie Count: 1223 Calories

Meal Plan 29

- Breakfast: Tuna and Egg Salad with Chili Mayo ~ **391 Calories**
- Lunch: Beef, Bell Pepper and Mushroom Kebabs ~ **379 Calories**
- Dinner: Pork with Dates Sauce ~ **240 Calories**
- Sides/Snacks: Cauliflower-Watercress Salad ~ **198 Calories**

Total Calorie Count: 1208 Calories

Meal Plan 30

- Breakfast: Western Omelet Quiche ~ **365 Calories**
- Lunch: Roasted Pork Stuffed with Ham and Cheese ~ **387 Calories**
- Dinner: Pork with Mushroom Bowls ~ **250 Calories**
- Sides/Snacks: Baked Potato with Thyme ~ **224 Calories**

Total Calorie Count: 1226 Calories

Meal Plan 31

- Breakfast: Pepper and Cheese Frittata ~ **201 Calories**
- Lunch: Barbecued Pork Chops ~ **342 Calories**
- Dinner: Baked Zucchini with Cheese and Chicken ~ **348 Calories**
- Sides/Snacks: Sweet Butternut & Ginger and Pumpkin Pie ~ **325 Calories**

Total Calorie Count: 1216 Calories

Meal Plan 32

- Breakfast: Soft Banana Bread ~ **399 Calories**
- Lunch: Buffalo Chicken Salad Wrap ~ **300 Calories**
- Dinner: Almond-Crusted Zucchini Chicken Stacks ~ **308 Calories**
- Sides/Snacks: Ginger Snaps & Hot Marinated Shrimp ~ **231 Calories**

Total Calorie Count: 1238 Calories

Meal Plan 33

- Breakfast: Turkey Bacon and Spinach Crepes ~ **391 Calories**
- Lunch: Chicken Sliders ~ **224 Calories**
- Dinner: Baked Chicken Wrapped in Smoked Salmon ~ **356 Calories**
- Sides/Snacks: Bean Soup ~ **258 Calories**

Total Calorie Count: 1229 Calories

Meal Plan 34

- Breakfast: Omelet with Mushrooms and Cheese ~ **299 Calories**
- Lunch: Chili Shrimp with Scallions Rice ~ **240 Calories**
- Dinner: Asparagus and Lemon Salmon ~ **434 Calories**
- Sides/Snacks: Lemon Zest Pudding ~ **231 Calories**

Total Calorie Count: 1204 Calories

Meal Plan 35

- Breakfast: Morning Herbed Eggs ~ **273 Calories**
- Lunch: Creamy Chicken with Caramelized Leeks ~ **359 Calories**
- Dinner: Baked Chicken Legs with Tomato Sauce ~ **385 Calories**
- Sides/Snacks: Cashew and Carrot Muffins ~ **245 Calories**

Total Calorie Count: 1262 Calories

Meal Plan 36

- Breakfast: Rosemary Eggs with Peppers ~ **272 Calories**
- Lunch: Creamy Smoky Pork Chops ~ **240 Calories**
- Dinner: Meatballs and Sauce ~ **435 Calories**
- Sides/Snacks: Pork Beef Bean Nachos ~ **269 Calories**

Total Calorie Count: 1216 Calories

Meal Plan 37

- Breakfast: Ham and Egg Casserole ~ **310 Calories**
- Lunch: Beef Burgers with Lettuce and Avocado ~ **400 Calories**
- Dinner: Bacon Topped Turkey Meatloaf ~ **326 Calories**
- Sides/Snacks: Shrimps Ceviche & Vegan Rice Pudding ~ **248 Calories**

Total Calorie Count: 1284 Calories

Meal Plan 38

- Breakfast: Breakfast Quinoa Cakes ~ **199 Calories**
- Lunch: Garlic Pork and Kale ~ **350 Calories**
- Dinner: Chicken with Potatoes Olives and Sprouts ~ **397 Calories**
- Sides/Snacks: Smoked Salmon, Bacon and Egg Salad ~ **321 Calories**

Total Calorie Count: 1267 Calories

Meal Plan 39

- Breakfast: Scrambled Eggs with Tofu and Mushrooms ~ **385 Calories**
- Lunch: Green Bean and Broccoli Chicken Stir Fry ~ **311 Calories**
- Dinner: Baked Cheesy Chicken Tenders ~ **312 Calories**
- Sides/Snacks: Baby Spinach Salad & Hoisin Meatballs ~ **204 Calories**

Total Calorie Count: 1212 Calories

Meal Plan 40

- Breakfast: Chili Omelet with Avocado ~ **322 Calories**
- Lunch: Pork and Pumpkin Chili ~ **289 Calories**
- Dinner: Coconut Fried Shrimp with Cilantro Sauce ~ **341 Calories**
- Sides/Snacks: Pork Beef Bean Nachos ~ **269 Calories**

Total Calorie Count: 1221 Calories

Meal Plan 41

- Breakfast: Omelet with Mushrooms and Cheese ~ **299 Calories**
- Lunch: Pork Chops with Thyme and Apples ~ **240 Calories**
- Dinner: Creamy Chicken Fried Rice ~ **319 Calories**
- Sides/Snacks: Cheesy Chicken Soup with Spinach ~ **381 Calories**

Total Calorie Count: 1239 Calories

Meal Plan 42

- Breakfast: Zucchini and Pepper Caprese Gratin ~ **283 Calories**
- Lunch: Pork Patties ~ **332 Calories**
- Dinner: Cumin Pork and Beans ~ **291 Calories**
- Sides/Snacks: Cauliflower Soup with Crispy Bacon ~ **333 Calories**

Total Calorie Count: 1239 Calories

Meal Plan 43

- Breakfast: Blueberry Waffles ~ **347 Calories**
- Lunch: Pimiento Cheese Pork Meatballs ~ **393 Calories**
- Dinner: Gingered Grilled Chicken ~ **293 Calories**
- Sides/Snacks: Chickpea and Kale Soup ~ **221 Calories**

Total Calorie Count: 1254 Calories

Meal Plan 44

- Breakfast: Arugula Pesto Egg Scramble ~ **392 Calories**
- Lunch: Tamari Chicken Thighs and Capers ~ **329 Calories**
- Dinner: Mackerel and Orange Medley ~ **300 Calories**
- Sides/Snacks: Coriander Seeds Cabbage ~ **252 Calories**

Total Calorie Count: 1273 Calories

Meal Plan 45

- Breakfast: Hash Brown Vegetable Casserole ~ **363 Calories**
- Lunch: Teriyaki Chicken Wings ~ **296 Calories**
- Dinner: Chicken and Chorizo Traybake ~ **305 Calories**

- Sides/Snacks: Moroccan Sweet Potato Soup ~ **260 Calories**

Total Calorie Count: 1224 Calories

Meal Plan 46

- Breakfast: Spiced Oatmeal ~ **200 Calories**
- Lunch: Thyme Chicken with Mushrooms and Turnip ~ **394 Calories**
- Dinner: Hawaiian Chicken ~ **340 Calories**
- Sides/Snacks: Bell Peppers Cakes & Parmesan Artichokes ~ **269 Calories**

Total Calorie Count: 1200 Calories

Meal Plan 47

- Breakfast: Crabmeat Frittata with Onion ~ **345 Calories**
- Lunch: Tilapia Broccoli Platter ~ **362 Calories**
- Dinner: Cabbage and Beef Steaks ~ **331 Calories**
- Sides/Snacks: Parsley Red Potatoes ~ **257 Calories**

Total Calorie Count: 1295 Calories

Meal Plan 48

- Breakfast: Apple Pancakes ~ **378 Calories**
- Lunch: Turkey and Vegetable Casserole ~ **364 Calories**
- Dinner: Balsamic Chili Roast ~ **265 Calories**
- Sides/Snacks: Quinoa and Scallops Salad ~ **221 Calories**

Total Calorie Count: 1228 Calories

Meal Plan 49

- Breakfast: Bacon and Cheese Cloud Eggs ~ **287 Calories**
- Lunch: Pork and Sweet Potatoes with Chili ~ **320 Calories**
- Dinner: Lemon-Parsley Chicken Breast ~ **317 Calories**
- Sides/Snacks: Turkey Ginger Soup ~ **318 Calories**

Total Calorie Count: 1242 Calories

Meal Plan 50

- Breakfast: Apple Quinoa Muffins ~ **200 Calories**
- Lunch: Beef Sausage and Okra Casserole ~ **400 Calories**
- Dinner: Lemon and Garlic Scallops ~ **351 Calories**
- Sides/Snacks: Spinach and Brussels Sprout Salad ~ **311 Calories**

Total Calorie Count: 1262 Calories

Meal Plan 51

- Breakfast: Arugula Pesto Egg Scramble ~ **392 Calories**
- Lunch: Broccoli and Carrot Turkey Bake ~ **385 Calories**
- Dinner: Chicken Relleno Casserole ~ **265 Calories**
- Sides/Snacks: Apple Crisp & Cherry Clafouti ~ **240 Calories**

Total Calorie Count: 1282 Calories

Meal Plan 52

- Breakfast: Bacon and Artichoke Omelet ~ **347 Calories**
- Lunch: Garlic Mushroom Chicken ~ **331 Calories**
- Dinner: Chicken and Sausage Gumbo ~ **303 Calories**
- Sides/Snacks: Fat-Free Fries ~ **260 Calories**

Total Calorie Count: 1241 Calories

Meal Plan 53

- Breakfast: Broccoli, Egg and Pancetta Gratin ~ **399 Calories**
- Lunch: Asparagus and Beef Shirataki ~ **398 Calories**
- Dinner: Cod Salad with Mustard ~ **258 Calories**
- Sides/Snacks: Lemon Zest Pudding ~ **231 Calories**

Total Calorie Count: 1286 Calories

Meal Plan 54

- Breakfast: Zucchini Skillet Cakes ~ **271 Calories**
- Lunch: Pimiento Cheese Pork Meatballs ~ **393 Calories**
- Dinner: Cumin Pork and Beans ~ **291 Calories**
- Sides/Snacks: Jalapeno Vegetable Frittata Cups ~ **335 Calories**

Total Calorie Count: 1290 Calories

Meal Plan 55

- Breakfast: Tuna and Egg Salad with Chili Mayo ~ **391 Calories**
- Lunch: Beef, Bell Pepper and Mushroom Kebabs ~ **379 Calories**
- Dinner: Mushroom and Beef Stir-Fry ~ **249 Calories**
- Sides/Snacks: Rosemary Feta Cheese Bombs ~ **279 Calories**

Total Calorie Count: 1298 Calories

Meal Plan 56

- Breakfast: Bacon and Blue Cheese Cups ~ **380 Calories**
- Lunch: Saffron Shrimp ~ **210 Calories**
- Dinner: Mustard Chicken with Rosemary ~ **315 Calories**
- Sides/Snacks: Salmon Apple Salad Sandwich ~ **315 Calories**

Total Calorie Count: 1220 Calories

Meal Plan 57

- Breakfast: Sesame and Poppy Seed Bagels ~ **352 Calories**
- Lunch: Thyme Chicken with Mushrooms and Turnip ~ **394 Calories**
- Dinner: Citrus Pork ~ **270 Calories**
- Sides/Snacks: Pesto Veggie Pinwheels ~ **241 Calories**

Total Calorie Count: 1257 Calories

Meal Plan 58

- Breakfast: Ratatouille Egg Bake ~ **248 Calories**
- Lunch: Turnip and Pork Packets with Grilled Halloumi ~ **399 Calories**
- Dinner: Pork and Salsa ~ **270 Calories**
- Sides/Snacks: Sweet Corn Soup ~ **310 Calories**

Total Calorie Count: 1227 Calories

Meal Plan 59

- Breakfast: Beef Breakfast Casserole ~ **379 Calories**
- Lunch: Spinach Chicken ~ **288 Calories**
- Dinner: Pizzaiola Steaks ~ **320 Calories**
- Sides/Snacks: Spinach Salad with Goat Cheese and Nuts ~ **240 Calories**

Total Calorie Count: 1227 Calories

Meal Plan 60

- Breakfast: Pepper and Cheese Frittata ~ **201 Calories**
- Lunch: Rosemary Buttered Pork Chops ~ **363 Calories**
- Dinner: Lemon and Garlic Scallops ~ **351 Calories**
- Sides/Snacks: Crispy Garlic Baked Potato Wedges ~ **324 Calories**

Total Calorie Count: 1239 Calories

Meal Plan 61

- Breakfast: Mushroom Frittata ~ **227 Calories**
- Lunch: Baked Chicken ~ **557 Calories**
- Dinner: Pineapple Glazed Chicken ~ **198 Calories**
- Sides/Snacks: Bacon and Gorgonzola Salad ~ **239 Calories**

Total Calorie Count: 1271 Calories

Meal Plan 62

- Breakfast: Omelet with Mushrooms and Cheese ~ **299 Calories**
- Lunch: Seared Scallops with Apricot Orzo Salad ~ **380 Calories**
- Dinner: Nutmeg Salmon and Mushrooms ~ **250 Calories**
- Sides/Snacks: Cauliflower Soup with Crispy Bacon ~ **333 Calories**

Total Calorie Count: 1262 Calories

Meal Plan 63

- Breakfast: Jackfruit Vegetable Fry ~ **236 Calories**
- Lunch: Stewed Pork with Cauliflower and Broccoli ~ **456 Calories**
- Dinner: Paprika Pork and Scallions ~ **271 Calories**
- Sides/Snacks: Fiery Shrimp Cocktail Salad ~ **241 Calories**

Total Calorie Count: 1204 Calories

Meal Plan 64

- Breakfast: Eggplant and Tomato Gratin ~ **213 Calories**
- Lunch: Shrimp and Orzo ~ **328 Calories**
- Dinner: Paella with Chicken, Leeks, and Tarragon ~ **388 Calories**
- Sides/Snacks: Caprese Salad Stacks Anchovies ~ **292 Calories**

Total Calorie Count: 1221 Calories

Meal Plan 65

- Breakfast: Berry Hemp Seed Breakfast ~ **400 Calories**
- Lunch: Lemon Pepper and Salmon ~ **464 Calories**
- Dinner: Mussels Curry with Lime ~ **260 Calories**
- Sides/Snacks: Bell Peppers Cake ~ **120 Calories**

Total Calorie Count: 1244 Calories

Meal Plan 66

- Breakfast: Hash Brown Mix ~ **221 Calories**
- Lunch: Stewed Pork with Cauliflower and Broccoli ~ **456 Calories**
- Dinner: Hawaiian Chicken ~ **340 Calories**
- Sides/Snacks: Grilled Avocado Caprese Crostini ~ **278 Calories**

Total Calorie Count: 1295 Calories

Meal Plan 67

- Breakfast: Cottage Pancakes ~ **345 Calories**
- Lunch: Tamari Chicken Thighs and Caper ~ **329 Calories**
- Dinner: Pan-Seared Squids and Sausage ~ **334 Calories**
- Sides/Snacks: Green Salad with Feta and Blueberries ~ **201 Calories**

Total Calorie Count: 1209 Calories

Meal Plan 68

- Breakfast: Crespelle al Mascarpone ~ **369 Calories**

- Lunch: Thyme Chicken with Mushrooms and Turnip ~ **394 Calories**
- Dinner: Pesto Chicken Breasts with Red Squash ~ **230 Calories**
- Sides/Snacks: Moroccan Sweet Potato Soup ~ **260 Calories**

Total Calorie Count: 1253 Calories

Meal Plan 69

- Breakfast: Mushroom and Cheese Lettuce Cups ~ **281 Calories**
- Lunch: Taco Casserole ~ **240 Calories**
- Dinner: Kabobs with Peanut Curry Sauce ~ **530 Calories**
- Sides/Snacks: Mushroom Sausages ~ **188 Calories**

Total Calorie Count: 1239 Calories

Meal Plan 70

- Breakfast: Roasted Red Pepper and Pesto Omelet ~ **314 Calories**
- Lunch: Stir Fry Ground Pork ~ **267 Calories**
- Dinner: Coconut Fried Shrimp with Cilantro Sauce ~ **341 Calories**
- Sides/Snacks: Refried Beans with Baked Tortilla or Pita Chips ~ **310 Calories**

Total Calorie Count: 1232 Calories

Meal Plan 71

- Breakfast: Zucchini Skillet Cakes ~ **271 Calories**
- Lunch: Shrimp Quesadillas ~ **299 Calories**
- Dinner: Chicken with Potatoes Olives and Sprouts ~ **397 Calories**
- Sides/Snacks: Smoked Mackerel Lettuce Cups ~ **234 Calories**

Total Calorie Count: 1201 Calories

Meal Plan 72

- Breakfast: Zucchini and Pepper Caprese Gratin ~ **283 Calories**
- Lunch: Seared Scallops with Apricot Orzo Salad ~ **380 Calories**
- Dinner: Pork Chops with Green Beans and Avocado ~ **321 Calories**
- Sides/Snacks: Spinach Salad with Pancetta and Mustard ~ **267 Calories**

Total Calorie Count: 1251 Calories

Meal Plan 73

- Breakfast: Wester Omelet Quiche ~ **365 Calories**
- Lunch: Chili Shrimp with Scallions Rice ~ **240 Calories**
- Dinner: Pork Sausage Sauerkraut ~ **355 Calories**
- Sides/Snacks: Vegetable Beef Stew ~ **321 Calories**

Total Calorie Count: 1281 Calories

Meal Plan 74

- Breakfast: Soft Banana Bread ~ **399 Calories**
- Lunch: Pork and Pumpkin Chili ~ **289 Calories**
- Dinner: Pumpkin and Black Beans Chicken ~ **354 Calories**
- Sides/Snacks: Zucchini and Leek Turkey Soup ~ **235 Calories**

Total Calorie Count: 1277 Calories

Meal Plan 75

- Breakfast: Spiced Oatmeal ~ **200 Calories**
- Lunch: Country Spareribs with White Beans ~ **390 Calories**
- Dinner: Pork Stew with Shallots ~ **261 Calories**
- Sides/Snacks: Baked Eggplant Chips with Salad and Aioli ~ **377 Calories**

Total Calorie Count: 1228 Calories

Meal Plan 76

- Breakfast: Scrambled Eggs with Mushrooms and Spinach ~ **291 Calories**
- Lunch: Pesto Chicken Cacciatore ~ **371 Calories**
- Dinner: Red Wine Beef Roast and Vegetables ~ **300 Calories**
- Sides/Snacks: Jalapeno Vegetable Frittata Cups ~ **335 Calories**

Total Calorie Count: 1297 Calories

Meal Plan 77

- Breakfast: Rosemary Eggs with Peppers ~ **272 Calories**
- Lunch: Chicken with Noodles ~ **210 Calories**
- Dinner: Peach-Mustard Pork Shoulder ~ **583 Calories**
- Sides/Snacks: Honey Granola ~ **150 Calories**

Total Calorie Count: 1215 Calories

Meal Plan 78

- Breakfast: Mexican Eggs ~ **395 Calories**
- Lunch: Chicken Sliders ~ **224 Calories**
- Dinner: Roasted Lemon Swordfish ~ **280 Calories**
- Sides/Snacks: Halloumi and Cheddar Sticks ~ **361 Calories**

Total Calorie Count: 1260 Calories

Meal Plan 79

- Breakfast: Hash Brown Vegetable Breakfast Casserole ~ **363 Calories**
- Lunch: Parmesan Chicken Meatballs ~ **363 Calories**
- Dinner: Pancetta, Beef and Broccoli Bake ~ **361 Calories**
- Sides/Snacks: Cheesy Mashed Sweet Potato Cakes ~ **126 Calories**

Total Calorie Count: 1213 Calories

Meal Plan 80

- Breakfast: Ham and Egg Casserole ~ **310 Calories**
- Lunch: Cauliflower Beef and Casserole ~ **391 Calories**
- Dinner: Saucy Chicken Legs with Vegetables ~ **264 Calories**
- Sides/Snacks: Cashew and Carrot Muffins ~ **245 Calories**

Total Calorie Count: 1210 Calories

Meal Plan 81

- Breakfast: Eggplant and Tomato Gratin ~ **213 Calories**
- Lunch: Broccoli and Carrot Turkey Bake ~ **385 Calories**
- Dinner: Tandoori Chicken ~ **290 Calories**
- Sides/Snacks: Leafy Greens and Cheddar Quesadillas ~ **320 Calories**

Total Calorie Count: 1208 Calories

Meal Plan 82

- Breakfast: Crespelle al Mascarpone ~ **369 Calories**
- Lunch: Braised Chicken with Tomato and Garlic ~ **353 Calories**
- Dinner: Turmeric Chicken Wings with Ginger Sauce ~ **253 Calories**
- Sides/Snacks: Pesto Veggie Pinwheels ~ **241 Calories**

Total Calorie Count: 1218 Calories

Meal Plan 83

- Breakfast: Creamy Oatmeal ~ **368 Calories**
- Lunch: Pancetta and Cheese Stuffed Chicken ~ **336 Calories**
- Dinner: grilled Swordfish with Lemon, Capers, and Olives ~ **270 Calories**
- Sides/Snacks: Pork Beef Bean Nachos ~ **269 Calories**

Total Calorie Count: 1243 Calories

Meal Plan 84

- Breakfast: Asparagus and Crabmeat Frittata ~ **340 Calories**
- Lunch: Olive Capers Chicken ~ **433 Calories**
- Dinner: Feta and Mozzarella Chicken ~ **343 Calories**
- Sides/Snacks: Vegan Rice Pudding ~ **148 Calories**

Total Calorie Count: 1264 Calories

Meal Plan 85

- Breakfast: Apple Quinoa Muffins ~ **200 Calories**
- Lunch: Oaxacan Chicken ~ **343 Calories**
- Dinner: Sriracha Tuna Kabobs ~ **467 Calories**
- Sides/Snacks: Lentil Sweet Bars ~ **214 Calories**

Total Calorie Count: 1224 Calories

Meal Plan 86

- Breakfast: Avocado and Tempeh Tacos ~ **219 Calories**
- Lunch: Marinated Fried Chicken ~ **389 Calories**
- Dinner: Coconut Chicken and Mushrooms ~ **300 Calories**
- Sides/Snacks: Spinach Chips with Avocado Hummus ~ **348 Calories**

Total Calorie Count: 1256 Calories

Meal Plan 87

- Breakfast: Bacon and Cheese Cloud Eggs ~ **287 Calories**
- Lunch: Herby Veggies and Chicken Cacciatore ~ **391 Calories**
- Dinner: Baked Cheesy Chicken Tenders ~ **312 Calories**
- Sides/Snacks: Mini Teriyaki Turkey Sandwiches ~ **252 Calories**

Total Calorie Count: 1242 Calories

Meal Plan 88

- Breakfast: Beef Breakfast Casserole ~ **379 Calories**
- Lunch: Beef Cheese and Egg Casserole ~ **400 Calories**
- Dinner: Mushroom and Beef Stir-Fry ~ **249 Calories**
- Sides/Snacks: Grilled Fruit ~ **260 Calories**

Total Calorie Count: 1288 Calories

Meal Plan 89

- Breakfast: Arugula Pesto Egg Scramble ~ **392 Calories**
- Lunch: Honey Spiced Cajun Chicken ~ **312 Calories**
- Dinner: Baked Chicken Wrapped in Smoked Salmon ~ **356 Calories**
- Sides/Snacks: Raspberry and Goat Cheese Focaccia Bites ~ **171 Calories**

Total Calorie Count: 1231 Calories

Meal Plan 90

- Breakfast: Cauliflower-Based Waffles ~ **336 Calories**

- Lunch: BBQ Pulled Chicken ~ **410 Calories**
- Dinner: Scallops and Rosemary Potatoes ~ **211 Calories**
- Sides/Snacks: Salmon Apple Salad Sandwich ~ **315 Calories**

Total Calorie Count: 1272 Calories

Meal Plan 91

- Breakfast: Cheddar and Chive Souffles ~ **288 Calories**
- Lunch: Ham and Cheese Stuffed Chicken ~ **343 Calories**
- Dinner: Spiced Winter Pork Roast ~ **288 Calories**
- Sides/Snacks: Wonton Soup ~ **320 Calories**

Total Calorie Count: 1239 Calories

Meal Plan 92

- Breakfast: Coconut Crepes with Vanilla Cream ~ **326 Calories**
- Lunch: BBQ Beef Sliders ~ **400 Calories**
- Dinner: Bacon-Topped Turkey Meatloaf ~ **326 Calories**
- Sides/Snacks: Toasted Orzo Pasta ~ **160 Calories**

Total Calorie Count: 1212 Calories

Meal Plan 93

- Breakfast: Egg Avocado Toast ~ **236 Calories**
- Lunch: Feta and Kale Chicken Bake ~ **359 Calories**
- Dinner: Stuffed Chicken Breasts ~ **361 Calories**
- Sides/Snacks: Sausage and Pesto Salad with Cheese ~ **311 Calories**

Total Calorie Count: 1267 Calories

Meal Plan 94

- Breakfast: Cottage Pancakes ~ **345 Calories**
- Lunch: Baked Chicken Nuggets ~ **373 Calories**
- Dinner: Almond-Crusted Zucchini Chicken Stacks ~ **308 Calories**
- Sides/Snacks: Quinoa and Scallops Salad ~ **221 Calories**

Total Calorie Count: 1247 Calories

CONCLUSION

When you boil the fad diet, macronutrients, and meal plan down to its simplest form, weight loss can be boiled down to one basic rule: Consume less calories than you expend each day. This is the main part of the 1,200-calorie diet, which is an eating pattern that is supposed to assist boost weight reduction by restricting your intake to no more than 1,200 calories per day.

This is the main part of the 1,200-calorie diet. Whether you do this by filling up on meals that are low in calories or by increasing the amount of time you spend exercising, there is no denying that reducing the total number of calories you consume each day will assist in the process of weight loss.

The strategy does not include any risks and is created to make it simpler for you to lose weight and, more significantly, to maintain your weight loss over an extended period of time. This is not a diet plan that will put you in a situation where you can regain the weight that you lost on the program once you stop following it and start eating normally again. It is more of a long-term diet plan that will not only help you lose the weight you don't want in a reasonable amount of time but will also allow you to keep it off.

The New Dr. Nowzaradan Diet Plan and Cookbook for Beginners

A Healthy Collection of Succulent
1200-Calorie Recipes and Affordable Meal Plans
for Every Age and Gender

Juan Smith

INTRODUCTION

There is more to losing weight than finding a surgeon, being approved for surgery, and, finally, having the procedure. For many, developing positive habits and breaking away from destructive old habits can be very challenging. You will need to cope with stress and daily struggles without reaching for food, but making these changes does get easier over time.

If you've never exercised before, you may be pleasantly surprised to find that you enjoy the activity and the stress relief that comes along with it. Taking one hour a day out of your busy life to exercise may provide multiple benefits.

It isn't enough to limit the number of calories you take in daily. Many aspects of your life will need to change: how you think about food, how you cook, and even how you dress will change during the weight loss process.

Finding support from friends, family, and even fellow weight loss surgery patients will be instrumental in your success. Finding someone willing to listen or someone who understands what you are going through is an invaluable part of the process.

It is safe to say that your life will be dramatically different after your surgery, mostly in very positive ways. As your body shrinks, you will feel better, look better, have more energy, and be a much healthier person than you ever imagined. If you doubt how much better you will feel after your weight loss, pick up a sack of potatoes at the grocery store the next time you are shopping and see how long it takes before your arms get tired. You will be losing that weight many times, and no longer carrying those extra pounds with every step will feel fantastic.

None of these changes will happen without hard work, but the rewards are well worth the effort. Fitting into smaller sizes, improving your self-confidence, and going up a flight of stairs or out for a walk without being exhausted will be just a few of the rewards of your weight loss. While weight loss surgery isn't going to make all of your troubles go away, it may make health problems such as high blood pressure, sleep apnea, and type 2 diabetes disappear.

Things you may have avoided in the past will become far more accessible as you lose weight. Imagine going to a movie and fitting comfortably into the movie seat or taking a vacation to a sunny beach and wearing a bathing suit without feeling self-conscious. As you work toward your weight loss goal, you will be meeting other purposes, such as being able to run and play with your children or walking from one actual end of the mall to the other without a second thought.

CHAPTER 1. THE 1200-CALORIE DIET

It is a diet plan that guarantees getting rid of the most dangerous health problems patients face. Now, for the first time, all your food will be cooked according to the 1200-calorie plan. Its ingredients include only a few simple, interesting, and healthy ingredients: replace highly addictive and unhealthy food; avoid drinking, smoking, or chewing tobacco before and after surgery. Ditch the usual fat and sugar-filled foods and replace them with foods that are not only healthy but are also very delicious.

Why go for a 1200-calorie recipe now?

Avoid unnecessary, expensive obesity surgery.

The kindest, healthiest, and the only permanent solution is here, that too for half the price!

You can eat 1200-calorie per day, even after your weight loss surgery.

Live with your loved ones without being an outsider.

You can cook delicious and nutritious foods by yourself.

You can have complete peace of mind that YOUR diet will be safe and healthy.

Cook delicious, healthy, and easy-to-make foods.

The other diets are not just expensive and dangerous; they are detrimental to the patient's health. The diet advertised on the television will not only deprive you of all rights, but it will also cause you significant health problems.

The main ingredient of the 1200-calorie diet is a special shake which is composed of:

- Low in fat, oil, and sugar.
- Very low in cholesterol.
- Low in salt.
- Very high in protein.

High in calcium, potassium, and magnesium - which typically play an important role in reducing blood pressure, body fat, and cholesterol.

Since the ingredients work in harmony to provide incredible health benefits, you will see the following results:

- No more artificial colors and flavors. Improve your appearance, general health, and happiness.
- It can be done at home.
- You can easily make the diet yourself.
- It will work only if you follow it.

The 1200-calorie diet is an individual diet plan that has been designed to not just help you lose weight but also perform an excellent weight loss surgery alternative. It promotes a diet with less than 1200-calorie without any side effects.

Doctors recommend their overweight and obese patients create and follow their 1200-calorie diet. Since it is a self-made diet, you will also be in total control of your diet.

However, the 1200-calorie diet plan is not for those who want to lose more than a few pounds and then give up. It is for patients who wish to remove excess weight and all its future risks permanently.

CHAPTER 2. FOLLOWING THE 1200-CALORIE DIET

There are no tagged in the 1200-calorie diet plan. The basic strategy is straightforward and straightforward. Your entire caloric consumption must be less than or equal to 1,200 calories per day in order to stay within the diet plan's restrictions. Muffin Top, Lose It, Cron-o-meter, FatSecret, and SparkPeople are just a few of the apps that may help you actually keep track of how many calories you eat.

Because the diet is more essential for weight loss than for weight maintenance, it is critical that you set a weight goal for yourself and take care to avoid losing muscle mass when losing weight. You have the option of raising your calorie intake after you have reached your goal weight; nevertheless, you should maintain your healthy eating habits to keep your weight under control.

It is my responsibility to advise you that if you choose to follow this diet, you will likely consume less calories per day than you may think if you are accustomed to eating a lot of calories. This is due to the fact that your body may be compelled to feel hunger while taking the supplement. This possible health danger is another reason why you should see a doctor before starting a diet.

To counteract the sensations of hunger that are prevalent while dieting, it is important to eat meals that are both healthy and will keep you feeling full for a long amount of time. Eat a little quantity of healthy and satiating meals to satisfy your appetite.

Watermelon, salad, grapefruit, vegetables, fruits with a high water content, and other healthy meals are just a few of the numerous possibilities available.

The plan allows you to have snacks in between each of your three meals, as well as eating six times per day with snacks in between those meals. It will also allow you to participate in less intense activity, which will help you attain your weight reduction goal.

Check to determine whether your 1200-calorie meal plan includes a healthy and well-balanced selection of meals when following this diet plan. This is necessary to ensure that you do not have any nutritional deficiencies and that you drink enough water on a regular basis to stay hydrated and maintain good hunger control.

Things to Keep in Mind

Cereals: Whole wheat, millet, ragi, amaranth, oats, and barley are high-fiber, multi-nutrient grains to include in your diet. Use these different flours to add diversity to your meals. Breakfast would be better served with a bowl of multigrain cereal rather than refined, sugar-coated, rose-flavored cereal. It doesn't mean you shouldn't eat refined grains; rather, it implies you should only do so on rare occasions.

Polished rice, which includes Idlu, Doa, and Uttaram, is one refined grain that is ideal for picking as a healthy diet alternative. To prepare a high-fiber salad, replace it for arugula and top white bread with a significant number of raw veggies.

These are essential for our bodies' growth, repair, and maintenance, as well as our hormones, blood, and immune systems. Eating meals with at least one type of protein may help you consume less cereal. Dal, besan, ou, raneer, and shee are all examples of vegetable sources of protein. Choose lower calorie alternatives to paneer and cheese, which are both rich in fat calories. In compared to beef, organ meats, and pig, chicken, fish, and eggs are the healthiest non-vegetarian protein sources, in that order.

Fats: They are very necessary and should not be excluded from your diet. You can control how many calories you consume by controlling how much you eat, and you can do so without sacrificing taste or losing any of the health advantages that come with it.

Even while refined vegetable oils are healthful, you should not restrict yourself to just one kind. Ghee and clarified butter contain the same amount of calories and fat as vegetable oil, however clarified butter and ghee have a greater saturated fat content. 1tr/day is ok.

Vegetables: Finally, a cuisine that will satiate your hunger to the utmost degree possible. Hungry? For a warm and salty snack, eat a carrot, boil your veggies, combine them, and create a soup out of them, or juice your vegetables for a cold and refreshing drink. 3 serving each day is recommended.

A leafy vegetable serving weighs 150 grams, whereas any other vegetable serving weighs 100 grams.

However, you have no need to be concerned about your weight since you are free to eat as much as you want. The satsh onlu is reserved for root and tuber delicacies like potato, sweet potato, and others.

They are actually and really capable of providing you with the same amount of calories as their part of a meal.

Fruit: These create a delicious dessert. Take two servings of 100-150 grams each of banana and mango (when in season).

Milk and milk-based products: Each meal should include some kind of milk, such as skim milk, fat-free dahi, or skim milk ricotta. You might also use ricotta made from skim milk. In fact, a late-night need for anything sweet may be satisfied with a fat-free milk ruddling. Regardless of how many calories you wish to eat, be sure you are not depriving yourself of the taste of food in any manner. Eat seasonally, try new cuisines, and consume your meals in their whole. Maintaining your health will not actually and only help you maintain your present weight, but will also give you a radiant complexion and lots of energy.

CHAPTER 3. CAN IT HELP YOU LOSE WEIGHT?

The development of a calorie deficit is necessary for effective weight loss. Some medical professionals say that cutting caloric intake by 500 to 750 calories per day is the most efficient strategy to lose weight in the short term. Adults in another research were assigned to one of three weight-loss programs: 500 calories per day, 1,200–1,500 calories per day, or 1,500–1800 calories per day. Those who maintained a diet of 1,200–1,500 calories per day for a year lost an average of an actual 15 pounds (6.8 kg). On the other hand, 23 percent of the 4,588 persons who were enrolled in the research and were eating a 1,200-calorie diet dropped out.

While early weight reduction on a low-calorie diet like a 1,200-calorie diet is generally swift and considerable, studies have shown that it is usually followed by bigger weight gain, some of which is connected with diets that entail just minor calorie restriction.

In another study on 57 overweight or obese people, researchers found that the participants gained back 50 percent of the weight they lost over a period of 10 months, on average.

Low-calorie diets promote metabolic changes that store energy and impede weight loss, which explains why. these changes include an increase in hunger, a loss of lean body mass, and a decrease in the quantity of real calories burnt, all of which make maintaining a healthy weight more difficult in the long run.

As a result, many health professionals now propose eating patterns that employ just a slight decrease in calorie intake to facilitate weight loss while reducing the detrimental metabolic adaptations associated with low-calorie diets. These eating habits have been found to help people lose weight.

Increases the Weight Loss

The only method to effectively and really lose weight is to burn more calories throughout the day than you consume. This may be achieved by either increasing your regular physical activity or reducing the quantity of calories you eat. The majority of people may achieve a caloric deficit, which may assist in weight loss, by cutting their daily intake to only 1,200 calories. According to the actual results of a study conducted in Montreal, sticking to a low-calorie diet for a short length of time will help reduce belly fat and result in an average weight loss of 8%. Following a nutrient-dense 1,200-calorie diet may result in weekly weight loss of one to two pounds, but the exact amount of weight loss will depend on your metabolism and nutritional needs.

CHAPTER 4. BREAKFAST RECIPES

Recipe 1. Baked Beans

These beans are high in protein and fiber without any meat. If you are looking for a hearty and meatless dish, you've found it.

Serving Size: 8

Preparation Time: 30 minutes

Cooking Time: 4 hours 20 minutes

Ingredients:

- ¾ cup of dry pinto beans
- ¾ cup of dry red kidney beans
- ¾ cup of dry navy beans
- 5 cups of low-sodium vegetable stock
- 1 medium onion peeled and halved
- 1/3 cup of molasses
- 1 tablespoon of Dijon mustard
- 1 teaspoon of salt
- ½ cup of chopped canned tomatoes
- 1 tablespoon of apple cider vinegar

Directions:

- Soak beans overnight after picking and sorting.
- Preheat oven to 250°F.
- Drain beans and place in a large-sized pot with vegetable stock, then bring to a boil over high heat and simmer for 30 minutes.
- Drain and reserve stock.
- Place beans in a 2 ½ quart baking dish with onion.
- Mix remaining ingredients. Pour over beans, covering them completely, then cover dish and bake for 4 hours, checking every ½ hour and adding more reserved stock if needed.

Nutritional Information:

- Calories: 250
- Fat: 1g
- Protein: 13g
- Carbohydrates: 49g

Recipe 2. Beef and Spinach Stroganoff

I grew up actually eating a lot of beef stroganoff over egg noodles. Just by omitting the flour usually used to thicken the sauce, this recipe became low-carb. Serve this over a bed of mashed cauliflower or Shredded Cabbage Noodles, and you won't even be thinking about those egg noodles.

Serving Size: 2

Preparation Time: 10 minutes

Cooking Time: 10 minutes

Ingredients:

- 8 ounces of sirloin steak, cut into ½-inch-thick slices
- 1 teaspoon of sea salt
- 1 teaspoon of freshly ground black pepper
- 1 tablespoon of avocado oil or extra-virgin olive oil
- 1 cup of sliced white mushrooms
- ½ white onion, thinly sliced
- 2 garlic cloves, thinly sliced
- ¼ cup of low-carb dry white wine
- ½ cup of half-and-half
- ¼ cup of sour cream
- 1 teaspoon of smoked paprika, plus more for serving
- 4 cups of baby spinach
- 2 tablespoons of chopped fresh parsley

Directions:

- Season the sirloin with the salt and pepper.
- In a medium skillet, heat the oil. Add the beef slices and cook for about 5 minutes, flipping halfway through, or until they start to brown. Transfer to a plate and set aside.
- In the same medium-sized skillet, cook the mushrooms, onion, and garlic for 5 minutes, or until the onions begin to turn translucent. Add the wine and simmer for approximately about 2 minutes.
- Return the beef and any juices to the skillet and reduce the heat to medium-low. Add the half-and-half, sour cream, and paprika and simmer for 8 to 10 minutes, until the sauce has thickened, and the sirloin is fork-tender.
- Divide the spinach between two bowls and serve the beef and gravy on top. Garnish with parsley and a sprinkling of smoked paprika.

Nutritional Information:

- Calories: 245
- Fat: 11g
- Protein: 39g
- Carbohydrates: 41g

Recipe 3. Baked Mac and Cheese

This favorite comfort food is no longer a diet disaster. You can indulge your love for creamy pasta without sacrificing your weight loss goals.

Serving Size: 4

Preparation Time: 20 minutes

Cooking Time: 55 minutes

Ingredients:

- 2 cups of low-fat or fat-free ricotta cheese
- 1 ½ cups of skim milk, divided use
- 1 tablespoon of all-purpose flour
- 2 cups of elbow macaroni, cooked
- 1 ½ cups of low-fat or fat-free shredded mozzarella or Cheddar cheese
- 1 cup of dry breadcrumbs, toasted Salt and pepper, to taste

Directions:

- In a medium bowl, combine ricotta and ½ cup milk and blend until smooth.
- In a separate bowl, combine flour and ¼ cup milk, blend until smooth.
- Heat remaining milk in saucepan until steaming, add ricotta and flour combinations, whisk until smooth and thickened.
- Add pasta to milk and cheese mixture and toss.
- Pour into baking dish, top with remaining cheese and bake for 25 minutes.
- Sprinkle with breadcrumbs, bake for additional 5 minutes or until crumbs are browned.
- Add the prepared salt and pepper to taste, serve while hot.

Nutritional Information:

- Calories: 380
- Fat: 11g
- Protein: 35g
- Carbohydrates: 78g

Recipe 4. Eggplant Lasagna

Craving lasagna? Try this low-fat recipe that is hearty and filling without the fat and calories you don't want. Using eggplant instead of pasta noodles keeps the calorie content down, but increases the fiber and adds flavor.

Serving Size: 6

Preparation Time: 20 minutes

Cooking Time: 1 hour

Ingredients:

- 1 medium eggplant, cut into ¼ inch slices
- 2 tablespoons of lemon juice Cooking spray
- 2 cups of tomato sauce
- 1 can of whole tomatoes, chopped
- 2 cloves of garlic, minced
- ¼ teaspoon of red chili flakes
- 1 tablespoon of basil
- 1 tablespoon of oregano
- 1/3 cup of breadcrumbs
- ¼ cup of fat-free Parmesan cheese, grated
- 1 cup of fat-free ricotta cheese
- 1 cup of fat-free mozzarella cheese, shredded

Directions:

- Brush eggplant slices with lemon juice, place on baking sheet (after coating sheet with cooking spray). Cook until tender, approximately 10 minutes, turning after 5 minutes.
- Combine tomato sauce, chopped tomatoes, garlic, chili flakes, oregano, and basil in a bowl. Set aside.
- Combine Parmesan and breadcrumbs in a bowl. Set aside.
- Combine ricotta and mozzarella cheese in a bowl. Set aside.
- Coat 9-inch square pan with cooking spray. Begin with a layer of the sauce mixture, then the eggplant slices, then ricotta and mozzarella cheese mixture. Repeat until all ingredients are used.
- Spread bread crumb mixture over the top; bake for 45 minutes.

Nutritional Information:

- Calories: 170
- Fat: 0.5g
- Protein: 14g
- Carbohydrates: 24g

Recipe 5. Ground Pork Wonton Ravioli

Low-fat ravioli have the same great taste when wonton wrappers are used instead of pasta and are stuffed with a tasty pork and shrimp blend.

Serving Size: 6

Preparation Time: 30 minutes

Cooking Time: 30 minutes

Ingredients:

- 8 ounces of ground pork
- 4 ounces of shrimp

- 1 green onion, finely chopped
- 2 garlic cloves, minced
- 1-inch fresh ginger root, peeled and minced
- 1 egg white
- 1 teaspoon of cornstarch
- 1 teaspoon of garlic chili paste
- Juice of ¼ of a lemon
- 1 tablespoon of low-sodium soy sauce
- Pinch of salt and black pepper
- 1 tablespoon of ground shiitake mushrooms dried
- 2 drops of toasted sesame oil
- 3 large Savoy cabbage leaves, shredded fine
- 36 round wonton wrappers

Directions:

- Place all ingredients except the cabbage and wrappers into a food processor and grind to form a paste.
- Fold in shredded cabbage.
- Place a wonton wrapper on cutting board or counter. Put 1 tablespoon of prepared filling in the center of wonton.
- Brush cold water on edges of the wonton and cover with a second wonton. Carefully remove all air and seal edges.
- Poach in water or stock until they float.

Nutritional Information:

- Calories: 130
- Fat: 3g
- Protein: 5g
- Carbohydrates: 6g

Recipe 6. Herb-Roasted Eggplant

Roasted eggplant is simple to prepare and so versatile. The key to this dish is to ensure that the fresh herbs and olive oil are liberally coated over every inch of the fleshy side of the eggplant. Eat it alone or topped with your favorite spaghetti sauce and some cheese.

Serving Size: 4

Preparation Time: 20 minutes

Cooking Time: 1 hour 10 minutes

Ingredients:

- 2 eggplants
- Salt
- 4 tablespoons of extra-virgin olive oil
- 4 teaspoons of chopped garlic
- 2 teaspoons of chopped fresh rosemary
- 2 teaspoons of chopped fresh thyme
- Freshly ground black pepper

Directions:

- Preheat the oven to 400°F. Line a baking sheet with parchment paper.
- Cut the eggplants in half lengthwise. Cut deep slits in a diamond pattern on the cut side of each eggplant half. Sprinkle with salt and let the eggplant sit for 30 minutes until it releases any excess liquid. Squeeze the eggplant to actually remove as much liquid as possible.
- Drizzle the cut side of the pieces of eggplants with the prepared olive oil and season with garlic, rosemary, thyme, salt, and pepper, making sure that the seasonings get into the deep crevices.
- Place each half of the eggplant, cut-side down, on the prepared baking sheet and bake for approximately about 50 to 60 minutes, or until they are tender.

Nutritional Information:

- Calories: 204
- Fat: 9.2g
- Protein: 1.1g
- Carbohydrates: 15.7g

Recipe 7. Potato Pancakes

Potato pancakes don't have to be smothered in oil to be crispy. In this recipe the combination of a small amount of butter and a nonstick pan are enough to produce a tasty pancake without frying.

Serving Size: 4

Preparation Time: 10 minutes

Cooking Time: 15 minutes

Ingredients:

- 1 large potato, peeled and shredded
- ¼ yellow onion, grated
- 1 ounce of egg substitute Pinch nutmeg
- 2 tablespoons of flour
- 1 tablespoon of fat-free Parmesan cheese
- 1 tablespoon of dried chives
- 1 tablespoon of butter, melted
- Fresh ground black pepper

Directions:

- In a bowl, combine all ingredients to form a batter.
- Spray a nonstick skillet with cooking spray and heat over medium heat.

- Ladle ¼ cup of batter onto pan and cook until pancake is golden brown, approximately minutes, then flip and continue to cook about 4 more minutes.
- Serve with applesauce and low-fat sour cream.

Nutritional Information:

- Calories: 190
- Fat: 3.5g
- Protein: 3g
- Carbohydrates: 12g

Recipe 8. Seared Tuna with White Bean Salad

Love tuna but tired of tuna salad? Try this seared tuna for a new way to eat this diet-friendly fish.

Serving Size: 2

Preparation Time: 30 minutes

Cooking Time: 1 hour

Ingredients:

- 2 (4-ounce) fresh ahi tuna steaks
- 1 tablespoon of prepared basil pesto
- 1 teaspoon of canola oil
- Salt and pepper, to taste
- ½ red bell pepper, seeded and julienned
- ½ green bell pepper, seeded and julienned
- ¼ red onion, thinly julienned
- ¼ cup of shredded carrot
- ¼ cup of Kalamata olives
- ½ cup of plum tomatoes, seeded and diced
- ½ cup of prepared low-fat balsamic vinaigrette
- ½ cup of fresh basil leaves, torn

Directions:

- Rub tuna with pesto and let sit for 1 hour.
- Season tuna with salt and pepper, then place in hot oil and cook 1½ to 2 minutes per side for medium rare. Remove from pan and place on plate.
- Combine all remaining ingredients (except basil) and toss in hot pan for 30–45 seconds to heat through, then add basil and pour over tuna.

Nutritional Information:

- Calories: 390
- Fat: 15g
- Protein: 36g
- Carbohydrates: 25g

Recipe 9. Stewed Mussels and Clams with Tomatoes and Olives

This dish is both easy and quick, but has the flavor of a dish that took hours to prepare.

Serving Size: 4

Preparation Time: 10 minutes

Cooking Time: 20 minutes

Ingredients:

- ¾ pound of fresh mussels, shell on
- ¾ pound of fresh clams, shell on
- 2 tablespoons of canola oil
- 3 cloves of garlic, smashed
- ¼ cup of white wine
- 1 tablespoon of lemon juice
- ½ cup of black olives, pitted
- 1 cup of fresh plum tomatoes, diced
- 1 cup of low-sodium vegetable or seafood stock
- Zest of 1 lemon
- 1/8 teaspoon of red chili flakes
- 5 tablespoons of fresh parsley, chopped

Directions:

- Soak clams and mussels in cold running water to clean. Discard any open or broken shells.
- Heat oil in the prepared sauté pan over medium heat, add garlic and chili flakes.
- Steam for 5 to 8 minutes until shellfish are open.
- Pour into bowl, add parsley, and serve with crusty bread.

Nutritional Information:

- Calories: 250
- Fat: 12g
- Protein: 23g
- Carbohydrates: 10mg

Recipe 10. Tomato-Basil Poached Cod

Sweet tomatoes, fragrant basil, and spicy garlic infuse this mild fish with flavor. Serve with Mediterranean Zucchini Hummus, assorted raw vegetables, and the rest of the bottle of white wine for a refreshing summer supper.

Serving Size: 4

Preparation Time: 10 minutes

Cooking Time: 4 hours 20 minutes

Ingredients:

- ¼ cup of extra-virgin olive oil
- 1 tablespoon of minced garlic
- 1-pound of grape tomatoes halved
- ¼ cup of dry white wine
- Zest and juice of 1 lemon
- 1 cup of minced fresh basil
- 4 (6-ounce) cod fillets
- Sea salt
- Freshly ground black pepper

Directions:

- Oil and heat the pan. Add the garlic, tomatoes, and cook until the tomatoes soften.
- Add the white wine. Simmer for 2 minutes to cook off some of the alcohol.
- Flip, and cook until the cod flakes easily with a fork.

Nutritional Information:

- Calories: 252
- Fat: 4g
- Protein: 27.8g
- Carbohydrates: 31g

CHAPTER 5. LUNCH RECIPES

Recipe 11. Asian Flank Steak with Edamame and Soba

If you enjoy the flavors of Asia, this dish includes sesame, teriyaki, and chili paste.

Serving Size: 4

Preparation Time: 10 minutes

Cooking Time: 30 minutes

Ingredients:

- ¼ pound of soba noodles
- 1 teaspoon of canola oil
- 4 ounces of trimmed beef flank steak, sliced thinly across grain
- 1 ½ tablespoons of lime juice
- 1 ½ tablespoons of low-sodium teriyaki sauce
- 1 ½ tablespoons of garlic and chili paste
- ½ teaspoon of cornstarch
- ½ teaspoon of sesame oil
- ½ red pepper, julienned
- 2 green onions, diagonally cut
- 8 snow peas, cut into strips
- ¼ cup of shredded carrot
- 1 cup of frozen edamame, thawed
- 1 tablespoon of fresh minced ginger root
- ¼ cup of cilantro

Directions:

- Cook soba noodles according to package directions.
- While noodles are cooking, heat sauté pan with oil. Add steak to pan and cook until just done (approximately 2 minutes).
- Whisk lime juice, teriyaki, chili paste, ginger root, cornstarch, and sesame oil together to form a sauce.
- Add red pepper, onions, snow peas, and carrot to pan and add prepared sauce. Cook 2 minutes.
- Add beef and juices from plate back into pan. Add edamame, toss to heat through.
- Add soba noodles and toss. Garnish with fresh cilantro, and serve.

Nutritional Information:

- Carbohydrates: 31g
- Calories: 230
- Protein: 17g
- Fat: 4g

Recipe 12. Baked Vegetables

Simple healthy.

Serving Size: 8

Preparation Time: 5 minutes

Cooking Time: 25 minutes

Ingredients:

- 1 onion (sliced) into wedges
- 6 carrots (sliced)
- 4 potatoes (sliced)
- 6 chicken breast fillets (sliced) into cubes
- 1 teaspoon of thyme
- Pepper to taste
- ½ cup of water

Directions:

- Preheat your oven to 400°F.
- Toss onion, carrots and potatoes in a baking pan.
- Arrange chicken on top.
- In a bowl, combine thyme, pepper and water, add to the chicken and bake for 1 hour.
- Transfer to food container and refrigerate for up to 2 days.
- Reheat before serving.

Nutritional Information:

- Calories: 240
- Cholesterol: 13mg
- Carbohydrate: 25g
- Fat: 3.5g

Recipe 13. Buffalo Wings

Buffalo wings don't have to be greasy and deep fried to be tasty.

Serving Size: 4

Preparation Time: 20 minutes

Cooking Time: 50 minutes

Ingredients:

- 12 jumbo chicken wings, skin removed
- 1 tablespoon of black peppercorns
- 1 medium onion
- 1 stalk of celery
- 1 head of garlic, halved
- 1 batch Hot and Spicy Marinade

- 2 tablespoons of Creole seasoning or spicy rub

Directions:

- Place chicken wings in a heavy deep pot and add peppercorns, onions, celery, and garlic; cook for 12 minutes.
- Remove chicken from water and cool.
- Coat in Hot and Spicy Marinade and let sit overnight.
- Preheat oven to 350°F.
- Spray sheet pan with nonstick spray and lay wings in a single layer on pan, season with Creole and bake for 12 minutes. Serve with the prepared celery sticks and low-fat blue cheese dressing.

Nutritional Information:

- Calories: 230
- Fat: 5g
- Protein: 21g
- Carbohydrates: 12g

Recipe 14. Curried Chicken Meatballs with Rice

If you like curry, these chicken meatballs are a real treat. Packed with the protein you need, these meatballs also have the flavor you crave.

Serving Size: 4

Preparation Time: 10 minutes

Cooking Time: 20 minutes

Ingredients:

- 1 pound of lean ground chicken
- ½ cup of yellow onion, minced
- ¼ cup of cilantro, chopped
- 3 tablespoons of low-fat plain yogurt
- 3 tablespoons of flour
- ¼ teaspoon of cumin
- ¼ teaspoon of turmeric
- ¼ teaspoon of ground coriander
- ¼ teaspoon of garam masala
- 1 small serrano chili, seeded and diced
- 2 cloves of garlic, minced
- ¼ cup of egg substitute
- ½ recipe Coconut Curry Sauce

Directions:

- Combine all ingredients and mix well.
- Place meatballs on sprayed sheet pan and bake for 7 minutes.
- Place curry sauce in saucepan over medium heat and bring to a simmer.
- Coat cooked meatballs with curry sauce and serve over rice.

Nutritional Information:

- Calories: 210
- Fat: 10g
- Protein: 22g
- Carbohydrates: 9g

Recipe 15. Green Bean Casserole

This family favorite doesn't need fried onions to taste great. Breadcrumbs and fresh onions give this casserole great flavor without frying.

Serving Size: 8

Preparation Time: 15 minutes

Cooking Time: 25 minutes

Ingredients:

- ½ yellow onion, sliced thin
- 2 tablespoons of butter
- 1 cup of breadcrumbs
- ½ cup of low-fat Parmesan cheese
- 1 cup of low-fat or fat-free cream of mushroom soup
- ½ cup of skim milk
- 1 teaspoon of soy sauce
- Fresh ground black pepper
- 4 cups of cut green beans, frozen and thawed
- 1 tablespoon of dry thyme

Directions:

- Sauté onions in butter and add breadcrumbs and Parmesan.
- Cover with breadcrumbs and onion mixture and bake for 20–25 minutes.

Nutritional Information:

- Calories: 350
- Fat: 6g
- Protein: 6g
- Carbohydrates: 20g

Recipe 16. Nut-Crusted Chicken Breasts

It tastes like fried chicken, only it is low in fat and doesn't go anywhere near a fryer.

Serving Size: 4

Preparation Time: 25 minutes

Cooking Time: 20 minutes

Ingredients:

- 2 boneless, skinless chicken breasts, lightly pounded to even thickness
- ¼ cup of flour
- 3 ounces of liquid egg replacement
- Salt and pepper, to taste
- ¼ teaspoon of cinnamon
- ¼ teaspoon of dry thyme
- ¼ teaspoon of dry mustard
- 1/8 teaspoon of cayenne
- ½ cup of very finely chopped pistachios, walnuts, almonds, or pecans
- 2 tablespoons of canola oil
- 4 tablespoons of maple syrup
- 1 tablespoon of Dijon mustard

Directions:

- Lightly dust chicken in flour and coat in beaten egg replacement.
- In a medium bowl, combine salt and pepper, cinnamon, thyme, dry mustard, and cayenne with the chopped nuts.
- Dredge (dip) chicken into nut mixture and press to completely cover the chicken.
- Place oil in nonstick pan and heat over medium heat.
- Place chicken in pan and cook until nuts brown (2–3 minutes), flip and cook for 2–3 minutes on second side, then place chicken in oven for 5–7 minutes.
- Pour over chicken for the last 2 minutes in the oven.

Nutritional Information:

- Calories: 320
- Fat: 16g
- Protein: 20g
- Fiber: 2g

Recipe 17. Roast Pork Loin with Rosemary and Garlic

This pork loin is tasty enough to be served at a dinner party, but healthy enough to make an actual regular appearance on your dinner table.

Serving Size: 8

Preparation Time: 22 minutes

Cooking Time: 45 minutes

Ingredients:

- 3 tablespoons of chopped rosemary
- 4 cloves of garlic, minced
- 1 teaspoon of kosher salt, divided
- ½ teaspoon of black pepper
- 1 (2-pound) boneless center-cut pork loin roast, visible fat trimmed
- 4 teaspoons of extra-virgin olive oil, divided

Directions:

- In a small bowl, combine rosemary, garlic, salt, and pepper.
- Mix the pork with the rosemary mixture on the meat, bake for 30 minutes.
- Serve.

Nutritional Information:

- Calories: 290
- Fat: 18g
- Protein: 30g
- Carbohydrates: 1g

Recipe 18. Rosemary Braised Chicken with Mushroom Sauce

The word "sauce" should set off warning bells for dieters everywhere. Sauces are usually fatty, loaded with salt, or have enough calories to make a meal by themselves.

Serving Size: 4

Preparation Time: 15 minutes

Cooking Time: 30 minutes

Ingredients:

- 1 pound of boneless skinless chicken thighs
- 2 tablespoons of canola oil
- 2 slices of turkey bacon or turkey prosciutto
- 1 small shallot, diced
- ¼ cup of yellow onion, diced
- 1 clove of garlic, crushed
- 3 sprigs of fresh rosemary
- 3 ounces of fresh cremini mushrooms, quartered
- 1 portobello mushroom cap, halved and sliced
- 1 teaspoon of flour
- 1 cup of low-sodium vegetable stock
- ½ cup of red wine
- Salt and pepper, to taste

Directions:

- Lightly coat chicken with oil, place in deep-sided skillet over medium heat, and brown on all sides (approximately 5 minutes per side).

- Add bacon, shallots, onions, garlic, rosemary, and mushrooms, and sauté for 10 minutes.
- Add flour, stock, and red wine; cover and reduce liquid by half until thick and chicken is cooked (approximately 10 minutes).

Nutritional Information:

- Calories: 380
- Fat: 21g
- Protein: 33g
- Carbohydrates: 9g

Recipe 19. Steak Fajitas

This recipe is flavorful, the steak is super moist, and there is no added fat.

Serving Size: 8

Preparation Time: 5 minutes

Cooking Time: 25 minutes

Ingredients:

- 1 onion cut into strips
- 1 green bell cut into strips
- ½ teaspoon of thyme
- ½ teaspoon of mustard powder
- 1 teaspoon of black pepper
- 1 teaspoon of cumin
- 2 teaspoons of rosemary (dried)
- 2 teaspoons of chili powder
- 2 packets of natural sweetener
- 1 tablespoon of paprika
- 1 tablespoon of sea salt
- 1 pound of lean sirloin steak, cut into strips

Directions:

- Place the salt, paprika, sweetener, chili powder, dried rosemary, cumin, pepper, mustard powder, and dried thyme into a bowl and mix well to actually combine.
- Take out one tsp. of this mixture and reserve.
- Place a large skillet on the stove and heat to medium-high.
- Add the prepared onion and pepper to the skillet along with the spice mixture that you set to the side earlier. You need to cook the onion and peppers until they have softened up and the onions turn translucent.
- Take off heat and place in a bowl. Cover to keep warm.
- Into the same skillet, add half the seasoned steak and cook for about two minutes per side or until done to your liking. Place cooked steak onto a clean plate and cover until the rest of the steak gets done.
- Once all the steak strips are done, add everything back into the skillet and warm everything up for a few minutes. Spoon onto plates and enjoy.

Nutritional Information:

- Calories: 401
- Fat: 22.1g
- Protein: 104.7
- Carbohydrates: 6g

Recipe 20. Tuna Noodle Casserole

Craving comfort food but avoiding unwanted fat and calories? Try this version of an old favorite.

Serving Size: 6

Preparation Time: 20 minutes

Cooking Time: 40 minutes

Ingredients:

- 6 ounces of dried wide whole wheat egg noodles
- 2 teaspoons of canola oil
- ½ cup of softened, chopped sun-dried tomatoes, not oil packed
- 1 small onion, diced small
- 1 red bell pepper, diced small
- 1 clove of minced garlic
- 1 stalk of celery, diced
- 2 tablespoons of all-purpose flour
- 2 cups of skim milk
- ½ cup of fat-free mayonnaise
- 1 can of spring water — packed tuna, drained (or canned chicken)
- ½ cup of grated low-fat Swiss cheese
- 2 tablespoons of chopped fresh basil
- 1 tablespoon of lemon juice
- Salt and pepper, to taste
- 1/3 cup of toasted almonds

Directions:

- Preheat oven to 425°F.
- Cook pasta about 6 minutes, drain, rinse in cold water, and set aside.
- Heat pan and add oil and garlic. Cook vegetables and tomatoes for 3 minutes then add the milk and flour cook for 4 minutes.
- Stir in mayo, tuna, cheese, and basil.
- Season with lemon juice, salt, and pepper.
- Sprinkle with almonds and bake for 20 minutes. Let stand 5 minutes before serving.

Nutritional Information:

- Calories: 310
- Fat: 9g
- Protein: 23g
- Carbohydrates: 37g

CHAPTER 6. DINNER RECIPES

Recipe 21. African Chicken and Rice

Low-fat chicken recipes have a tendency to be dry and bland. To replace the flavor lost from fat, this recipe uses chilies, tomatoes, and chicken stock to increase the flavor and keep the chicken moist.

Serving Size: 6

Preparation Time: 20 minutes

Cooking Time: 35 minutes

Ingredients:

- ¼ teaspoon of dried thyme
- 1 cup of white rice, cooked
- 1 quart of low-sodium chicken stock
- 2 tablespoons of tomato paste
- 1 clove of garlic, crushed
- 1 cup of canned diced tomato
- 1 tablespoon of vegetable oil
- 1 medium onion, diced
- 2 tablespoons of ground dried shrimp
- ½ serrano chili, seeded and diced
- 2 pounds of boneless skinless chicken breast

Directions:

- Oil and heat the pan
- Mix thyme and garlic and rub mixture into the chicken.
- Add diced tomato, tomato paste, and onion to heated oil and cook the chicken for 3 minutes per side.
- Then add dried shrimp, stock, and chili and cook for 15 minutes.
- Serve chicken on the rice and garnish with sauce.

Nutritional Information:

- Calories: 410
- Fat: 8g
- Protein: 51g
- Carbohydrates: 32g

Recipe 22. Chicken and Veggie Unfried Rice

Craving fried rice but you know that any food that starts with the word "fried" can't be a good fit for your diet? Try this low-fat recipe that has all of the best parts of fried rice without the calories or fat you find in restaurants.

Serving Size: 4

Preparation Time: 20 minutes

Cooking Time: 20 minutes

Ingredients:

- 3 ounces of liquid egg replacement
- 2 chicken breasts, cut into thin strips
- 1 garlic clove, minced
- ¼ teaspoon of garlic chili paste
- ½ cup of frozen mixed vegetables, thawed
- ½ yellow onion, finely chopped
- ¼ cup of fresh bean sprouts
- 1 tablespoon of low-sodium soy sauce
- ½ teaspoon of sesame oil
- 2 cups of cooked brown rice, cold

Directions:

- Spray nonstick pan with spray; add liquid eggs and cook over low heat until a single sheet of cooked egg forms (like an omelet) — finish in oven if needed.
- Pull eggs out and allow to cool, then fold over and cut into strips.
- Oil and heat the pan, add garlic, chicken, and chili paste and cook 3 minutes.
- Add onion, frozen vegetables, and bean sprouts and cook another 2 minutes.
- Add rice, soy sauce, and sesame oil, toss to heat, then add in the egg strips last, tossing to combine. Serve hot.

Nutritional Information:

- Carbohydrates: 27g
- Fat: 3g
- Protein: 19g
- Calories: 220

Recipe 23. Pasta with Alfredo Sauce

This sauce is a low-fat version of a high-fat classic pasta dish.

Serving Size: 2

Preparation Time: 15 minutes

Cooking Time: 25 minutes

Ingredients:

- Nonfat cooking spray

- 2 cloves of garlic, minced
- 2 tablespoons of fat-free cream cheese
- 1 1/3 cups of skim milk
- 2 tablespoons of all-purpose flour
- 2 tablespoons of butter sprinkles (or butter substitute)
- 1 cup of fat-free or low-fat Parmesan cheese
- Black pepper, to taste
- 2 cups of cooked pasta of choice

Directions:

- Spray nonstick skillet with cooking spray. Add garlic over low heat and cook until tender.
- Add milk, cream cheese, and flour, whisking over medium heat; bring to a boil.
- Add butter sprinkles, Parmesan cheese, and black pepper, whisk until combined. Immediately add to pasta and toss to coat.

Nutritional Information:

- Calories: 440
- Fat: 1.5g
- Protein: 27g
- Carbohydrates: 60g

Recipe 24. Pork Shoulder Roast

This portion is large enough for a small dinner party. The roast will shrink by about half after cooking, leaving two to three pounds of flavorful but inexpensive pork roast.

Serving Size: 12

Preparation Time: 18 minutes

Cooking Time: 35 minutes

Ingredients:

- 2 tablespoons of fresh sage, chopped
- 2 tablespoons of fresh rosemary, picked and chopped
- 10 cloves of garlic, minced
- 1 tablespoon of fennel seeds, toasted
- 1 ½ tablespoons of kosher salt
- 1 tablespoon of black pepper
- 1 tablespoon of orange juice
- 2 cups of apple cider
- 1 pork shoulder roast, 4 to 5 pounds, tied by butcher
- 3 Granny Smith apples, cut in half and cored

Directions:

- Combine sage, rosemary, garlic, fennel, salt, pepper, orange juice, and apple cider in food processor and blend into a paste. Rub paste all over pork roast.
- Place apples in roasting pan, rest roast on top of them.
- Cover and cook for 6 hours on middle rack of oven. When internal temperature reaches 175°F and the meat shreds with a fork, remove from oven and allow to rest for 15 minutes.
- Shred meat with fork and serve.

Nutritional Information:

- Calories: 310
- Fat: 12g
- Protein: 38g
- Carbohydrates: 11g

Recipe 25. Pork Tenderloin with Cherry Sauce

Pork tenderloin is a great way to feed your family, because it is perfectly sized to make a meal for four. Tenderloin is also a very lean cut of pork, making it a great choice for your diet.

Serving Size: 4

Preparation Time: 10 minutes

Cooking Time: 28 minutes

Ingredients:

- 1 pound of pork tenderloin (not pork loin)
- ¼ teaspoon of salt
- ¼ teaspoon of freshly ground black pepper
- 2 sliced shallots
- 1 teaspoon of olive oil
- ½ cup of dried cherries
- 1 cup of low-sodium chicken stock
- 3 tablespoons of balsamic vinegar
- 1 teaspoon of tarragon
- ¼ cup of pomegranate juice

Directions:

- Lightly season the prepared pork with salt and pepper and sear in a large sauté pan.
- Oil the pan and add cherries cook for 2 minutes.
- Add the remaining of the prepared ingredients and bring to a boil. Slice pork and garnish with sauce.

Nutritional Information:

- Carbohydrates: 32g
- Protein: 26g
- Fat: 6g
- Calories: 280

CHAPTER 7. SOUP RECIPES

Recipe 26. Cheesy Cauliflower Soup

My father doesn't like vegetables, but he always asks for seconds of this soup.

Serving Size: 8

Preparation Time: 20 minutes

Cooking Time: 45 minutes

Ingredients:

- 3 tablespoons of olive oil
- ¾ cup of onions, finely chopped
- 5 cups of chicken broth
- 1 cup of water
- 1 medium cauliflower, cut into florets
- ⅛ teaspoon of rosemary
- 2 cups of cheddar cheese, shredded
- ⅛ teaspoon of thyme
- ¼ teaspoon of black pepper
- 2 tablespoons of butter, melted
- ¼ cup of whole flour

Directions:

- Oil and heat the pan; add onions and cook over medium heat until softened, about 5 minutes.
- Add broth, water, cauliflower, rosemary, thyme, and pepper. Cover; cook over low heat for approximately about 30 minutes, or until cauliflower is tender. Remove from heat.
- Using a potato masher, mash cauliflower mixture until cauliflower is broken into small pieces; return to heat.
- In a small-sized bowl, combine melted butter and flour; mix well, then add to soup, cooking over low heat and stirring until soup is thickened to desired consistency.
- Add cheese, one cup at a time, stirring until cheese is melted. Serve.

Nutritional Information:

- Calories 252
- Total Fat 14g
- Total Carbohydrate 24g
- Protein 0g

Recipe 27. Chicken and Bean Soup

This soup was love at first bite for me. I usually use veggie bacon in place of regular bacon as it becomes soft in soup.

Serving Size: 4

Preparation Time: 15 minutes

Cooking Time: 40 minutes

Ingredients:

- 1 tablespoon of olive oil
- ½ cup of onion, finely chopped
- 1 clove of garlic, finely chopped
- 1 can of chicken broth, with roasted vegetable and herb flavoring
- ½ cup of water
- 1 cup of canned great northern beans, rinsed and drained
- ¾ cup of chicken, cooked and finely chopped
- ¼ teaspoon of black pepper
- 1 strip of veggie bacon, cooked and finely crumbled

Directions:

- In a prepared medium saucepan, heat oil; add onion and garlic, cooking over low heat until softened, about 5 minutes.
- Boil water and broth in a pan.
- Add remaining ingredients; cook for 30 minutes. Stir occasionally.

Nutritional Information:

- Calories 225.7
- Total Fat 5.7g
- Total Carbohydrate 39g
- Protein 4.6g

Recipe 28. Chicken Barley Soup

A nourishing, hearty soup that really leaves you satisfied. Be sure to let this soup simmer for a couple hours so the barley becomes nice and tender. This soup will be even softer the second day, as the barley will continue to soften overnight.

Serving Size: 8

Preparation Time: 20 minutes

Cooking Time: 1 hour

Ingredients:

- 1-pound of ground chicken

- 2 (14-ounce) cans chicken broth
- 1 cup of vegetable juice blend (such as V8)
- 4 cups of water
- 1 cup of carrots, peeled and thinly sliced
- ½ cup of cabbage, finely shredded
- ½ cup of green pepper, diced
- 1 cup of onion, finely chopped
- 2 cloves of garlic, minced
- 2 teaspoons of seasoned salt
- ¾ cup of barley, uncooked

Directions:

- Cook the prepared ground chicken in a large saucepan over medium heat, stirring often, until the chicken is browned and crumbly. Drain fat
- Stir in the barley as you add the broth, juice, water, carrots, cabbage, green pepper, onion, and garlic. Season with seasoned salt. Cover; simmer over low heat for 1 12 to 2 hours, or until barley is cooked; stir the mixture on occasion.

Nutritional Information:

- Calories 90
- Total Fat 3g
- Total Carbohydrate 11 g
- Protein 5g

Recipe 29. Chicken Noodle Soup

Using home cooked chicken with homemade broth will add depth of flavor to this soup. Even if you only have one cup of homemade broth to add along with canned broth it will help create that homemade flavor for this lovely "comfort" soup.

Serving Size: 8

Preparation Time: 30 minutes

Cooking Time: 1 hour 30 minutes

Ingredients:

- 1 tablespoon of olive or canola oil
- ¾ cup of onion, finely chopped
- ⅔ cup of carrots, shredded
- 4 cups of chicken broth
- 2 cups of water
- 1 tablespoon of dried celery flakes
- 1 bay leaf
- 1 cup of cooked chicken, finely chopped
- 1 tablespoon of parsley flakes
- 1 teaspoon of seasoned salt
- ¼ teaspoon of black pepper, or to taste
- 1 ½ cups of egg noodles, uncooked and broken into 3-inch pieces

Directions:

- In a large saucepan, add oil, carrots and onion then allow to cook for 5 minutes.
- Add water, bay leaf, celery flakes, broth, and chicken; cook for 1 hour, stirring occasionally.
- Stir in parsley, seasoned salt, pepper, and noodles; cover and continue cooking over low heat for 25 minutes. Remove bay leaf before serving.

Nutritional Information:

- Calories 220
- Total Fat 5g
- Total Carbohydrate 24g
- Protein 18g

Recipe 30. Cream of Broccoli Soup

If you love broccoli, this is the soup for you. Blended smooth, it goes down easy, is flavorful, and goes great with your favorite sandwich.

Serving Size: 6

Preparation Time: 15 minutes

Cooking Time: 45 minutes

Ingredients:

- 4 cups of broccoli florets
- 1 cup of onion, chopped
- 1 tablespoon of celery flakes
- 1 clove of garlic, chopped
- 1 medium potato, peeled and diced
- 1 (14-ounce) chicken broth
- 2 cups of milk
- 1 ½ cups of cheddar cheese, shredded
- ¼ teaspoon of thyme
- ½ teaspoon of salt
- ¼ teaspoon of white pepper

Directions:

- Place broccoli, onion, celery flakes, garlic, potato, and chicken broth in a medium saucepan; bring to a boil; decrease heat, cover, and simmer over low heat for thirty minutes.
- Once the veggies have been pureed, put them back into the pot and add the milk, cheese, thyme, salt, and pepper.
- Carry on heating the cheese over a low heat while tossing it often until the cheese has melted.

Nutritional Information:

- Calories 168
- Total Fat 7g
- Total Carbohydrate 15g
- Protein 5g

Recipe 31. Cream of Potato Soup

This wonderfully versatile recipe can be easily changed to accommodate your tastes. It can be enjoyed as a simple potato soup, or other ingredients can be added, such as ham, cheese, or vegetables. For a smoother soup, just put it in a blender to puree or mash lightly.

Serving Size: 6

Preparation Time: 15 minutes

Cooking Time: 45 minutes

Ingredients:

- 1 tablespoon of butter
- 1 cup of onion, finely chopped
- 3 cups of diced potatoes
- 1 cup of sharp cheddar cheese, shredded (optional)
- 3 cups of chicken broth
- ¼ teaspoon of black pepper
- ½ teaspoon of salt
- ½ teaspoon of garlic powder
- ¼ cup of whole flour
- 1 ½ cups of milk

Directions:

- Heat the butter in apan. Add the prepared onion; stir and cook until onions are softened.
- Add potatoes, chicken broth, pepper, salt, and garlic powder, plus ham if desired.
- Cover; cook over a heat of low heat until potatoes are tender and easily fall apart, about 40 minutes.
- Add cheese if desired; stir just until melted and smooth. Serve.

Nutritional Information:

- Calories 225.7
- Total Fat 5.7g
- Total Carbohydrate 39g
- Protein 4.6g

Recipe 32. Creamy Chicken Vegetable Soup

This recipe was actually given to me by a dental assistant—she often made this soup for her in-laws when they began needing soft foods. They loved it, and so will you!

Serving Size: 6

Preparation Time: 20 minutes

Cooking Time: 1 hour 45 minutes

Ingredients:

- 2 tablespoons of olive oil
- ½ cup of onions, finely chopped
- ½ cup of carrots, thinly sliced or shredded
- ½ cup of potatoes, diced
- ½ cup of green beans
- ½ cup of peas
- 1 cup of chicken, finely chopped
- 1 (14-ounce) can chicken broth
- ¼ teaspoon of black pepper
- 1 ¼ cups of milk
- 1 (10¾-ounce) can cream of celery soup
- 1 (10¾-ounce) can cream of cheddar cheese soup

Directions:

- In a large-sized saucepan, heat oil; add onions and carrots; cook for 5 minutes. Add potatoes, green beans, peas, chicken, broth, and pepper. Cover, and cook over a heat of low heat for 1½ hours, or until vegetables are soft; stir occasionally.
- Add celery soup, milk and cheddar cheese soup; stir and continue cooking until heated throughout.

Nutritional Information:

- Calories 128
- Total Fat 3.6g
- Total Carbohydrate 15.6g
- Protein 7.6g

Recipe 33. French Onion Soup

French onion soup has such great flavor yet has only a few ingredients. This soup is wonderfully easy to throw together for a quick lunch.

Serving Size: 6

Preparation Time: 30 minutes

Cooking Time: 30 minutes

Ingredients:

- ½ cup of dry red wine
- 4 cups of chicken broth
- 1 teaspoon of garlic, finely chopped
- 6 slices of French bread, 1-inch thick
- 1 tablespoon of olive oil
- 6 tablespoons of Parmesan cheese, freshly grated
- 2 cups of sweet onions, finely chopped

Directions:

- Oil and heat the pan with onions, Add wine, broth, and garlic; cover and cook for 25 minutes.
- Meanwhile, toast bread until lightly browned; place one piece of toast in bottom of individual soup bowls; sprinkle each toast with 1 tablespoon Parmesan cheese.
- Pour soup over toast to serve.

Nutritional Information:

- Calories 190
- Total Fat 9g
- Total Carbohydrate 21g
- Protein 7g

Recipe 34. Ham and Bean Soup

You can never go wrong by warming up with this classic soup on a cold day. Eating it with corn bread on the side makes for a perfect, simple, meal.

Serving Size: 8

Preparation Time: 25 minutes

Cooking Time: 5 hours

Ingredients:

- ½ (16-ounce) package navy beans
- (14-ounce) cans chicken broth
- 2 cups of water
- 1 cup of carrots, thinly sliced
- 1 cup of onion, finely chopped
- 2 cloves of garlic, sliced
- 1 (14-ounce) can diced tomatoes, with juice
- ½ teaspoon of black pepper
- 1 ½ teaspoons of seasoned salt
- 1 cup of green cabbage, finely chopped
- 1 (5-ounce) can smoked ground ham

Directions:

- Wash navy beans according to package directions.
- Bring one quart of the prepared water to a boil in a pot that is big enough to hold it. Turn off the heat, add the beans, cover, and let them rest for one hour so that they may soften up. After that, drain them.
- Add the ham, cabbage, broth, water, carrots, onion, garlic, tomatoes, pepper, seasoned salt, and seasoned salt, along with the seasoning packet. Cook the beans, covered, over a low heat for three to four hours, or until they are extremely soft. Mix it up every so often.

Nutritional Information:

- Calories 177
- Total Fat 2g
- Total Carbohydrate 26g
- Protein 14g

CHAPTER 8. SNACKS RECIPES

Recipe 35. Creamed Peas

For a softer dish yet, puree just before serving.

Serving Size: 4

Preparation Time: 10 minutes

Cooking Time: 25 minutes

Ingredients:

- ⅔ cup of chicken broth
- 2 cups of green peas
- 2 tablespoons of butter
- ⅓ cup of half-and-half
- 2 tablespoons of flour
- ¼ teaspoon of black pepper
- ¼ teaspoon of salt
- 2 tablespoons of Parmesan cheese, grated (optional)

Directions:

- In a medium saucepan, add broth and peas; bring to near boiling. Reduce heat cook for 25 minutes.
- In a small-sized bowl, combine half-and-half and flour; add to the peas mixture, cook and stir until thickened.
- Add the pepper and salt, plus Parmesan cheese if desired, stirring to combine.

Nutritional Information:

- Calories 150
- Total Fat 6.2g
- Total Carbohydrate 19g
- Protein 5.9g

Recipe 36. Creamed Spinach

This is a traditional recipe for creamed spinach—the kind you remember from days gone by.

Serving Size: 8

Preparation Time: 10 minutes

Cooking Time: 10 minutes

Ingredients:

- (10-ounce) packages frozen spinach, thawed, finely chopped
- 2 tablespoons of butter
- 1 small clove of garlic, finely chopped
- 2 tablespoons of onion, finely chopped
- Sauce:
- 2 tablespoons of butter
- ⅛ teaspoon of nutmeg
- 2 tablespoons of whole flour
- 1 cup of milk
- ¼ teaspoon of salt
- ⅛ teaspoon of black pepper

Directions:

- Oil and heat the pan; add onion and garlic; stir and cook until softened, about 5 minutes. Add spinach; stir gently to combine and transfer to a serving bowl.
- Meanwhile, in a small saucepan, melt butter over low heat; add flour, milk, salt, pepper, and nutmeg; stir until thickened to desired consistency.
- Mix sauce and spinach. Serve.

Nutritional Information:

- Calories 188
- Total Fat 9.02g
- Total Carbohydrate 11.94g
- Protein 6.66g

Recipe 37. Egg Salad Sandwich

A light and lovely classic egg salad sandwich. You can turn this into curried egg salad by adding ½ teaspoon sweet curry powder, or try adding some shredded cheese, and cooked peas.

Serving Size: 4

Preparation Time: 15 minutes

Cooking Time: 1 hour

Ingredients:

- ½ cup of mayonnaise
- 2 tablespoons of pickle relish
- 1 teaspoon of prepared mustard
- ¼ teaspoon of salt
- ¼ teaspoon of black pepper
- 8 hard-cooked eggs, peeled and chopped
- 1 tomato, peeled and sliced (optional)
- portobello mushrooms

Directions:

- In a medium-sized bowl, combine mayonnaise, relish, mustard, salt and pepper.
- Add chopped eggs; mix gently. Refrigerate to chill.
- Spoon chilled egg salad into portobello mushrooms; top with the prepared tomato slices if desired.

Nutritional Information:

- Calories 220
- Total Fat 9.5g
- Total Carbohydrate 10g
- Protein 12.8g

Recipe 38. Gelatin with Peaches and Cottage Cheese

Our family has enjoyed this cool side dish for decades. It is especially good on a warm summer day. For an even softer gelatin dish, puree the cottage cheese and peaches before folding them into the gelatin.

Serving Size: 6

Preparation Time: 15 minutes

Cooking Time: 20 minutes

Ingredients:

- 1 (.3-ounce) package cherry flavored gelatin
- 1 cup of small curd cottage cheese
- 1 cup of peaches, sliced or diced

Directions:

- Prepare gelatin according to package instructions; refrigerate to chill.
- Meanwhile, cut peach slices into bite sized pieces.
- When gelatin is almost set, fold in cottage cheese and peaches.
- Return to refrigerator and chill until firm.

Nutritional Information:

- Calories 220
- Total Fat 2g
- Total Carbohydrate 16g
- Protein 20g

Recipe 39. Ham Salad Sandwich

The smoked ham in this recipe turns a basic ham salad into a tasty sandwich.

Serving Size: 4

Preparation Time: 15 minutes

Cooking Time: 30 minutes

Ingredients:

- (5-ounce) cans ground smoked ham, drained
- 2 hard cooked eggs, finely chopped
- ½ cup of mayonnaise
- 2 tablespoons of sweet pickle relish
- ½ teaspoon of onion powder
- 1 teaspoon of prepared mustard
- ¼ teaspoon of black pepper
- ½ cup of cheddar cheese, shredded (optional)
- 4 grilled portobello mushrooms, halved

Directions:

- In a prepared small bowl, combine mayonnaise, pickle relish, onion powder, mustard and pepper; stir until well blended.
- Pour mayonnaise mixture over ham and eggs, adding cheese if desired. Mix well; refrigerate to chill.
- Spoon ham salad into portobello mushrooms to serve.

Nutritional Information:

- Calories 293
- Total Carbohydrate 5g
- Total Fat 6.5g
- Protein 14g

Recipe 40. Hot Shredded Chicken Sandwich

This family favorite is cooked in broth, while some hot shredded chicken recipes use a can of creamed soup to create a creamier sauce. If you prefer to use soup, just use half the amount of broth and leave out the seasoned salt. Either way, this is an enjoyable sandwich.

Serving Size: 8

Preparation Time: 10 minutes

Cooking Time: 15 minutes

Ingredients:

- 3 ½ cups of cooked chicken, finely chopped or 1 (28-ounce) can chicken
- 1 ¾ cups of chicken broth, divided
- ½ sleeve round buttery crackers, crushed
- 1 teaspoon of seasoned salt
- ¼ teaspoon of black pepper
- 1 (10 ¾-ounce) can low-sodium cream of mushroom soup (optional)
- 8 portobello mushrooms, halved, grilled

Directions:

- In a medium saucepan, add chicken, 1½ cups broth, cracker crumbs, seasoned salt and pepper; stir and cook over low heat.
- Continue cooking, stirring frequently, until heated throughout and chicken is moist and slightly juicy, but not so wet that it will make the mushrooms soggy; add more broth if it becomes too dry while cooking.

- Spoon hot chicken into portobello mushrooms; serve.

Nutritional Information:

- Calories 201
- Total Fat 6.5g
- Total Carbohydrate 25.1g
- Protein 32.6g

Recipe 41. Marinated Tomato Slices

A pretty looking dish, this is a simple way to enjoy the fruits of summer. Eat this with bread or rolls, if you like, so you can soak up the tasty sauce.

Serving Size: 8

Preparation Time: 20 minutes

Cooking Time: 3 hours

Ingredients:

- 4 large tomatoes
- ¼ cup of olive oil
- 1 tablespoon of lemon juice
- 1 teaspoon of sugar
- ½ teaspoon of salt
- ½ teaspoon of oregano
- 1 tablespoon of parsley

Directions:

- Peel the tomatoes and cut into ½-inch slices; layer in an oblong shallow serving dish.
- In a small bowl, combine salt, oregano, lemon juice, oil, sugar, and parsley mix well.

Nutritional Information:

- Calories 58
- Total Fat 3.7g
- Total Carbohydrate 5.9g
- Protein 0.7g

Recipe 42. Potato Salad

A traditional summer side dish, I usually put several hard-boiled eggs in it as my parents sometimes eat a small dish of potato salad as a simple lunch. I use veggie bacon because it becomes soft in salad dressing while still giving that lovely bacon taste.

Serving Size: 8

Preparation Time: 10 minutes

Cooking Time: 30 minutes

Ingredients:

- 4 medium potatoes, cooked, peeled, and diced
- 4 hard cooked eggs, peeled and chopped
- 2 pieces of veggie bacon, crisp cooked and crumbled
- 1 teaspoon of onion powder
- ½ cup of mayonnaise
- ¼ cup of Ranch dressing
- 1 ½ teaspoons of vinegar
- 2 teaspoons of sugar
- 1 teaspoon of prepared mustard
- 1 tablespoon of chives
- 1 tablespoon of Parmesan cheese, grated
- ½ teaspoon of seasoned salt
- ¼ teaspoon of black pepper

Directions:

- In a large bowl, place cooled diced potatoes, chopped eggs, and veggie bacon crumbles.
- In a medium bowl, add mayonnaise, Ranch dressing, vinegar, sugar, chives, Parmesan cheese, seasoned salt and pepper; stir until well blended.
- Pour mayonnaise dressing mixture over potato mixture; stir gently to combine; cover, refrigerate.

Nutritional Information:

- Calories 197
- Total Fat 11 g
- Total Carbohydrate 18.9 g
- Protein 5.8 g

Recipe 43. Soft Cauliflower Salad

A lovely, light soft salad.

Serving Size: 4

Preparation Time: 20 minutes

Cooking Time: 10 minutes

Ingredients:

- 3 cups of cauliflower florets
- 4 cups of water
- 1 bay leaf
- Dressing:
- ⅛ teaspoon of thyme or rosemary
- 2 tablespoons of balsamic or white wine vinegar
- ½ teaspoon of sugar
- 1 clove of garlic, finely chopped
- ⅛ teaspoon of black pepper
- ½ teaspoon of basil
- ⅓ cup of olive oil
- ½ teaspoon of oregano

Directions:

- Boil 4 cups of water; add cauliflower and bay leaf.
- Cover: cook over low heat until cauliflower is soft; drain, remove bay leaf; place cauliflower in a medium bowl and refrigerate to cool.
- Meanwhile, in a small-sized bowl, combine olive oil, garlic, vinegar, sugar, basil, oregano, thyme, and pepper, whisk until well blended.
- Drizzle dressing over cauliflower; toss gently to combine; cover and refrigerate to chill.

Nutritional Information:

- Calories 125
- Total Fat 6.7g
- Total Carbohydrate 14.4g
- Protein 4.9g

Recipe 44. Turkey Bacon Brussels Sprouts

These Turkey bacon Brussel sprouts uses the rendered fat from the Turkey bacon to add a dash of flavor to your generally bitter Brussel sprouts. To enhance the flavor consider adding a bit of Apple Cider Vinegar and topping with crispy Turkey bacon bits.

Serving Size: 4

Preparation Time: 20 minutes

Cooking Time: 1 hour 25 minutes

Ingredients:

- 1 pound of brussels sprouts, trimmed, halved
- 2 tablespoons of butter
- 2 ounces of thick-cut Turkey bacon, fried and chopped
- 2 cloves of garlic, minced
- ¼ teaspoon of salt
- ¼ teaspoon of pepper

Directions:

- Preheat the water bath to 183°F.
- Seal and place in water bath all the ingredients. Cook 1 hour.
- Set to bake until nicely roasted (about 5 minutes). Enjoy!

Nutritional Information:

- Protein 4g
- Total Fat 20.2g
- Total Carbohydrate 10.8g
- Calories 230

CHAPTER 9. MEAL PLANS

Meal Plan 1

- Breakfast: Baked Mac and Cheese ~ **380 Calories**
- Lunch: Buffalo Wings ~ **230 Calories**
- Dinner: Pasta with Alfredo Sauce ~ **440 Calories**
- Sides/Snacks: Creamed Peas ~ **150 Calories**

Total Calorie Count: 1200 Calories

Meal Plan 2

- Breakfast: Tomato-Basil Poached Cod ~ **252 Calories**
- Lunch: Green Bean Casserole ~ **350 Calories**
- Dinner: Chicken and Veggie Unfried Rice ~ **220 Calories**
- Sides/Snacks: Ham and Bean Soup + Hot Shredded Chicken Sandwich ~ **378 Calories**

Total Calorie Count: 1200 Calories

Meal Plan 3

- Breakfast: Seared Tuna with White Bean Salad ~ **390 Calories**
- Lunch: Steak Fajitas ~ **401 Calories**
- Dinner: Creamy Beef Stroganoff with Mushrooms ~ **351 Calories**
- Sides/Snacks: Marinated Tomato Slices ~ **58 Calories**

Total Calorie Count: 1200 Calories

Meal Plan 4

- Breakfast: Stewed Mussels and Clams with Tomatoes and Olives ~ **250 Calories**
- Lunch: Rosemary Braised Chicken with Mushroom Sauce ~ **380 Calories**
- Dinner: Chipotle Shredded Pork ~ **260 Calories**
- Sides/Snacks: Chicken Barley Soup + Egg Salad Sandwich ~ **310 Calories**

Total Calorie Count: 1200 Calories

Meal Plan 5

- Breakfast: Potato Pancakes ~ **190 Calories**
- Lunch: Roast Pork Loin with Rosemary and Garlic ~ **290 Calories**
- Dinner: Seared Salmon with Peppercorn Sauce ~ **280 Calories**
- Sides/Snacks: Cheesy Cauliflower Soup + Creamed Spinach ~ **440 Calories**

Total Calorie Count: 1200 Calories

Meal Plan 6

- Breakfast: Baked Beans ~ **250 Calories**
- Lunch: Nut-Crusted Chicken Breasts ~ **320 Calories**
- Dinner: Slow-Roasted Pesto Salmon ~ **282 Calories**
- Sides/Snacks: Creamy Chicken Vegetable Soup + Gelatin with Peaches and Cottage Cheese ~ **348 Calories**

Total Calorie Count: 1200 Calories

Meal Plan 7

- Breakfast: Ground Pork Wonton Ravioli ~ **130 Calories**
- Lunch: Curried Chicken Meatballs with Rice ~ **210 Calories**
- Dinner: Ranch-Seasoned Crispy Chicken Tenders ~ **462 Calories**
- Sides/Snacks: Cream of Broccoli Soup + Turkey Bacon Brussels Sprouts ~ **398 Calories**

Total Calorie Count: 1200 Calories

CONCLUSION

This diet plan is without a doubt effective, and it works really well for reducing weight. Consult your physician before beginning the diet plan, and ask for a calorie reduction in order to achieve a more well-rounded diet, as well as the addition of any kind of dietary supplement that actually contains nutrients that are essential for the body.

A diet with 1,200 calories per day is considered a low-calorie diet plan since it provides less calories than your body requires on a daily basis.

Weight is not the only or even the best indicator of overall health. It is actually not necessary for a person to get healthier only by reducing their body weight. In other cases, having a lower weight might even make a person less healthy, particularly if they consume food that isn't good for them or don't get enough essential nutrients in their diet.

Also, sticking to a very low-calorie diet may be challenging, especially for those who already have trouble meeting their daily food requirements. It is essential for a person to choose a diet and exercise routine that they will be able to maintain for the rest of their life, regardless of the method of weight reduction that they pick.

A dietitian or nutritionist may assist with the creation of a customized diet and nutrition plan that includes the appropriate amount of indulgent foods and nutrient-dense foods.

HIGH PROTEIN LOW CARB DR. NOW RECIPES

Avoid eating fat and make weight loss a fact!

Juan Smith

CHAPTER 1. RECIPES

Recipe 1. Asparagus Casserole

In this recipe, we pour creamy cheese sauce and sprinkle crunchy breadcrumbs on top of fresh asparagus spears. This dish is loaded with cheesy and savory flavors that you love. Make sure that you blanch the asparagus and not overcook it so that they'd still have the bright green color that make this dish look more appetizing. Enjoy your Asparagus Casserole that serves 10!

Serving Size: 10

Preparation Time: 20 minutes

Cooking Time: 45 minutes

Total Time: 1 hour 5 minutes

Ingredients:

- 3 tablespoons of butter, divided
- ½ cup of panko breadcrumbs
- 3 pounds of asparagus spears, trimmed and sliced
- 1 tablespoon of garlic, chopped
- 2 tablespoons of all-purpose flour
- 2 cups of whole milk
- Salt to taste
- ½ cup of mozzarella cheese, shredded
- 5 ounces of cream cheese

Directions:

- Preheat your oven to 450 degrees F.
- Oil and heat the butter in a pan and add breadcrumbs and set aside.
- Prepare a bowl filled with water near the stove. Add ice cubes to the bowl. Boil a pot of water.
- Plunge the asparagus in the medium-sized bowl of ice water. Drain. Spread the blanched asparagus on a baking pan.
- Add the remaining butter. Cook the garlic for approximately about 1 minute. Mix the flour and milk and boil.
- Pour this mixture on top of the asparagus.
- Coat evenly. Bake in the oven for approximately about 15 minutes.

Nutritional Value: Calories 327 | Carbohydrates 8.3 g | Fat 16 g | Protein 12 g

Recipe 2. Bacon and Parsnip Chicken Bake

This recipe is healthy, delicious, and perfect for diet! It is a simple side dish that is ideal for a large holiday feast or a straightforward meal! Enjoy your Bacon and Parsnip Chicken Bake that serves 4!

Serving Size: 4

Preparation Time: 30 minutes

Cooking Time: 60 minutes

Total Time: 1 hour 20 minutes

Ingredients:

- 6 bacon slices cut into pieces
- 1 cup of chopped up scallions
- 1 pound of ground turkey
- 1 cup of heavy cream
- 2 tablespoons of butter
- 2 ounces of cream cheese, softened
- 1 1/4 cup of grated
- 1/2 pound of parsnips, diced
- Pepper Jack

Directions:

- Preheat oven to 390 F. Place bacon in a skillet, cook it until golden and crispy, approximately about 6 minutes, and then put aside. Melt butter and sauté parsnips in the skillet until soft and lightly brown. Cook the chicken for 8 minutes. Incorporate heavy cream, cream cheese, and two-thirds of Pepper Jack cheese into the skillet.
- Mix the ingredients on moderate heat, frequently stirring, for approximately about 7 minutes. Spread the mixture onto an oven dish, pour the heavy cream mixture over it, and sprinkle bacon and scallions. Serve.

Nutritional Value: Calories 351 | Carbohydrates 9 g | Fat 56 g | Protein 30 g

Recipe 3. Baked Mac and Cheese

The flavor is quite impressive! This recipe is very colorful and delicious. This dish is loaded with cheesy and savory flavors that you love. Enjoy your Baked Mac and Cheese that serves 4!

Serving Size: 4

Preparation Time: 20 minutes

Cooking Time: 55 minutes

Total Time: 1 hour 15 minutes

Ingredients:

- 2 cups of low-fat or fat-free ricotta cheese
- 1 ½ cups of skim milk, divided use
- 1 tablespoon of all-purpose flour
- 2 cups of elbow macaroni, cooked
- 1 ½ cups of low-fat or fat-free shredded mozzarella or Cheddar cheese
- 1 cup of dry breadcrumbs, toasted salt, and pepper, to taste

Directions:

- In a medium bowl, combine ricotta and ½ cup milk and blend until smooth.
- In a separate bowl, combine flour and ¼ cup milk, blend until smooth.
- Heat remaining milk in saucepan until steaming, add ricotta and flour combinations, whisk until smooth and thickened.
- Add pasta to milk and cheese mixture and toss.
- Bake for 25 minutes.
- Sprinkle with breadcrumbs, bake for approximately about additional 5 minutes or until crumbs are browned.
- Season with pepper and salt, serve while hot.

Nutritional Value: Calories 380 | Carbohydrates 78 g | Fat 11 g | Protein 35 g

Recipe 4. Berries and Grilled Calamari

The flavor is quite impressive! This recipe is very colorful and delicious. This dish is loaded with cheesy and savory flavors that you love. Enjoy your Berries and Grilled Calamari that serves 4!

Serving Size: 4

Preparation Time: 10 minutes

Cooking Time: 5 minutes

Total Time: 15 minutes

Ingredients:

- ¼ cup of dried cranberries
- ¼ cup of extra virgin olive oil
- ¼ cup of olive oil
- ¼ cup of sliced almonds
- ½ lemon, juiced
- ¾ cup of blueberries
- 1 ½ pounds of calamari tube, cleaned
- 1 granny smith apple, sliced thinly
- 1 tablespoon of fresh lemon juice
- 2 tablespoons of apple cider vinegar
- 6 cups of fresh spinach
- Freshly grated pepper to taste
- Sea salt to taste

Directions:

- In a large-sized bowl, make the vinaigrette by mixing well the tablespoon of lemon juice, apple cider vinegar, and extra virgin olive oil. Turn on the grill to medium fire and let the grates heat up for approximately about a minute or two.
- In a large-sized bowl, add olive oil and the calamari tube. Season calamari generously with pepper and salt. Place seasoned and oiled calamari onto heated grate and grill until cooked or opaque.
- As you wait for the calamari to cook, you can combine almonds, cranberries, blueberries, spinach, and the thinly sliced apple in a large salad bowl. Toss to mix.
- Remove cooked calamari from grill and transfer on a chopping board. Cut into ¼-inch thick rings and throw into the salad bowl.
- Drizzle with prepared vinaigrette and toss well to coat salad. Serve and enjoy!

Nutritional Value: Calories 567 | Carbohydrates 30.6 g | Fat 24.5 g |

Recipe 5. Brown Rice Pilaf with Butternut Squash

Yummy and tasty. This is a good family recipe, which will also make a nice meal for a group of friends. Enjoy this delicacy. Enjoy your Brown Rice Pilaf with Butternut Squash that serves 3!

Serving Size: 3

Preparation Time: 15 minutes

Cooking Time: 50 minutes

Total Time: 1 hour 5 minutes

Ingredients:

- Pepper to taste
- A pinch of cinnamon
- 1 teaspoon of salt
- 2 tablespoons of chopped fresh oregano
- ½ cup of chopped fennel fronds
- ½ cup of white wine
- 1 ¾ cups of water + 2 tablespoon, divided
- 1 cup of instant or parboiled brown rice
- 1 tablespoon of tomato paste
- 1 garlic clove, minced
- 1 large onion, finely chopped

- 3 tablespoons of extra virgin olive oil
- 2 pounds of butternut squash, halved

Directions:

- In a large hole grater, grate squash. On medium low fire, place a large nonstick skillet and heat oil for approximately about 2 minutes. Add garlic and onions. Sauté for approximately about 8 minutes or until lightly colored and soft.
- Add 2 tablespoon water and tomato paste. Stir well to combine and cook for approximately about 3 minutes. Add rice, mix well to coat in mixture and cook for approximately about 5 minutes while stirring frequently. If needed, add squash in batches until it has wilted so that you can cover pan.
- Add remaining water and increase fire to medium high. Add wine, cover and boil. Once boiling, lower fire to an actual simmer and cook for approximately about 20 to 25 minutes or until liquid is fully absorbed. Stir in pepper, cinnamon, salt, oregano, and fennel fronds.
- Turn off fire, cover and let it stand for approximately about 5 minutes before serving.

Nutritional Value: Calories 147 | Carbohydrates 22.1 g | Fat 5.5 g | Protein 2.3 g

Recipe 6. Cabbage and Beef Steaks

It is an easy and exciting casserole for all low-carb dieters, containing layers of meat, vegetables, and cheese. It's a nutritious meal and a good dish for potlucks. Enjoy this delicious casserole with family and friends! Enjoy your Cabbage and Beef Steaks that serves 4!

Serving Size: 4

Preparation Time: 25 minutes

Cooking Time: 55 minutes

Total Time: 1 hour 20 minutes

Ingredients:

- 1 pound of chuck steak
- 1 head canon cabbage, grated
- 1/4 cup of olive oil
- 3 tablespoons of coconut flour
- 1 teaspoon of Italian mixed herb blend
- 1 cup of bone broth

Directions:

- Ziploc the coconut flour and the steak slices. Create little mounds of cabbage in a well-greased baking dish. Serve with olive oil.
- Then, remove the meat strips made of coconut flour Shake off any excess flour, and place 3-4 beef strips on each cabbage mound. Sprinkle with the Italian herb mix and drizzle it with the olive oil remaining. Roast for approximately about 30 minutes. Take the pan off and add the broth. Bake until the meat is cooked. Serve and enjoy!

Nutritional Value: Calories 331 | Carbohydrates 4.5 g | Fat 20 g | Protein 23 g

Recipe 7. Cheesy Baked Beans

A delicious twist for a busy morning. Enjoy your Cheesy Baked Beans that serves 2!

Serving Size: 2

Preparation Time: 5 minutes

Cooking Time: 16 minutes

Total Time: 21 minutes

Ingredients:

- 4 large eggs
- 2 ounces of smoked gouda, chopped
- Everything bagel seasoning
- Kosher salt and pepper to taste

Directions:

- Break eggs into a bowl and separate them. Beat the whites until stiff.
- Mix the yolks with Everything Bagel seasoning, salt, and pepper until well combined.
- Fold in the chopped Smoked Gouda gently.
- Pour the mixture into small egg muffin tins, approximately about 1 tablespoon of mixture for each muffin.
- Place the tins into a single layer in the air fryer and bake for approximately about 14 minutes at 400 degrees.
- When they are done, carefully remove egg muffin cups with a fork and place them on a plate.
- Top with a pinch of Everything Bagel seasoning and some pepper before serving.

Nutritional Value: Calories 188 | Carbohydrates 8 g | Fat 6 g | Protein 44 g

Recipe 8. Chicken Momos

As we all know, chicken is a versatile ingredient. We've created a version of Chicken Momos that's packed with flavor and prepared using the healthy steaming technique using this wonderful quality. Enjoy your Chicken Momos that serves 12!

Serving Size: 12

Preparation Time: 25 minutes

Cooking Time: 1 hour and 35 minutes

Total Time: 2 hours

Ingredients:

- 4.2 ounces of refined flour
- ¼ teaspoon of baking powder
- 1 cup of minced chicken
- ½ tablespoon of saltwater
- 1 tablespoon of oil
- ½ cup of finely chopped onions
- ¼ teaspoon of black pepper powder
- ½ teaspoon of soya sauce
- ¼ teaspoon of vinegar
- ½ teaspoon of garlic paste
- Salt, to taste

Directions:

- Combine the chicken, onions, pepper powder, soy sauce, vinegar, garlic paste, salt, and oil in a mixing dish. Combine baking powder, flour, and saltwater.
- Separate the dough into tiny pieces and shape each into a flat disc.
- Fill each of these discs halfway with the chicken mixture and bring the sides together to seal the package. Steam all the Momos for approximately about 10 minutes in a steamer. Red chili sauce should be served with the chicken Momos.

Nutritional Value: Calories 226 | Carbohydrates 9g | Fat 3.9g | Protein 9g

Recipe 9. Cilantro-Lime Shrimp and Peppers

Here's a super-speedy meal that you can have on the table within minutes. What makes this dish sing is the freshly squeezed lime juice and cilantro at the end—so don't skimp on that! I like to serve this with my Chili and Cumin Fried Cauliflower "Rice" for a delicious spicy dinner. Enjoy your Cilantro-Lime Shrimp and Peppers that serves 2!

Serving Size: 2

Preparation Time: 10 minutes

Cooking Time: 30 minutes

Total Time: 40 minutes

Ingredients:

- 2 tablespoons of avocado oil or extra-virgin olive oil
- 1 white onion, thinly sliced
- 2 garlic cloves, thinly sliced
- 1 pound of medium shrimp, peeled and deveined
- ¼ cup of chopped fresh cilantro
- ½ red bell pepper, thinly sliced
- Juice of 2 limes
- ½ teaspoon of sea salt
- ½ teaspoon of red pepper flakes
- ½ green bell pepper, sliced
- ¼ cup of crumbled Cotija or feta cheese
- 1 avocado, sliced

Directions:

- Oil and heat the pan and add onion, bell peppers, and garlic and stir-fry until the vegetables begin to soften. Add the shrimp to the skillet and cook, tossing with the vegetables, until the shrimp are pink and firm.
- Stir in the cilantro, lime juice, salt, and red pepper flakes.
- Evenly divide the shrimp and vegetables between two bowls. Top each serving with 2 tablespoons Cotija and half the avocado and serve.

Nutritional Value: Calories 352 | Carbohydrates 21g | Fat 19g | Protein 7g

Recipe 10. Coconut and Lemongrass Turkey Soup

Yummy and tasty. This is a good family recipe, which will also make a nice meal for a group of friends. Enjoy this delicacy. Enjoy your Coconut and Lemongrass Turkey Soup that serves 5!

Serving Size: 5

Preparation Time: 15 minutes

Cooking Time: 40 minutes

Total Time: 55 minutes

Ingredients:

- 1 teaspoon of finely sliced lemongrass
- 1 teaspoon of ground ginger
- 1 garlic clove, minced
- 1 tablespoon of fresh cilantro, chopped
- 1 tablespoon of dried basil

- Juice of 1 lime
- 1 tablespoon of coconut oil
- 1 cup of diced white onion
- 12 ounces of skinless turkey breast, diced
- ½ cup of low-fat chicken broth
- ½ cup of water
- 1 cup of snow peas

Directions:

- Crush the lemongrass, ginger, garlic, cilantro, basil, and lime juice in a mortar and pestle to form a paste. Heat the prepared coconut oil in a skillet over medium-high heat and stir-fry the paste for approximately about 1 minute. Add the onions and turkey to the skillet and coat evenly with the paste to brown.
- Cook for 6 hours after adding water and the broth plus the snow peas to the soup 15 minutes. Top with scallions and fresh cilantro if desired.

Nutritional Value: Calories 287 | Carbohydrates 9 g | Fat 5 g | Protein 16 g

Recipe 11. Creamed Peas

The flavor is quite impressive! This recipe is very colorful and delicious. This dish is loaded with cheesy and savory flavors that you love. Enjoy your Creamed Peas that serves 4!

Serving Size: 4

Preparation Time: 10 minutes

Cooking Time: 25 minutes

Total Time: 35 minutes

Ingredients:

- ⅔ cup of chicken broth
- 2 cups of green peas
- 2 tablespoons of butter
- ⅓ cup of half-and-half
- 2 tablespoons of flour
- ¼ teaspoon of black pepper
- ¼ teaspoon of salt
- 2 tablespoons of Parmesan cheese, grated (optional)

Directions:

- In a medium saucepan, add broth and peas; bring to near boiling. Reduce heat.
- Cover; cook on low heat for approximately about 25 minutes, or until peas are tender. Add butter.
- In a small-sized bowl, combine half-and-half and flour; add to the peas mixture, cook and stir until thickened.
- Add the pepper and salt, plus Parmesan cheese if desired, stirring to combine.

Nutritional Value: Calories 150 | Carbohydrates 19 g | Fat 6.2 g | Protein 5.9 g

Recipe 12. Crispy Pollock and Gazpacho

It is an easy and exciting casserole for all low-carb dieters, containing layers of meat, vegetables, and cheese. It's a nutritious meal and a good dish for potlucks. Enjoy this delicious casserole with family and friends! Enjoy your Crispy Pollock and Gazpacho that serves 3!

Serving Size: 3

Preparation Time: 10 minutes

Cooking Time: 15 minutes

Total Time: 25 minutes

Ingredients:

- 85 grams of whole-wheat bread, torn into chunks
- 4 tablespoons of olive oil
- 4 pieces of Pollock fillets, skinless
- 4 large tomatoes, cut into chunks
- 3/4 cucumber, cut into chunks
- 2 tablespoons of sherry vinegar
- 2 garlic cloves, crushed
- 1/2 red onion, thinly sliced
- 1 yellow pepper, deseeded, cut into chunks

Directions:

- Preheat the oven to 200C, gas to 6, or fan to 180C. Over a baking tray, scatter the chunks of bread. Toss with 1 tablespoon of the prepared olive oil and bake for approximately about 10 minutes, or until golden and crispy. Meanwhile, mix the cucumber, tomatoes, onion, pepper, crushed garlic, sherry vinegar, and 2 tablespoons of the olive oil; season well.
- Heat a non-stick large frying pan. Add the remaining prepared 1 tablespoon of the olive oil and heat. When the prepared oil is already hot, add the fish; cook for approximately about 4 minutes or until golden. Flip the fillet; cook for approximately about additional 1 to 2 minutes or until the fish cooked through. In a mixing bowl, quickly toss the salad and the croutons; divide among 4 plates and then serve with the fish.

Nutritional Value: Calories 296 | Carbohydrates 19 g | Fat 13 g | Protein 27 g

Recipe 13. Ginger Sesame Pork Soup

This healthy, easy-to-prepare, broth-based soup will quickly become a weeknight favorite you can have on the table in less than 30 minutes. Ginger offers many incredible health benefits for the body, including anti-inflammatory properties, so don't hesitate to garnish your soup with some extra fresh ginger before eating. Use the leftover bok choy stems for a quick stir-fry dinner or add them to your favorite soup. Enjoy your Ginger Sesame Pork Soup that serves 2!

Serving Size: 2

Preparation Time: 10 minutes

Cooking Time: 25 minutes

Total Time: 35 minutes

Ingredients:

- ½ tablespoon of avocado oil or extra-virgin olive oil
- 1 teaspoon of sesame oil
- 8 ounces of ground pork
- 2 small carrots, diced
- 1 ½ teaspoons of minced peeled fresh ginger
- 4 cups of chicken stock
- 2 tablespoons of soy sauce
- 1 cup of halved sugar snap peas
- 1 cup of thinly sliced bok choy leaves
- Sea salt
- Freshly ground black pepper
- ½ jalapeño, seeded and thinly sliced
- ½ cup of chopped fresh cilantro
- Juice of 1 lime

Directions:

- In a soup pot, heat both oils over medium-high heat. Add the pork, carrots, and ginger and cook for approximately about 5 to 7 minutes, frequently stirring, until the pork begins to brown.
- Reduce the heat to low, add the sugar snap peas, cover, simmer for approximately about 10 minutes, add the bok choy leaves and season with pepper and salt to taste.
- Divide between two bowls and serve each garnished with jalapeño, cilantro, and lime juice.

Nutritional Value: Calories 236 | Carbohydrates 5g | Fat 1.8g | Protein 7g

Recipe 14. Gingered Honey Salmon

This recipe is made with well-done salmons. This recipe is healthy, delicious, and perfect for diet! It is a simple side dish that is ideal for a large holiday feast or a straightforward meal! Enjoy your Gingered Honey Salmon that serves 6!

Serving Size: 6

Preparation Time: 10 minutes

Cooking Time: 15 minutes

Total Time: 25 minutes

Ingredients:

- 1/3 cup of orange juice
- 1/3 cup of reduced-sodium soy sauce
- 1/4 cup of honey
- 1 green onion, chopped
- 1 teaspoon of ground ginger
- 1 teaspoon of garlic powder
- 1 salmon of fillet (1-1/2 pounds and 3/4 inch thick)

Directions:

- Place salmon in upside-down, 9-inch round (2-1/2-quart) glass baking dish (pie dish); pour orange juice over.
- In a small bowl, stir together soy sauce, honey, green onions, ginger, and garlic powder.
- Drizzle soy mixture over salmon.
- Bake at 400 degrees, uncovered, for approximately about 20 to 25 minutes or until fish flakes with a fork and is tender.

Nutritional Value: Calories 237 | Carbohydrates 15 g | Fat 10 g | Protein 20 g

Recipe 15. Glazed Miso Cod with Baby Bok Choy

If you haven't tried miso yet, you're in for a surprise. It is fermented soybean paste that is salty, funky, and barely sweet. It lends a delicious quality to nearly everything it touches. Start with white miso paste for a mild flavor. Pretty soon, you'll find yourself whisking it into everything from salads to ice cream. (Yes, for real!) You can find it refrigerated in the grocery store, often next to the tofu, tempeh, and specialty vegan foods. Enjoy your Glazed Miso Cod with Baby Bok Choy that serves 4!

Serving Size: 4

Preparation Time: 8 minutes

Cooking Time: 15 minutes

Total Time: 23 minutes

Ingredients:

- 2 tablespoons of toasted sesame oil, divided
- 2 tablespoons of white miso
- 2 tablespoons of low-sodium soy sauce, divided
- 2 tablespoons of freshly squeezed lime juice
- Pinch red pepper flakes
- 1 tablespoon of minced fresh ginger
- 2 or 3 drops of liquid stevia
- 4 (6-ounce) cod fillets
- 2 pounds of baby bok choy, halved lengthwise
- 1 teaspoon of minced garlic

Directions:

- Combine the miso, ginger, 1 tablespoon of sesame oil, 1 tablespoon of soy sauce, lime juice, and liquid stevia.
- Coat the cod fillets in the mixture and put them in a baking dish.
- Transfer the baking dish to the oven, and bake for approximately about 10 to 12 minutes, or until the fish flakes easily with a fork.
- Meanwhile, heat a large skillet over medium-high heat until hot, then pour in the remaining 1 tablespoon of oil, and tilt to coat the bottom.
- Place the bok choy in the skillet, cut side down. It will pop and splatter, so stand back a bit at first. Sear the bok choy until well browned, about 4 minutes.
- Add the red pepper and garlic then remove from the heat.
- Drizzle with the remaining 1 tablespoon of soy sauce, and toss gently to disburse the garlic, red pepper flakes, and soy sauce.
- Serve the cod with the bok choy on the side.

Nutritional Value: Calories 296 | Carbohydrates 19 g | Fat 13 g | Protein 27 g

Recipe 16. Ham and Bean Soup

Yummy and tasty. This is a good family recipe, which will also make a nice meal for a group of friends. Enjoy this delicacy. Enjoy your Ham and Bean Soup that serves 8!

Serving Size: 8

Preparation Time: 25 minutes

Cooking Time: 5 hours

Total Time: 5 hours 25 minutes

Ingredients:

- ½ (16-ounce) package of navy beans
- (14-ounce) cans of chicken broth
- 2 cups of water
- 1 cup of carrots, thinly sliced
- 1 cup of onion, finely chopped
- 2 cloves of garlic, sliced
- 1 (14-ounce) can of diced tomatoes, with juice
- ½ teaspoon of black pepper
- 1 ½ teaspoons of seasoned salt
- 1 cup of green cabbage, finely chopped
- 1 (5-ounce) can of smoked ground ham

Directions:

- Wash navy beans according to package directions. Bring one quart of the prepared water to a boil in a pot that is big enough to hold it. Turn off the heat, add the beans, cover, and let them rest for one hour so that they may soften up. After that, drain them.
- Add the ham, cabbage, broth, water, carrots, onion, garlic, tomatoes, pepper, seasoned salt, and seasoned salt, along with the seasoning packet. Cook the beans, covered, over a low heat for approximately about three to four hours, or until they are extremely soft. Mix it up every so often. The beans should be mashed with a potato masher until about half of the beans are broken up, and then they should be stirred to combine.

Nutritional Value: Calories 177 | Carbohydrates 26 g | Fat 2 g | Protein 14 g

Recipe 17. Herbed Chicken Paprikash

The flavor is quite impressive! This recipe is very colorful and delicious. This dish is loaded with cheesy and savory flavors that you love. Enjoy your Herbed Chicken Paprikash that serves 4!

Serving Size: 4

Preparation Time: 12 minutes

Cooking Time: 30 minutes

Total Time: 42 minutes

Ingredients:

- 4 (8-ounce) chicken leg quarters, skin removed
- 1 teaspoon of olive oil
- 1/3 cup of dry white wine
- 1/3 cup of chicken broth
- 1 small onion, peeled and sliced thinly
- 2/3 cup of sliced fresh button mushrooms
- 1/2 teaspoon of dried oregano
- 1/4 teaspoon of dried thyme

- 1/4 teaspoon of dried basil
- 1/8 teaspoon of dried rosemary
- 1/4 cup of finely grated carrots
- 4 cups of chopped fresh baby spinach
- 2 tablespoons of white whole-wheat flour
- 2 tablespoons of water
- 2 teaspoons of ground paprika
- 2 tablespoons of plain nonfat yogurt

Directions:

- Put the oregano, thyme, basil, and rosemary into a small bowl and stir to combine—heat a large nonstick skillet over medium heat.
- Oiled both sides of your chicken with oil and sprinkle evenly with herb mixture.
- Put your chicken in the skillet and cook on both sides until browned, roughly approximately about 2 minutes per side.
- Boil the chicken broth and add wine, Add onion, mushrooms, and carrots; cover and simmer for 8 minutes.
- Then add spinach cook for 2 minutes. Remove chicken from your pan and place it on the serving plate. Cover to keep warm.
- Mix flour plus water in a small bowl; whisk to remove any lumps
- Cook on medium heat then stirs until the mixture thickens, add paprika and yogurt.
- Pour sauce over chicken. Serve immediately.

Nutritional Value: Calories 236 | Carbohydrates 5g | Fat 1.8g | Protein 7g

Recipe 18. Jackfruit Vegetable Fry

A delicious twist for a busy day. The result is tender, juicy, and flavorful. Enjoy your Jackfruit Vegetable Fry that serves 6!

Serving Size: 6

Preparation Time: 5 minutes

Cooking Time: 5 minutes

Total Time: 10 minutes

Ingredients:

- 2 finely chopped small onions
- 2 cups of finely chopped cherry tomatoes
- 1/8 teaspoon of ground turmeric
- 1 tablespoon of olive oil
- 2 seeded and chopped red bell peppers
- 3 cups of seeded and chopped firm jackfruit
- 1/8 teaspoon of cayenne pepper
- 2 tablespoons of chopped fresh basil leaves
- Salt

Directions:

- In a greased skillet, sauté the onions and bell peppers for about 5 minutes.
- Add the tomatoes then stir.
- Cook for approximately about 2 minutes.
- Then add the jackfruit, cayenne pepper, salt, and turmeric.
- Cook for approximately about 8 minutes.
- Garnish the meal with basil leaves.
- Serve warm.

Nutritional Value: Calories 236 | Carbohydrates 5g | Fat 1.8g | Protein 7g

Recipe 19. Lamb Chops with Lemon and Mint Asparagus

The flavor is quite impressive! This recipe is very colorful and delicious. This dish is loaded with cheesy and savory flavors that you love. Enjoy your Lamb Chops with Lemon and Mint Asparagus that serves 4!

Serving Size: 4

Preparation Time: 10 minutes

Cooking Time: 15 minutes

Total Time: 25 minutes

Ingredients:

- 3 tablespoons of chopped fresh oregano
- Juice of 1 ½ lemons, divided
- ¼ cup plus 2 tablespoons of extra-virgin olive oil, divided, plus more for drizzling
- 4 tablespoons of grated garlic, divided
- 2 teaspoons of salt, divided
- 2 ½ teaspoons of freshly ground black pepper, divided
- 8 (3-to 4-ounce) bone-in lamb loin chops
- 1 pound of asparagus, trimmed
- 1 ½ teaspoons of chopped fresh mint

Directions:

- In a resealable plastic bag, mix the oregano, juice of 1 lemon, ¼ cup of olive oil, 3 tablespoons of garlic, 1 teaspoon of salt, and 2 teaspoons of pepper. Add the lamb chops, seal the bag, and refrigerate for approximately about at least 4 (and up to 12) hours.
- Then let it rest at room temperature for 20 minutes. Oil and heat the pan. Cook for approximately about 4–6 minutes per side. Move to a dish and relax.

- Wipe the skillet clean and reheat the remaining 1 tablespoon olive oil. Sauté asparagus for 4–5 minutes, until fork-tender. Add the remaining sauce and 1 tablespoon of garlic and sauce. Add the mint, remaining lemon juice, 1 teaspoon of salt, and ½ teaspoon of pepper.

Nutritional Value: Calories 384 | Carbohydrates 28g | Fat 8g | Protein 11g

Recipe 20. Loaded Shrimp Pasta

Asparagus, peas, and mushrooms are delicious in this everything-but-the-kitchen-sink dish, but you can prepare the recipe using any vegetables you have on hand. With its sumptuous blend of sweet, savory, bitter, and acidic, get ready for this pasta to become a new favorite meal. Enjoy your Loaded Shrimp Pasta that serves 4!

Serving Size: 4

Preparation Time: 10 minutes

Cooking Time: 15 minutes

Total Time: 25 minutes

Ingredients:

- 8 ounces of whole-wheat pasta
- 4 tablespoons of oil
- 1 teaspoon of jarred minced garlic
- 1 pound of shrimp, peeled and deveined
- 1 bunch of asparagus, cut into 1-inch pieces
- 1 lemon, halved
- 1 cup of fresh or frozen spinach
- 1 cup of canned or frozen green peas
- 1 cup of cherry or grape tomatoes, halved
- 1 cup of sliced mushrooms

Directions:

- Boil water with pasta for 20 minutes.
- Oil and heat the pan and garlic. Add the mushrooms, spinach, shrimp, peas, asparagus, and tomatoes cook for 10 minutes.
- Add the pasta to the pan of shrimp and vegetables.
- Serve

Nutritional Value: Calories 296 | Carbohydrates 19 g | Fat 13 g | Protein 27 g

Recipe 21. Lobster Casserole

Enjoy this delicious casserole with family and friends! Enjoy your Lobster Casserole that serves 4!

Serving Size: 4

Preparation Time: 26 minutes

Cooking Time: 55 minutes

Total Time: 1 hour 21 minutes

Ingredients:

- 3 tablespoons of butter
- 1 pound of lobster meat, bite-sized pieces
- 3 tablespoons of all-purpose flour
- 3/4 teaspoon of dry mustard
- salt and pepper to taste
- 1 cup of heavy cream
- 1/2 cup of milk
- 3 slices of bread, crust removed

Directions:

- Place a medium sized pot on low heat. Add butter and melt. Add the lobster meat and sauté until it begins to change color. Avoid cooking too fast or too long as this will cause the lobster meat to toughen. In the same used saucepan, combine the remaining butter, flour, salt, pepper, and dry mustard. Keep aside.
- Add the flour, salt, and the pepper and dry mustard to the remaining butter in the same pot. Stir well. Slowly whisk in the milk and cream. Continue cooking while stirring continuously for approximately about five minutes until the mixture thickens. Add in the lobster meat back to the pot. Cut the bread into small and tiny pieces and toss it into the sauce, stirring constantly.
- Place dish in preheated oven and bake for approximately about 20 to 25 minutes until it bubbles and turns to a delicate brown color.

Nutritional Value: Calories 316 | Carbohydrates 30 g | Fat 12 g | Protein 17 g

Recipe 22. Mustard Maple Chicken with Potato Wedges

Yummy and tasty. This is a good family recipe, which will also make a nice meal for a group of friends. Enjoy this delicacy. Enjoy your Mustard Maple Chicken with Potato Wedges that serves 6!

Serving Size: 6

Preparation Time: 17 minutes

Cooking Time: 45 minutes

Total Time: 1 hour 2 minutes

Ingredients:

- 2 pounds of boneless, skinless chicken thighs

- 6 medium gold potatoes, scrubbed & cut into 8 wedges per potato
- 1/4 cup of pure maple syrup
- 2 tablespoons of apple cider vinegar
- 2 tablespoons of olive oil
- 2 tablespoons of mustard
- 1/2 teaspoon of freshly ground black pepper
- 11/2 teaspoons of all-purpose seasoning

Directions:

- Combine maple syrup, vinegar, oil, mustard, and pepper in a large gallon-sized zip-top bag. Add chicken to the marinade bag.
- Preheat oven to 400°F. Oil a large 9" × 13" baking dish and set aside. Remove chicken from the refrigerator and set aside. Bake seasoned potatoes for 15 minutes.
- Add chicken, then marinade to the pan and return to the middle rack in the oven. Bake for approximately about 20–30 minutes until potato wedges are tender and the chicken has an internal temperature of 165°F and is no longer pink inside.
- Remove from oven and serve immediately.

Nutritional Value: Calories 296 | Carbohydrates 19 g | Fat 13 g | Protein 27 g

Recipe 23. Pan-Seared Butter Scallops

Scallops cooked over high heat and basted with butter and garlic are just about as good as it gets for me. The texture of the scallops is like that of lobster, and they cost less, though they are still somewhat pricey. Splurge on extra-large diver scallops or sea scallops if you can. Prepare the Sautéed Zucchini with Mint and Pine Nuts in the same pan for a complete meal. Enjoy your Pan-Seared Butter Scallop that serves 4!

Serving Size: 4

Preparation Time: 5 minutes

Cooking Time: 10 minutes

Total Time: 15 minutes

Ingredients:

- 4 tablespoons of butter
- 2 tablespoons of extra-virgin olive oil
- 1 pound of large scallops
- Sea salt
- Freshly ground black pepper
- 2 teaspoons of roughly chopped garlic
- ¼ cup of roughly chopped fresh parsley

Directions:

- Heat a large skillet over high heat. Melt the butter and add the olive oil.
- When the butter and oil are hot, place the scallops in the pan, being sure not to crowd them.
- Oil and heat the pan with butter. Drizzle this over the scallops as they cook. Sear for approximately about 2 minutes on the first side. Carefully flip and sear on the second side for approximately about 2 more minutes or until the scallops are cooked through and opaque in the center.
- During your last minute of cooking this dish, add the garlic and parsley, and spoon the flavored oil and butter over the scallops.

Nutritional Value: Calories 147 | Carbohydrates 22.1 g | Fat 5.5 g | Protein 2.3 g

Recipe 24. Pistachio-Crusted Scallops

Scallops may seem like an intimidating type of seafood to cook at home, but it couldn't be easier to transform them into a sophisticated meal with a hot pan and a few other simple ingredients. Enjoy your Pistachio-Crusted Scallops that serves 4!

Serving Size: 4

Preparation Time: 9 minutes

Cooking Time: 15 minutes

Total Time: 24 minutes

Ingredients:

- ½ cup of shelled unsalted pistachios
- Zest of 1 medium lemon
- 1 pound of sea
- 2 tablespoons of extra-virgin olive oil
- ½ teaspoon of freshly ground black pepper
- ¾ teaspoon of kosher salt or sea salt

Directions:

- Pulse pistachios in a food processor until crumbs form. Toss the pistachio crumbs with the lemon zest and 14 teaspoon of salt in a small dish. Remove from the equation.
- Oil and heat the pan. Season the scallops with the remaining 12 teaspoon salt and black pepper on both sides. Add the scallops to the pan and cook for approximately about 2 to 3 minutes, or until browned,

before flipping and cooking for approximately about another 1 to 2 minutes, or until somewhat firm.
- Transfer the scallops to the pistachio crust-coated plate with tongs; flip and toss the scallops until they are evenly coated on both sides. Serve right away.

Nutritional Value: Calories 236 | Carbohydrates 5g | Fat 1.8g | Protein 7g

Recipe 25. Rosemary Braised Chicken with Mushroom Sauce

Yummy and tasty. This is a good family recipe, which will also make a nice meal for a group of friends. Enjoy this delicacy. Enjoy your Rosemary Braised Chicken with Mushroom Sauce that serves 4!

Serving Size: 4

Preparation Time: 15 minutes

Cooking Time: 30 minutes

Total Time: 45 minutes

Ingredients:

- 1 pound of boneless skinless chicken thighs
- 2 tablespoons of canola oil
- 2 slices of turkey bacon or turkey prosciutto
- 1 small shallot, diced
- ¼ cup of yellow onion, diced
- 1 clove of garlic, crushed
- 3 sprigs of fresh rosemary
- 3 ounces of fresh cremini mushrooms, quartered
- 1 portobello mushroom cap, halved and sliced
- 1 teaspoon of flour
- 1 cup of low-sodium vegetable stock
- ½ cup of red wine
- Salt and pepper, to taste

Directions:

- Lightly coat chicken with oil, place in deep-sided skillet over medium heat, and brown on all sides (approximately 5 minutes per side).
- Add bacon, shallots, onions, garlic, rosemary, and mushrooms, and sauté for approximately about 10 minutes. Add flour, stock, and red wine; cover and reduce liquid by half until thick and chicken is cooked (approximately 10 minutes).
- Serve

Nutritional Value: Calories 380 | Carbohydrates 9 g | Fat 21 g | Protein 33 g

Recipe 26. Rosemary Pork Roast

Using the vegetables in this dish as a roasting bed, they absorb the luscious flavors from the pork drippings. The vegetables can be served as is or puréed with the pan drippings as a rich gravy to complement the roast and the other vegetables. Enjoy your Rosemary Pork Roast that serves 4!

Serving Size: 4

Preparation Time: 45 minutes

Cooking Time: 3 hours

Total Time: 3 hours 45 minutes

Ingredients:

- 1 teaspoon of freshly ground black pepper
- ¼ cup of chopped fresh rosemary
- ¼ cup of chopped garlic
- 3 tablespoons of extra-virgin olive oil, divided
- 1 teaspoon of salt
- 2 cups of whole mushrooms, trimmed
- 2 cups of turnips, cut into cubes
- 1 head cabbage, cut into 8 wedges
- 1 (2- to 2 ½-pound) pork shoulder roast
- ¾ cup of water

Directions:

- In a mixing bowl, mix the pepper, garlic, rosemary, salt, and 2 tablespoons of olive oil into a paste. In a large baking dish, toss together the turnips, mushrooms, and cabbage. Season the vegetables with salt and pepper and drizzle with the remaining olive oil.
- Score the top of the pork roast in a crosshatch pattern and set it on top of the vegetable mixture. Generously rub the rosemary mixture over the entire surface of the roast. Add the water to the baking dish.
- Roast for approximately about 20 minutes. Cover with aluminum foil, reduce the oven temperature to 325°F, and cook for approximately about 3 hours or until the internal temperature reaches 160°F.

Nutritional Value: Calories 351 | Carbohydrates 30 g | Fat 9 g | Protein 31 g

Recipe 27. Salmon-Kale Summer Rolls

A new way of boosting your day's mood is to try the salmon-kale summer rolls. It entails a range of ingredients that are good for your health. Enjoy the Salmon-Kale Summer rolls. Enjoy your Salmon-Kale Summer Rolls that serves 4!

Serving Size: 4

Preparation Time: 30 minutes

Cooking Time: 55 minutes

Total Time: 1 hour 25 minutes

Ingredients:

- 5 large lacinato kale leaves
- 1 tablespoon of canola oil.
- 2 teaspoons of light brown sugar.
- 1 ½ cup of very thinly sliced English cucumbers
- 6 ounces of thinly sliced smoked salmon.
- 4 ½ tablespoon of rice vinegar, divided.
- ¾ teaspoon of kosher salt, divided.
- 8 round of rice paper sheets.
- 1 ½ very thinly sliced radishes
- 1 sliced avocado, 16 slices.

Directions:

- In a strainer, put rice. Rinse for 1 minute with cold water until clear.
- Move rice to a tiny cup, add 1 ½ cups of water. Cover and put over high heat to a boil.
- Reduce to medium-low heat and cook for approximately about 40 minutes. Remove from heat and allow 20 minutes to stand.
- Transfer to a medium-sized bowl and toss with sugar, 3 ½ vinegar tablespoon, and 1⁄2 salt teaspoon. Let it cool for about 20 minutes.
- Put kale in a bowl with olive oil, one tablespoon of vinegar, and 1⁄4 teaspoon of salt.
- Fill a large, shallow dish with warm water at a depth of 1 inch. Place one sheet of rice on the water; let stand only about 30 seconds until soft. Move to a smooth surface of the sheet.
- Arrange 1/8 of the radishes, 1/8 of the cucumbers, and two avocado pieces in a row across the wrapper center, leaving at every end a 1-inch margin. Finish with 1⁄4 cup of rice, pinch together grains as you seal.
- Add 1⁄4 cup of peanut and 3⁄4 ounce of salmon. Fold the ends of the sheet and roll up, jelly-roll mode. Push the seam gently to close.
- Place roll, seam side down, on a platter lined in a damp towel or paper, and cover with another damp towel of paper so that it is not dry.
- Repeat the rest of the ingredients cycle. Serve immediately.

Nutritional Value: Calories 306 | Carbohydrates 29 g | Fat 19 g | Protein 22 g

Recipe 28. Seafood Paella

Yummy and tasty. This is a good family recipe, which will also make a nice meal for a group of friends. Enjoy this delicacy. Enjoy your Seafood Paella that serves 4!

Serving Size: 4

Preparation: 16 minutes

Cooking Time: 25 minutes

Total Time: 41 minutes

Ingredients:

- 1 large head cauliflower
- 8 ounces of chorizo (or other smoked sausages)
- 8 ounces of large shrimp
- 12 live littleneck clams
- 12 live mussels
- 4 bone-in chicken thighs
- 1 cup of chicken stock (or seafood stock)
- 1 small white onion
- 1 teaspoon of saffron
- Pinch of ground black pepper
- Pinch of sea salt
- 2 tablespoons of coconut oil

Directions:

- Heat a large pan over medium heat and add coconut oil.
- Peel and chop the onion. Add to hot oiled pan and sauté until translucent, about 2 minutes.
- Add chicken thighs and brown for approximately about 5 minutes. Turn the chicken over and cook another 5 minutes.
- Rinse and clean clams and mussels and remove any beards with pliers. Peel and devein shrimp. Cut the chorizo into 1-inch slices. Set aside.
- Roughly chop cauliflower and shred in a food processor to make "rice." Or chop cauliflower.
- Add rice or minced cauliflower to chicken and sauté for approximately about 2 minutes. Add chorizo, clams, mussels, and shrimp. Add saffron and sauté for approximately about another 2 minutes.
- Add chicken or seafood stock and stir to combine. Turn up the heat and simmer. Cover and reduce heat to medium. Let simmer for approximately about 5 - 7 minutes, until liquid evaporates, shrimp is opaque, and mussels and clams open. Discard any that do not open. Plate and serve hot.

Nutritional Value: Calories 351 | Carbohydrates 30 g | Fat 9 g | Protein 31 g

Recipe 29. Spanish Rice Casserole with Cheesy Beef

A delicious twist for a busy day. This recipe is healthy, delicious, and perfect for diet! It is a simple side dish that is ideal for a large holiday feast or a straightforward meal! The result is tender, juicy, and flavorful. Enjoy your Spanish Rice Casserole with Cheesy Beef that serves 2!

Serving Size: 2

Preparation Time: 10 minutes

Cooking Time: 32 minutes

Total Time: 42 minutes

Ingredients:

- 2 tablespoons of chopped green bell pepper
- 1/4 teaspoon of Worcestershire sauce
- 1/4 teaspoon of ground cumin
- 1/4 cup of shredded Cheddar cheese
- 1/4 cup of finely chopped onion
- 1/4 cup of Chile sauce
- 1/3 cup of uncooked long grain rice
- 1/2-pound of lean ground beef
- 1/2 teaspoon of salt
- 1/2 teaspoon of brown sugar
- 1/2 pinch of ground black pepper
- 1/2 cup of water
- 1/2 (14.5 ounce) can of canned tomatoes
- 1 tablespoon of chopped fresh cilantro

Directions:

- Place a nonstick saucepan on medium fire and brown beef for approximately about 10 minutes while crumbling beef. Discard fat.
- Stir in pepper, Worcestershire sauce, cumin, brown sugar, salt, chile sauce, rice, water, tomatoes, green bell pepper, and onion. Mix well and cook for approximately about 10 minutes until blended and a bit tender.
- Transfer to an ovenproof casserole and press down firmly. Sprinkle cheese on top and cook for approximately about 7 minutes at 400 F preheated oven. Broil for approximately about 3 minutes until top is lightly browned.
- Serve and enjoy with chopped cilantro.

Nutritional Value: Calories 460 | Carbohydrates 35.8 g | Fat 17.9 g | Protein 37.8 g

Recipe 30. Spicy Carrot and Lime Soup

It is an easy and exciting casserole for all low-carb dieters, containing layers of meat, vegetables, and cheese. It's a nutritious meal and a good dish for potlucks. Enjoy this delicious casserole with family and friends! Enjoy your Spicy Carrot and Lime Soup that serves 2!

Serving Size: 2

Preparation Time: 15 minutes

Cooking Time: 7 hours

Total Time: 7 hours 15 minutes

Ingredients:

- 1 teaspoon of mustard seeds, crushed
- 1 teaspoon of fennel seeds, crushed
- 1 tablespoon of ground ginger
- 4 medium carrots, peeled and chopped
- 1 cup of diced red onion
- 1 lime, zest, and juice
- 2 cups of water
- 1 tablespoon of fresh oregano, chopped
- ½ cup of fat free Greek yogurt
- Freshly ground black pepper, to taste

Directions:

- Heat a non-stick skillet over medium-high heat. Add the crushed mustard seeds and fennel seeds and stir-fry for approximately about a minute. Add the ground ginger and cook for another minute.
- Add the carrots, onions, and lime juice and cook until the vegetables are softened, approximately about 5 minutes. Remove from the heat and transfer to the slow cooker pot.
- Add the water, lime zest and juice, and fresh oregano to the pot. Set the slow cooker to LOW for approximately about 7-8 hours or HIGH for approximately about 3-4 hours.
- Serve with ¼ cup of Greek yogurt swirled through and black pepper to taste.

Nutritional Value: Calories 224 | Carbohydrates 32 g | Fat 1 g | Protein 16 g

Recipe 31. Spinach and Brussels Sprout Salad

Try this recipe and you will forget about meat. So, there's no need to wait any longer since we've already outlined the procedures, you'll need to take to prepare this delectable dish. Enjoy this delicious casserole with family and friends! Enjoy your Spinach and Brussels Sprout Salad that serves 2!

Serving Size: 2

Preparation Time: 15 minutes

Cooking Time: 35 minutes

Total Time: 50 minutes

Ingredients:

- 1 pound of brussels sprouts, halved
- 2 tablespoons of olive oil
- Black pepper and salt to taste
- 1 tablespoon of balsamic vinegar
- 2 tablespoons of extra-virgin olive oil
- 1 cup of baby spinach
- 1 tablespoon of Dijon mustard
- 1/2 cup of hazelnuts

Directions:

- The oven should be heated at 400 F. Drizzle the Brussels sprouts with olive oil, then sprinkle with salt and black pepper and place them on a baking tray. Bake until they are tender, approximately about 20 minutes, turning them frequently.
- In a dry skillet over moderate temperature, toast the hazelnuts for approximately about 2 minutes, let them cool, and then cut them into smaller pieces. Move the Brussels sprouts into a salad bowl, including baby spinach. Mix until well-combined. In the bowl of a small serving dish, mix vinegar along with mustard and olive oil. Pour the dressing over the salad, and then top it with hazelnuts and serve.

Nutritional Value: Calories 311 | Carbohydrates 10 g | Fat 43 g | Protein 14 g

Recipe 32. Stout-Steamed Shellfish with Charred Onions

You can double the recipe on two pots and serve with some warm baguettes if you want this main course to serve 8. Enjoy your Stout-Steamed Shellfish with Charred Onions that serves 8!

Serving Size: 8

Preparation Time: 8 minutes

Cooking Time: 15 minutes

Total Time: 23 minutes

Ingredients:

- 2 tablespoons of grapeseed or vegetable oil
- 1 large onion
- 1 bay leaf
- 5 pounds of littleneck clams and mussels
- 1 head of garlic, halved crosswise
- 1 (12 ounces) bottle stout
- 1 (4-inch) piece kombu or 1 toasted nori sheet
- 6 tablespoons of unsalted butter
- Kosher salt, freshly ground pepper
- 5 sprigs of thyme

Directions:

- In a big wide pot, heat oil on high heat and cook the onions, occasionally stirring, for approximately about 6 - 8 minutes until the edges blacken.
- Allow the pot to slightly cool, add in thyme, garlic (cut side down), and butter, then cook on low heat for approximately about 3 minutes until the garlic is fragrant and golden.
- Add the stout, bay leaf, and kombu, then raise the heat to medium-high.
- Add in the shellfish and cover. Cook while shaking the pot frequently for approximately about 5 - 8 minutes until all the shellfish open, moving the shellfish onto a big bowl as they open.
- Throw away the ones that didn't open. Season the cooking broth with pepper and salt.
- Divide the shellfish into bowls and ladle the broth over them.

Nutritional Value: Calories 306 | Carbohydrates 29 g | Fat 19 g | Protein 22 g

Recipe 33. Strip Steak with Creamy Peppercorn Sauce

This recipe is all about this amazing creamy peppercorn sauce that is simple to prepare and full of flavor. This classic sauce can be used on any steak, chicken, or white fish. Add a side of sautéed mushrooms and onions to this recipe to replicate the full steakhouse experience. Enjoy your Strip Steak with Creamy Peppercorn Sauce that serves 2!

Serving Size: 2

Preparation Time: 10 minutes

Cooking time: 15 minutes

Total Time: 25 minutes

Ingredients:

- 1 (10-ounce) strip of steak
- 1 teaspoon of sea salt, plus more to taste
- 1 teaspoon of ground black pepper
- 1 tablespoon of avocado oil or extra-virgin olive oil
- 1 tablespoon of minced white onion
- 1 tablespoon of chopped fresh parsley
- 1 garlic clove, minced
- ⅓ cup of beef stock
- 2 tablespoons of low-carb white wine (optional)
- ¼ cup of heavy (whipping) cream
- ½ tablespoon of coarsely cracked black pepper
- 1 teaspoon of chopped fresh thyme leaves
- ½ teaspoon of Worcestershire sauce

Directions:

- Season the steak with the pepper and salt.
- Heat the oil in a pan and add the steak and cook for approximately about 3 to 5 minutes per side, until the desired doneness is reached. Set aside on a plate.
- Add the onion and garlic to the skillet and cook for approximately about 1 minute, or until fragrant.
- Reduce the heat to medium-low. Add the beef stock and wine (if using), scraping up the cooked bits on the bottom of the pan. Add the cream, cracked pepper, thyme, and Worcestershire sauce. Simmer for approximately about 3 minutes, or until the sauce just begins to thicken. Season with more salt to taste.
- Slice the steak across the grain into ¼-inch-thick slices. Divide between two plates, drizzle with the peppercorn sauce, and garnish with parsley.

Nutritional Value: Calories 351 | Carbohydrates 30 g | Fat 9 g | Protein 31 g

Recipe 34. Turkey and Quinoa Stuffed Peppers

It is an easy and exciting casserole for all low-carb dieters, containing layers of meat, vegetables, and cheese. It's a nutritious meal and also a good dish for potlucks. Enjoy your Turkey and Quinoa Stuffed Peppers that serves 6!

Serving Size: 6

Preparation Time: 25 minutes

Cooking Time: 55 minutes

Total Time: 1 hour 20 minutes

Ingredients:

- 3 large red bell peppers
- 2 teaspoons of chopped fresh rosemary
- 2 tablespoons of chopped fresh parsley
- 3 tablespoons of chopped pecans, toasted
- ¼ cup of extra virgin olive oil
- ½ cup of chicken stock
- ½ pound of fully cooked smoked turkey sausage, diced
- ½ teaspoon of salt
- 2 cups of water
- 1 cup of uncooked quinoa

Directions:

- On high fire, place a large saucepan and add salt, water and quinoa. Bring to a boil. Once boiling, reduce fire to a simmer, cover and cook until all water is absorbed around 15 minutes. Uncover quinoa, turn off fire and let it stand for another 5 minutes. Add rosemary, parsley, pecans, olive oil, chicken stock and turkey sausage into pan of quinoa. Mix well. Slice peppers lengthwise in half and discard membranes and seeds.
- In another boiling pot of water, add peppers, boil for approximately about 5 minutes, drain and discard water. Grease a prepared 13 x 9 baking dish and preheat oven to 350 F. Place boiled bell pepper onto preparation ared baking dish, evenly fill with the quinoa mixture and pop into oven. Bake for approximately about 15 minutes.

Nutritional Value: Calories 255 | Carbohydrates 21.6 g | Fat 12.4 g | Protein 14.4 g

Recipe 35. Viognier Steamed Clams with Parsnips and Bacon

Yummy and tasty. This is a good family recipe, which will also make a nice meal for a group of friends. Enjoy this delicacy. Enjoy your Viognier Steamed Clams with Parsnip and Bacon that serves 5!

Serving Size: 5

Preparation Time: 40 minutes

Cooking Time: 1 hour 30 minutes

Total Time: 2 hours 10 minutes

Ingredients:

- 1 pound of parsnips peeled
- 1 and 1/2 cups of viogniers
- 1/4 cup of virgin olive oil
- 6 ounces of thickly sliced bacon
- 1 minced shallot
- 2 tablespoons of unsalted butter

- 1 cup of heavy cream
- 4 dozen of scrubbed, rinsed littleneck clams
- 2 tablespoons of snipped chives
- oyster crackers to garnish
- freshly ground pepper
- salt

Directions:

- Preheat oven to 350 degrees, lace parsnips on a baking sheet, brush with olive oil, season with pepper and salt
- Roast for approximately about 40 minutes until tender, turning over twice, allow to slightly cool, then quarter and slice into 1/4 thick pieces lengthwise
- Cook bacon over moderate heat in a large skillet until crisp and well browned, drain on paper towels, wipe skillet
- Bring butter, shallot, and viognier to boil in skillet, add clams, cover, and cook for approximately about 6-8 minutes over high heat until they open; transfer clams to a large bowl with a slotted spoon
- Pour clam broth into a measuring cup, rinse out skillet, pour clam broth back into skillet slowly and stop when you reach grit underneath
- Add cream and boiled for approximately about 8 minutes until the liquid has reduced by half, puree the cream sauce in a blender if it separates, and transfers back to the skillet when smooth
- Add bacon, roasted parsnips, cooked clams, and chives to skillet, season with plenty pepper, cover, bring to boil
- Spoon into shallow bowls, sprinkle oyster crackers, serve immediately.

Nutritional Value: Calories 383 | Carbohydrates 11.6 g | Fat 19 g | Protein 9 g

Recipe 36. White Cabbage and Lentils with Relish

Try this recipe and you will forget about meat. So, there's no need to wait any longer since we've already outlined the procedures, you'll need to take to prepare this delectable dish. Enjoy this delicious casserole with family and friends! Enjoy your White Cabbage and Lentils with Relish that serves 4!

Serving Size: 4

Preparation Time: 5 minutes

Cooking Time: 1 hour 30 minutes

Total Time: 1 hour 35 minutes

Ingredients:

- 1 medium head of white cabbage, shredded
- 2 cups of boiling water
- Juice from 1 lemon
- Freshly ground black pepper, to taste
- ½ cup of lentils (canned or dried and soaked the night before)
- ½ small cucumber, diced
- 1 tablespoon of dried dill
- 1 cup of fat free Greek yogurt/sour cream

Directions:

- Add the cabbage, water and half the lemon juice to the slow cooker pot. Season generously with freshly ground black pepper.
- Add in enough water until it just covers the cabbage.
- Add the lentils and stir well.
- Set the slow cooker to a heat of LOW and cook for approximately about 1 ½ hours: the dish is ready when most of the prepared water has been soaked up.
- While the cabbage is cooking, make the cucumber and dill relish:
- Mix the cucumbers, dill, remaining lemon juice and Greek yogurt and set aside to chill.
- Serve the cabbage with the cucumber and dill relish spooned over the top.

Nutritional Value: Calories 159 | Carbohydrates 32 g | Fat 1 g | Protein 16 g

Recipe 37. Zucchini and Pepper Caprese Gratin

A quick and simple vegetarian zucchini, tomato, and mozzarella bake that serves two, four as an appetizer, or even as a side dish. My Roman friends taught me this traditional Italian dish. If served as a main dish, nothing beats crusty bread that has been manually pulled from the loaf and a green salad with vinaigrette dressing made with lemon and/or lime. It is a simple side dish that is ideal for a large holiday feast or a straightforward meal! Alternating rows of thinly sliced tomato, potato, and zucchini are baked with tomato sauce, Italian seasonings, and olive oil. Enjoy your Zucchini and Pepper Caprese Gratin that serves 4!

Serving Size: 4

Preparation Time: 20 minutes

Cooking Time: 50 minutes

Total Time: 1 hour 10 minutes

Ingredients:

- 2 zucchinis, sliced
- 1 red bell pepper chopped
- Salt and black pepper to taste
- 1 cup of ricotta cheese, crumbled
- 4 ounces of fresh mozzarella, sliced
- 2 tomatoes, sliced
- 2 tablespoons of butter
- 1/4 teaspoon of xanthan gum
- 1 cup of heavy whipped cream

Directions:

- Bake at 370 F. Creates an even layer of bell peppers and zucchinis in a baking dish that has been greased with the bell peppers and zucchinis overlapping. Sprinkle salt and pepper on top, and then sprinkle with Ricotta cheese. Repeat the process of layering a second time.
- Mix butter, xanthan gum, and whipping cream in a microwave for approximately about two minutes, stir it until completely mixed and then sprinkle over the vegetables. Then, top with the remaining ricotta. The gratin is baked for 30 mins or until the top is golden brown. Remove from oven and layer it with fresh mozzarella and tomato slices. Bake for approximately about another 5-10 minutes. Slice into thin slices and serve them warm.

Nutritional Value: Calories 283 | Carbohydrates 5.6 g | Fat 22 g | Protein 16 g

CONCLUSION

The Dr. Nowzaradan diet, or Dr. Now diet, is a 1,000-1,200 calorie diet designed to promote fast weight reduction in patients before having weight loss surgery.

While effective for weight loss, the diet can be very tough to follow long-term owing to its rigidity and potential side effects like low energy, poor sex drive, and irritability.

A better alternative to losing weight is to gradually adopt healthy lifestyle choices that you can keep up over time, such increasing your consumption of fruits and vegetables, prioritizing sleep, and being physically active. Particularly after sticking to the Now diet for a while to reach your goal weight.

AND A HUGE BONUS FOR YOU...
LOW-CALORIE KETO DIET
COOKBOOK

**A MOUTH WATERING COLLECTION OF LOW CARB RECIPES
WITH LESS THAN 1200 CALORIE
TO ACTIVATE KETOSIS AND BURN EXCESS FAT
WITHOUT FEELING DIETING**

Juan Smith

CHAPTER 1. ALL ABOUT KETO EXPLAINED

A ketogenic, or keto, diet is a low-carb high-fat (LCHF) diet and stands out among popular regimens. Unlike many diet trends and fads, it's straightforward and easy to follow once you get to grips with it. High carb foods cause your body to produce insulin and glucose; it is the sensitive interaction between them, which is described in detail later, which controls a weight loss process called ketosis. So, your success on the keto diet depends on how successful you are with managing ketosis, and this depends on how disciplined you are in limiting your high-carb food intake.

- Glucose: A simple sugar that converts energy from the food we eat to fuel our body.
- Insulin: A hormone our pancreas secretes to transport glucose (energy) through our bloodstream to our cells.

Since the dawn of civilization in East Africa, glucose has been a human's primary source of energy; it is what we use to fuel our body, fight off competition, evolve and stay alive! On a regular diet today, especially one followed by a modern human, glucose converts to fat in our actual bodies at a rate faster than what occurred in the bodies of our distant ancestors: we are larger than them, physically. Indeed, science tells us that modern humans living today are eating too many high carbohydrate foods. This excess carb consumption means our bodies are storing glucose in the fatty deposits around our body more than it should or has done historically: we are fat! Fortunately, we humans have evolved an intelligent body. Our body doesn't use this excess supply of glucose caused by a generic, unhealthy Westernized diet as energy because it has no need to if we're constantly eating foods high in carbs. So, our body doesn't need it and simply stores it away as fat to be used when our dietary habit changes: a change on the keto diet that we call ketosis.

Science tells us that carbs are our number-one source of energy, and while this may be true, carbs do not come without their drawbacks. The keto diet eliminates these problems by substituting carbs with healthy fats and some protein. But the amount of carbs we substitute on the diet depends on our dietary preference and which variation of the diet we follow.

Keto Calorie Budget

Importantly, the keto diet is based on the nutritional science of a daily calorie budget, which varies for male and females. Humans consume calories every day, whether we know it or not. Food, such as carbs, contains calories: calories provide energy. This is true whether you're following a keto diet or not. Science tells us two things:

- The keto diet prescribes a calorie intake lower than one on a non-keto diet.
- This calorie intake varies between men and women.

The American Medical Association recommends the following general daily calorie intake for men and women following a keto diet. Note, this is a general recommendation and doesn't consider your weight, height, BMI and overall medical history and condition. They will calculate a daily calorie budget most suitable for you. Alternatively, you can use an online calculator to do the calculation yourself, although I don't recommend this option because my experience suggests that most people calculate it incorrectly.

The science behind the calorie intake is that the amount of energy stored inside your body is equal to the energy in minus energy out. This can be represented mathematically by the following equation:

This relationship implies that if you, as an active human being, burn more calories by doing physical work such as exercise, regulating core bodily function/processes, than you intake daily, you will lose weight. This is the traditional weight loss model, but it is basic. Translated to the keto diet, your focus and priority whilst on the diet is to minimize 'energy in' (by limiting calorie intake) to your body so that ketosis forces it to burn calories from its existing 'energy stored'. So, your focus on the diet is to manipulate the energy that comes into your body by changing what you eat: by avoiding high-carb foods. But this is where it might get a little complicated: the difference between keto and a normal diet is that keto focuses on intentionally splitting this daily calorie budget across three common macronutrient groups: carbs, proteins and fats.

In other words, each version of the keto diet apportions a specific percentage to each group. So, every form of keto diet, and there are four main types described below, is based on this fundamental science of a daily calorie budget. Each type must have a specific calorie budget assigned to it for the diet to work and this budget is divided differently across the three macro food groups, depending on which type of diet you choose to follow. Without one, the diet would not work; it is what all knowledge of the diet rests on and is top of the list of your 'things to do before starting a keto diet'.

- Standard Ketogenic Diet (SKD): It is the one highly recommended by nutritionists and advertised online. It is based on splitting your daily calorie budget into a macronutrient ratio of 75% fat, 20% protein and 5% carbs.
- High-Protein Ketogenic Diet: This involves eating more protein and is based on splitting your daily calorie budget into a macronutrient ratio of 60% fat, 35% protein and 5% carbs.
- Targeted Ketogenic Diet (TKD): This a good choice for athletes who use up their glycogen reserves quickly and involves consuming more carbs than on a SKD.
- Cyclical Ketogenic Diet (CKD): Your carb intake varies on this variety. You dedicate two days a week to high-carb consumption and five days being ketogenic: low-carb intake.

While a standard keto diet is encouraged amongst beginners, it's important to also consider the other three, especially if one better fits your medical history, lifestyle, and body. I recommend all beginners start with the SKD. Many keto dieters achieve excellent results with it right off the bat—some of them exceed expectations! Usually, though, it takes most people a little time to adapt to its challenges. Starting something new is not an easy thing for us humans to do and the keto diet is no exception. All types of keto diet require patience and perseverance. Be careful, though, a lot of misinformation surrounds it, some of which is described in this book.

CHAPTER 2: FUNDAMENTALS OF THE KETOGENIC DIET

The ketogenic diet offers a solution to such a problem as it offers carb-restricted alternatives for a daily meal. It basically challenged the existing norms and practices and propagated the idea of a carb-free lifestyle. Carbohydrates are known as an instant and cheapest source of energy, and even today, many millions of people rely on carb-rich food to meet their energy needs. However, the ketogenic diet provided an alternative which was earlier never thought of.

History of the Ketogenic Diet

The rise of the ketogenic diet dates to the 1920 to 1930s as a food therapy for epilepsy, a brain-related disease. Unlike other medicated treatments, ketogenic diet worked due to its long-lasting impact. It emerged as a good alternative to fasting, which was earlier used to treat epilepsy. But the idea of keto therapy soon faced failure due to a lack of research and extensive use of medications.

However, in 1921, Rollin Woodyatt revived the idea of the ketogenic diet and brought its benefits back into the spotlight when is spotted the three important compounds being produced in the bodies of those who either fast or eat low-carb and high-fat diet. Soon Russel Wilder termed such a diet "Ketogenic" due to its known effects of producing a high amount of ketones in the body. From that point on, the concept of ketosis prevailed. It was, however, got to the public attention as late as 1997 when Charlie Abraham's epilepsy was treated using a complete Ketogenic Diet plan. The interest of the scientific community and ordinary individuals in the study of ketogenic study came to the rise by 2007; the idea spread to up to 45 countries around the world. People actively sought this diet plan not only to treat specific diseases but also to reduce weight and avoid cardiovascular disease.

The Phases of the Ketogenic Diet:

The dietary changes never come with quick results. Our body always takes enough to process the change and then work accordingly. Switching from a carb-dependent lifestyle to a low-carb one is one huge change for our bodies. That is why the ketogenic diet's result appears after at least three to four weeks. The early time period is utilized by the body to adapt to the changes, get into ketosis, and maintain sufficient energy levels. And once the ketosis is initiated and you have completely switched to the ketogenic diet, the real challenge starts from there! And then comes the next stage. A dieter experiences different effects on the body during these phases. So, here is how you can divide the whole keto journey!

Stage 1:

So, the first phase only begins when you manage to initiate this process in the body. Let me just tell you how it will turn out for you in this first phase. Initially, it takes extra effort to force your liver to produce ketones. It is only possible when you burn and deplete the existing glycogen reserves. And that is the challenging part. Because to do so, you need to abandon all the carbs and adopt an active lifestyle to burn more calories every day. The dieter may experience mild discomfort during this phase, but with determination, strong will, and an expert's opinion, he can get through this part once the dieter gets over this keto flu or the feeling of discomfort that marks the end of phase 1.

Phase 1:

To avoid developing an electrolyte imbalance in the body, add more minerals to your diet. Eat leafy green vegetables and low-carb juicy veggies to consume magnesium, potassium, and phosphorous.

Lastly, if you are not familiar with the keto substitutes and their taste, then it is best not to use them at this stage. Start with basic low-carb recipes that you already know and like in taste. Remember, the specific goal of this phase is to get you one step closer to the ketogenic lifestyle. So, if there is anything that can put you off track, you should probably avoid it.

Stage 2: Keto-Adaption

Once your body switches to actual ketosis for energy production, the keto-adaption phase starts. Up till now, the body only has taken a turn to ketogenesis to produce ketones and release energy, but it takes a little while for other systems and organs to start working on this new fuel. In this phase, the other parts of the body learn to live on ketosis. So, in this phase, you will need to do everything that will help each cell to metabolize according to the new lifestyle.

During this phase, all those symptoms of ketosis that a person feels during the early days start to disappear. And he will start feeling better. A new positive energy kicks in, which makes the keto dieter feel more active and alive. Unlike the 'getting into ketosis' phase, the keto-adaptation is not short-lived; it all depends on your body and your effort. But once you get through this part, living on the ketogenic diet gets easier.

The human body longs for stability, routine, and balance, and it makes that happen through homeostasis. So, when you externally change the conditions or dietary factors, the body gradually starts changing according to it, and a point comes when it fully shapes itself according to those changes. And that's what happens during this phase. So, to make your body more flexible to the keto lifestyle, you need to be strategic about your carb intake. Unlike the first phase, now you need to periodically shift in and out of ketosis. It will help to instantly switch to the available source of energy to meet its need. This is the phase in which adding a few carbs to the diet might not affect the metabolism.

Carb Cycling

In the carb cycling technique, you can have some good quality carbs once a week. Select a day and pick some healthy carb sources like whole grains and sweet potatoes to have on this cheat day. By refeeding carbs occasionally, you can refill the depleted glycogen reserves in the muscles, and that can help strengthen them.

On this cheat day, you can eat roughly about 15-25 per cent of protein, 60-70 per cent of carbohydrates, and 15 per cent of fats in the diet. Whereas for the rest of the week, you need to get back on track and should only eat a low-carb diet. Yes, you can have some carb-rich fruits and vegetables on this day, but this day is not an excuse to stuff yourself with a pizza, cakes, or ice cream.

Targeted Keto Diet

This technique is suitable for those who regularly carry out high-intensity exercises. The diet and the carbohydrate intake are then adjusted around the workout schedule. So, instead of carb cycling on a random, once-in-a-week basis, in this approach, you can get to have carbs on the day of your exercise. In this way, all the excess calories will be used by the muscles. A dieter can have up to 50 grams of carbohydrates about 30 minutes before the exercise. Unlike the cyclic ketogenic diet, in this approach, you need to look for simpler and refined carbs. So that they are broken down instantly, and the energy is then utilized by the muscle cells. But set a limit to this intake and avoid over-consumption. This practice is only to provide a temporary break to your body from ketosis.

How you manage the keto-adaption period depends on your lifestyle. No matter which approach you select for yourself, remember that this going in and out of ketosis is as crucial as the diet itself in order to reach metabolic flexibility. At the end of the keto-adaption phase, you will start noticing prominent changes in your health, from weight to body mass index, your focus, attention span, memory, metabolism, everything gets better.

Stage 3: Metabolic Flexibility

The last of the ketogenic transition is termed the phase of metabolic flexibility. It is the time when your body overcomes all the challenges and masters the art of keto-adaptation. By this time, your body gets more flexible in adjusting itself according to the given fuel source. Now it knows how to work best through ketosis and how to use it for its own advantages. It also learns to adjust its metabolic pathways according to the energy source available, whether it's fat or glucose as a fuel. So now you don't need to stay strictly Keto all the time. You can continue with the carb-cycling while being on the ketogenic diet. Add exercise, healthy fats, and keto supplements to maintain the rate of ketosis in the body.

Even if you mistakenly consume some grains or carbs during this phase, your body won't even respond to it as it is adjusted itself to run on fat-sourced energy. However, a person can also lose metabolic flexibility when he starts eating a high-carb diet again on a regular basis. So, even when you are on a cyclic ketogenic diet, make sure to continue eating healthy and keep the balance of the nutrients in between the two consecutive keto-eating periods.

The Ketosis Process

The word ketosis comes from the word "ketone," it is described as the process during which fats are broken in the body to produce energy and Ketones. A high level of ketosis means a greater amount of ketones. In the absence of complex carbohydrates, the fats are forced to break down and produce ketones which are highly beneficial for active metabolism. To make this all happen, a special meal plan is required, known as the "Ketogenic diet." It describes a sum whole of all the eatables which are low in carbs and high in fats. Thus, allowing the body to extract energy directly from fats and not from glucose. The diet plan is prescribed to treat several diseases like diabetes, epilepsy, obesity, and heart problems. However, there are certain complexities related to this diet, and it should always be opted with the guidance of a professional nutritionist, at least at the beginning when it is essential to learn about the basics of ketosis and the right approach to switch to a ketogenic balanced diet.

CHAPTER 3: RECIPES

Recipe 1. Almond Halibut and Vegetable Curry

Make this delicious curry dish whenever you are craving seafood that has a bit of a fiery kick to it. Use the freshest vegetables possible for the tastiest results.

Serving Size: 4

Preparation Time: 25 minutes

Cooking Time: 1 hour

Total Time: 1 hour and 25 minutes

Ingredients:

For the base:

- 4 cups of carrot juice
- 1 cup of celery, chopped
- 1 cup of onion, chopped
- ¼ cup of ginger, peeled and chopped
- 1 cup of carrots, chopped
- 4 cloves of garlic, chopped
- 2 tablespoons of extra virgin olive oil
- 3 tablespoons of thai yellow curry paste
- 1 cup of unsweetened coconut milk
- 3 cups of bell peppers and squash, mixed together and chopped
- dash of sea salt
- dash of black pepper

For the halibut:

- ½ cup of almonds, cut into slivers
- 4, 4 ounces halibut fillets, skinless
- dash of sea salt
- 1 egg white
- 2 tablespoons of extra virgin olive oil
- basil leaves, chopped and for garnish

Directions:

- In a pot set over low to medium heat, add in 2 tablespoons of the extra virgin olive oil. Add in the chopped carrots, chopped celery, chopped onion, chopped ginger, and chopped cloves of garlic. Stir well to mix. Cook for approximately about 10 to 15 minutes or until soft.
- Increase the heat of the stove to medium to high heat. Add in the Thai curry paste. Cook for 3 minutes or until caramelized.
- Add in the carrot juice and bring to a boil.
- Strain the curry base through a sieve into a bowl. Toss out the solids. Transfer back into the pot. Add in the coconut milk and mixed chopped vegetables. Stir well to mix.
- Dip the tops of the halibut fillets in the beaten egg whites. Press into the ground almonds and place onto a plate with the crust side facing up.
- In a large-sized skillet set over medium to high heat, add in the remaining two tablespoons of extra virgin olive oil. Add in the halibut fillets with the crust side facing down and cook for approximately about 4 minutes. Flip and transfer onto a baking sheet.
- Place into the prepared preheated oven to bake for approximately about 5 minutes or until the halibut fillets are opaque.
- Remove and serve the fillets with a garnish of basil.

Nutritional Value: Calories 742 | Carbohydrates 57.6 g | Fat 39.6 g | Protein 38.6 g

Recipe 2. Beef and Bell Pepper Frittata

Yummy and tasty. This is a good family recipe, which will also make a nice meal for a group of friends. Enjoy this delicacy.

Serving Size: 4

Preparation Time: 30 minutes

Cooking Time: 55 minutes

Total Time: 1 hour 25 minutes

Ingredients:

- 1 tablespoon of butter
- 12 ounces of ground sausage made from beef
- 1/4 cup of shredded cheddar
- 12 whole eggs
- 1 cup of sour cream
- 2 bell peppers red cut into pieces
- black pepper and salt to taste

Directions:

- Preheat the oven to 350 F. Crack eggs in a blender. Add the salt, sour cream, and pepper. Then, at a low speed, blend the ingredients. Set aside. Add the beef sausage, and cook until golden brown, continually stirring and breaking the lumps into tiny pieces for approximately about 10 minutes.

- Sprinkle bell peppers on top, pour the egg mixture all over, and sprinkle top cheddar cheese. Place the skillet in the oven for approximately about at least 30 mins or so until the eggs are set, and the cheese melts. Take the frittata out, cut it into slices and serve warm with salad.

Nutritional Value: Calories 321 | Carbohydrates 6.5 g | Fat 49 g | Protein 33 g

Recipe 3. Bell Pepper Cream Pan with Pumpkin

The creamy sauce is delicious and keeps you full for a long time. The pumpkin also contributes to this: it contains few calories, but many vitamins, e.g., A, B1, B2, B6, C, and E, folic acid, and minerals such as sodium, potassium, calcium, phosphorus, magnesium, iron, and zinc. In addition, due to the high potassium content, pumpkin has a mildly dehydrating effect and stimulates digestion.

Serving Size: 4

Preparation Time: 22 minutes

Cooking Time: 30 minutes

Total Time: 52 minutes

Ingredients:

- 2 red onions
- 1 clove of garlic
- 600 grams of sliced turkey
- 2 tablespoons of oil
- 290 ml of soy cream or cooking cream
- 190 ml of water
- 2 tablespoon of Worcester sauce
- 2 tablespoon of tomato paste
- 2 red peppers
- 750 grams of pumpkin pulp (e.g., Hokkaido or butternut)
- chili powder
- salt
- 2 tablespoons of parsley (fresh or frozen)

Directions:

- Weigh the pumpkin and prick the skin with a fork. Bring to the boil in a saucepan with a bit of water and simmer over mild heat for approximately about 15 minutes.
- Cut the onions and garlic. Clean and dice the peppers. First, fry the onion cubes and garlic together with the turkey slices in a bit of oil. Then add the pepper cubes and deglaze with the soy cream or cooking cream and water. Stir in tomato paste and Worcester sauce, season with salt and chili, and let reduce.
- Drain the pumpkin and cut it into bite-sized cubes. Add this to the sliced meat in the pan and let simmer for approximately about 3 to 5 minutes until the pumpkin has the desired consistency. Sprinkle with parsley and serve.

Nutritional Value: Calories 241 | Carbohydrates 1.1 g | Fat 17.7 g | Protein 18.8 g

Recipe 4. Butternut Squash Soup

Yummy and tasty. This is a good family recipe, which will also make a nice meal for a group of friends. Enjoy this delicacy.

Serving Size: 4

Preparation Time: 31 minutes

Cooking Time: 1 hour

Total Time: 1 hour 31 minutes

Ingredients:

- 1 medium-large butternut squash (about 2 cups diced)
- 2 cups of chicken stock (or veggie stock)
- 1/2 cup of coconut milk (optional)
- 1/2 onion (white, yellow, or sweet)
- 1/2 large carrot
- 1/2 celery stalk
- 1 cinnamon stick
- Ground black pepper, to taste
- Celtic sea salt, to taste
- 2 tablespoons of coconut oil (or bacon fat)
- 2 tablespoons of bacon fat (or coconut oil)

Directions:

- Heat oven to 375 degrees F. Heat medium cast iron pan over medium-high heat. Add bacon fat to a hot oiled pan.
- Peel squash and remove seeds. Dice and add to the hot oiled pan with salt and pepper to taste. 3 to 4 minutes, or until golden. Place pan in oven and roast until browned on all sides, approximately about 15 minutes.
- Heat medium pot over medium-low heat. Add coconut oil to the hot pot.
- Peel and dice onion, celery, and carrot. Add to hot oiled pot with cinnamon stick, salt, and pepper to taste.

- Remove squash from the oven and let cool slightly. Add food processor or high-speed blender and process until puréed.
- Add chicken broth to the pot.
- Stir in squash purée and simmer for approximately about 10 minutes.
- Blend the mixture and stir in coconut milk (optional). Transfer to serving dish. Sprinkle with cracked black pepper. Serve hot.

Nutritional Value: Calories 460 | Carbohydrates 35.8 g | Fat 17.9 g | Protein 37.8 g

Recipe 5. Carrot Cake Quinoa

A delicious twist for a busy day. This recipe is healthy, delicious, and perfect for diet! It is a simple side dish that is ideal for a large holiday feast or a straightforward meal! The result is tender, juicy, and flavorful.

Serving Size: 16

Preparation Time: 15 minutes

Cooking Time: 15 minutes

Total Time: 30 minutes

Ingredients:

- 1 tablespoon of flaxseed meal + 3 tablespoon water
- 1/4 cup of pure maple syrup
- 1 teaspoon of cinnamon
- 1 teaspoon of baking powder
- 1/2 cup of cashew butter or nut/seed butter of choice
- 1/2 cup of quinoa flakes
- 3/4 cup of shredded carrots
- 1 medium banana mashed
- 1/2 teaspoon of nutmeg
- 1/2 cup of rolled oats
- 1 flax egg
- 1/4 teaspoon of salt
- 1 teaspoon of vanilla extract

Directions:

- Place the flaxseed meal in a small bowl, add water and whisk well. Set aside.
- Combine the banana cashew butter, vanilla, and syrup in a large bowl, add the flaxseed meal mixture and mix well.
- Add the quinoa flakes, baking powder, oats, spices, and salt and stir well. Add shredded carrots.
- Place 2 tablespoon of the dough into the prepared baking sheets, continue with the dough until no more dough.
- Place the baking sheets in the heated oven and bake until golden brown for approximately about 17 minutes.
- Remove from preheated oven and let it cool on the pan for approximately about 5 minutes before placing on a wire rack to cool down completely. Serve warm and enjoy!

Nutritional Value: Calories 108 | Carbohydrates 12 g | Fat 5 g | Protein 2 g

Recipe 6. Cheese Soup with Mushrooms

A spicy soup with a delicious cheese flavor. In addition, there are protein and iron as well as vitamin D. Parmesan also naturally contains the flavor enhancer glutamate. This arises during ripening and provides an intense aroma. Don't worry, and this glutamate won't harm you. On the contrary, it helps the cheese to sustainably satisfy the taste buds and protect you from food cravings for a long time. So, this soup is not only a treat for the body, but really for all the senses.

Serving Size: 4

Preparation Time: 18 minutes

Cooking Time: 30 minutes

Total Time: 48 minutes

Ingredients:

- 2 onions
- 150 grams of cocktail tomatoes
- 350 grams of mushrooms
- 3 tablespoons of oil
- 2 cloves of garlic
- 750 ml of vegetable broth
- 250 ml of white wine
- 200 grams of Parmesan or Emmentaler cheese, grated
- 200 ml of soy cream or cooking cream
- Salt
- Pepper
- Nutmeg (as desired)
- 4 tablespoons of chives, chopped
- 12 borage flowers (if available)

Directions:

- Finely dice the onions, quarter the mushrooms, dice the tomatoes and finely chop the garlic.
- Sweat the onion cubes in a bit of oil, add the garlic. Deglaze with the wine and stock, simmer for approximately about 7 minutes.

- In the meantime, fry the mushrooms in a bit of oil, add the tomatoes and fry for approximately about a few minutes: salt and pepper.
- Dissolve the cheese in the soup, pour over the soy cream or cooking cream. Beat the soup with a hand blender until frothy, season with salt, pepper, and nutmeg to taste.
- Serve the soup with the tomato and mushroom vegetables and sprinkle with chives and the borage flowers.

Nutritional Value: Calories 742 | Carbohydrates 57.6 g | Fat 39.6 g | Protein 38.6 g

Recipe 7. Cheesy Mashed Sweet Potato Cakes

It is an easy and exciting casserole for all low-carb dieters, containing layers of meat, vegetables, and cheese. It's a nutritious meal and a good dish for potlucks. Enjoy this delicious casserole with family and friends!

Serving Size: 4

Preparation Time: 10 minutes

Cooking Time: 30 minutes

Total Time: 40 minutes

Ingredients:

- ¾ cup of breadcrumbs
- 4 cups of mashed potatoes
- ½ cup of onions
- 2 cups of grated mozzarella cheese
- ¼ cup of fresh grated parmesan cheese
- 2 large cloves finely chopped
- 1 egg
- 2 teaspoons of finely chopped parsley
- Salt and pepper to taste

Directions:

- Line your baking sheet with foil. Wash, peel and cut the prepared sweet potatoes into 6 pieces. Arrange them inside the baking sheet and drizzle a small amount of oil on top before seasoning with salt and pepper.
- Cover with a baking sheet and bake it for approximately about 45 minutes. Once cooked transfer them into a mixing bowl and mash them well with a potato masher.
- To the sweet potatoes in a bowl add green onions, parmesan, mozzarella, garlic, egg, parsley, and breadcrumbs. Mash and combine the mixture together using the masher.
- Put the remaining ¼ cup of the breadcrumbs in a place. Scoop a teaspoon of mixture into your palm and form round patties around ½ and inch thick.
- Oil and heat the pan to cook the patties in batches 4 or 5 per session and cook each side for approximately about 6 minutes until they turn golden brown. Using a spoon or spatula flip them. Add oil to prevent burning.

Nutritional Value: Calories 126 | Carbohydrates 15 g | Fat 6 g | Protein 3 g

Recipe 8. Chicken Casserole

The chicken can be prepared and enjoyed in thousands of different ways. But sometimes, it is industrially deformed to the point that only the word "chicken" on the packaging enables us to know what it is … it's a shame! So, give yourself the pleasure of a real chicken and enjoy without excess.

Serving Size: 4

Preparation Time: 25 minutes

Cooking Time: 1 hour 10 minutes

Total Time: 1 hour 35 minutes

Ingredients:

- 1 whole chicken, cut into 8 pieces
- 2 tablespoons of olive oil
- 1 onion, chopped
- 2 garlic cloves, crushed
- 1 green and red pepper, cut into strips
- 1 large canned of chopped tomatoes
- 4 large potatoes, cut into four pieces, each of them
- ½ cup of white wine
- 6 ounces of black olives, stoned
- 1 bay leaf
- Salt and pepper

Directions:

- Warm up olive oil in a large saucepan. Place the chicken pieces and fry until golden brown on all sides. Add the green and red peppers and tomatoes. Re-add the chicken to the pan.
- Pour the white wine and add the thyme and bay leaf. Add potatoes and black olives.
- Bring to the boil and reduce to low heat. Cook and simmer for approximately about 45 minutes. Stir occasionally. Serve immediately and enjoy it.

Nutritional Value: Calories 355 | Carbohydrates 6 g | Fat 31 g | Protein 20 g

Recipe 9. Chicken Souvlaki

A delicious twist for a busy day. This recipe is healthy, delicious, and perfect for diet! It is a simple side dish that is ideal for a large holiday feast or a straightforward meal! The result is tender, juicy, and flavorful.

Serving Size: 4

Preparation Time: 10 minutes

Cooking Time: 5 minutes

Total Time: 15 minutes

Ingredients:

- 4 pieces (6-inch) pitas, cut into halves
- 2 cups of roasted chicken breast skinless, and sliced
- 1/4 cup of red onion, thinly sliced
- 1/2 teaspoon of dried oregano
- 1/2 cup of Greek yogurt, plain
- 1/2 cup of plum tomato, chopped
- 1/2 cup of cucumber, peeled, chopped
- 1/2 cup (2 ounces) feta cheese, crumbled
- 1 tablespoon of olive oil, extra-virgin, divided
- 1 tablespoon of fresh dill, chopped
- 1 cup of iceberg lettuce, shredded
- 1 1/4 teaspoons of minced garlic, bottled, divided

Directions:

- In a large-sized mixing bowl, combine the yogurt, cheese, 1 teaspoon of the olive oil, and 1/4 teaspoon of the garlic until well mixed. Oil and heat the pan.
- Add the remaining 1 teaspoon garlic and the oregano: sauté for approximately about 20 seconds. Add the chicken; cook for approximately about 2 minutes or until the chicken are heated through. Put 1/4 cup chicken into each pita halves. Top with 2 tablespoons yogurt mix, 2 tablespoons lettuce, 1 tablespoon tomato, and 1 tablespoon cucumber. Divide the onion between the pita halves.

Nutritional Value: Calories 414 | Carbohydrates 38 g | Fat 6.4 g | Protein 32.3 g

Recipe 10. Cream of Mushroom Soup

Yummy and tasty. This is a good family recipe, which will also make a nice meal for a group of friends. Enjoy this delicacy.

Serving Size: 4

Preparation Time: 15 minutes

Cooking Time: 30 minutes

Total Time: 45 minutes

Ingredients:

- 3 cups of vegetable broth (or chicken broth)
- 1 can (13.5 ounces of) full-fat coconut milk
- 4 cups of mushrooms (white, baby Bella, etc.)
- 1/2 onion (yellow or white)
- 1 garlic clove
- 1 teaspoon of ground white pepper (or ground black pepper)
- 2 teaspoons of Celtic Sea salt
- 2 tablespoons of bacon fat (or coconut oil)

Directions:

- Oil and heat the pan, Add 1 tablespoon fat to the hot pot.
- Slice 1 cup mushrooms and add to pot. Add remaining fat to the hot pot. Reduce heat to medium.
- Peel and chop onions and garlic. Add to hot oiled pot and sauté until fragrant and lightly browned, approximately about 5 minutes. Add whole mushrooms to the pot and sauté until lightly browned and tender, approximately about 8 to 10 minutes.
- Transfer mushrooms, onion, and garlic to a food processor or high-speed blender with vegetable broth, coconut milk, salt, and pepper. Process until smooth, approximately about 1 to 2 minutes. Or add vegetable broth, coconut milk, salt, and pepper to pot and purée with an immersion blender. Heat pot over medium heat. Add reserved sliced mushrooms to the pot and stir to combine. Bring to simmer and heat through approximately about 8 to 10 minutes.
- Transfer to serving dish and serve hot.

Nutritional Value: Calories 302 | Carbohydrates 15.7 g | Fat 8.9 g | Protein 18 g

Recipe 11. Eggplant Lasagna

The flavor is quite impressive! This recipe is very colorful and delicious. This dish is loaded with cheesy and savory flavors that you love.

Serving Size: 6

Preparation Time: 20 minutes

Cooking Time: 1 hour

Total Time: 1 hour 20 minutes

Ingredients:

- 1 medium eggplant, cut into ¼ inch slices
- 2 tablespoons of lemon juice
- 1 cup of fat-free mozzarella cheese, shredded
- Cooking spray
- 2 cups of tomato sauce
- 1 can of whole tomatoes, chopped
- ¼ cup of fat-free Parmesan cheese, grated
- 2 cloves of garlic, minced
- ¼ teaspoon of red chili flakes
- 1 tablespoon of basil
- 1/3 cup of breadcrumbs
- 1 cup of fat-free ricotta cheese
- 1 tablespoon of oregano

Directions:

- Brush eggplant slices with lemon juice, place on baking sheet (after coating sheet with cooking spray). Cook until tender, approximately about 10 minutes, turning after approximately about 5 minutes.
- Combine chili flakes, chopped tomatoes, oregano, garlic, tomato sauce, and basil in a bowl. Set aside. Combine Parmesan and breadcrumbs in a bowl. Set aside.
- Combine ricotta and mozzarella in a bowl. Set aside.
- Coat 9-inch square pan with cooking spray. Begin with a layer of the sauce mixture, then the eggplant slices, then ricotta and mozzarella cheese mixture. Bake for approximately about 45 minutes.

Nutritional Value: Calories 170 | Carbohydrates 24 g | Fat 0.5 g | Protein 14 g

Recipe 12. Eight Layer Casserole

It's a nutritious meal and a good dish for potlucks.

Serving Size: 12

Preparation Time: 30 minutes

Cooking Time: 1 hour 15 minutes

Total Time: 1 hour 45 minutes

Ingredients:

- 1 pound of frozen home-style egg noodles
- 2 pounds of ground beef
- 2 cans (15 ounces of each) tomato sauce
- 1 tablespoon of dried minced onion
- 2 teaspoons of sugar
- 2 teaspoons of Italian seasoning, dried basil, and dried parsley flakes
- 1-1/2 teaspoons of garlic powder
- 1 teaspoon of salt
- 1/2 teaspoon of pepper
- 1 package (8 ounces) cream cheese, softened
- 1 cup (8 ounces) sour cream
- 1/2 cup of milk
- 2 packages (10 ounces of each) frozen chopped spinach, thawed and squeezed dry
- 1 cup of shredded compound of Monterey Jack cheese
- 1 cup of shredded cheddar cheese

Directions:

- Cook noodles following the instruction of the package.
- Oil and heat the pan then cook beef until there is not pink anymore; and then drain. Add sugar, tomato sauce, seasonings, and onion. Allow to boil. Decrease heat; cover while simmering for approximately about around 10 minutes. Combine in a small bowl with sour cream, milk, and cream cheese.
- In a greased baking dish of 13 x 9-inch, place half of the noodles; have 3 cups meat mixture to top. Layer in order with cream cheese mixture, spinach and remaining meat mixture then noodles. Have cheeses to sprinkle (dish will be full).
- . Allow 10 minutes to rest before serving.

Nutritional Value: Calories 382 | Carbohydrates 9.7 g | Fat 13 g | Protein 15 g

Recipe 13. Grilled Chicken Wings

Tasty and yummy.

Serving Size: 10

Preparation Time: 40 minutes

Cooking Time: 30 minutes

Total Time: 1 hour 10 minutes

Ingredients:

- 4 ears fresh corn, halved
- 2 tablespoon of cider vinegar
- 1 pieces of chipotle pepper in adobo, finely chopped
- Zest and lime of 1 pc lime
- 1 tablespoon of dark brown sugar
- ¼ cup of cilantro, chopped
- Kosher salt and black pepper to taste
- 2 teaspoons of Worcestershire sauce
- ½ cup of ketchup
- 2 tablespoon of olive oil, divided
- 3 pounds of chicken wings, split
- 1 ounce of feta cheese, crumbled

- ½ cup of sour cream

Directions:

- Preheat the grill on medium.
- Combine sugar, ketchup, Worcestershire sauce, cider vinegar, and chopped chipotle in a small bowl.
- Mix sour cream, crumbled feta, freshly chopped cilantro, lime zest and juice until combined. Set aside both sauces.
- Toss chicken wings with a tablespoon of oil, plus some salt and pepper.
- Grill chicken wings for 12 minutes, covered, until charred and cooked through, turning occasionally. Pop the corn on the grill as well.
- Baste both the chicken wings and corn with some prepared Worcestershire mixture while grilling, reserve the remaining in a small bowl.
- Transfer the wings and the corn in a serving platter and serve with the sour cream mixture and the remaining Worcestershire mixture.

Nutritional Value: Calories 742 | Carbohydrates 57.6 g | Fat 39.6 g | Protein 38.6 g

Recipe 14. Keto Pizza Casserole

It is an easy and exciting casserole for all low-carb dieters, containing layers of meat, vegetables, and cheese.

Serving Size: 6

Preparation Time: 20 minutes

Cooking Time: 43 minutes

Total Time: 1 hour 3 minutes

Ingredients:

- 1 pound of ground Italian sausage
- 1 red bell pepper, chopped
- ½ medium white onion, finely chopped
- 1 cup of sliced cremini mushrooms
- 6 garlic cloves, minced
- Salt and black pepper to taste
- 2 tablespoons of Italian seasoning
- 1 can of diced tomatoes, not drained
- 1 cup of ricotta cheese
- 2 cups of grated mozzarella cheese
- 1 cup of grated Parmesan cheese
- 1 cup of sliced pepperonis
- ½ cup of sliced black olives

Directions:

- Preheat oven to 375 degrees F. Then, using cooking spray, butter a casserole dish. Cook sausage in a medium-sized skillet over medium heat for approximately about 10 minutes or until brown. Transfer to a plate. Stir-fry bell pepper, onion, mushrooms, garlic, and cook for about 3 minutes or until tender; season with salt, black pepper, and Italian seasoning.
- In this order, spread half each of sausage, vegetables, tomatoes, ricotta cheese, mozzarella cheese, Parmesan cheese, pepperonis, and olives. Layer a second time in the same manner. Cover with foil and bake for 20 minutes

Nutritional Value: Calories 434 | Carbohydrates 6 g | Fat 26 g | Protein 42 g

Recipe 15. Mixed Seafood Lasagna

This is going to be the highlight of your next dinner!

Serving Size: 6

Preparation Time: 30 minutes

Cooking Time: 50 minutes

Total Time: 1 hour 20 minutes

Ingredients:

- 15 ounces of milk
- 1 garlic clove, minced
- 2 bay leaves
- 2 ounces of butter, melted
- 1 teaspoon of mustard
- 2 ounces of white flour
- A pinch of salt and black pepper
- 14 ounces of no-cook lasagna noodles
- 2 tablespoons of tarragon, chopped
- 14 ounces of mixed salmon, cod, and mussels, chopped
- A handful spinach, chopped
- 5 ounces of cheddar, grated
- 3 ounces of parmesan, grated

Directions:

- Oil and heat the milk add the bay leaves and the garlic, stir, and bring to a simmer. Heat a pot with the butter over medium heat, add the flour, whisk for about 2 minutes, and take the heat. Discard bay leaves from the milk, add to pan with the butter and whisk well. Add salt, pepper, and the mustard, whisk well again, and leave aside.
- In a bowl, mix fish, seafood, tarragon, and spinach with some sauce and stir. Continue with the layers

until you finish all the ingredients, sprinkle the cheddar and the parmesan, bake at 360 degrees F for approximately about 40 minutes, cool down a bit, slice and serve. Enjoy!

Nutritional Value: Calories 460 | Carbohydrates 35.8 g | Fat 17.9 g | Protein 37.8 g

Recipe 16. Penne and Sausage Casseroles

This casserole featuring mushrooms, sausage, and cheese is always a hit.

Serving Size: 2

Preparation Time: 20 minutes

Cooking Time: 50 minutes

Total Time: 1 hour 10 minutes

Ingredients:

- 1 - 1/2 pounds of uncooked penne pasta
- 1 pound of Johnsonville Ground Mild Italian sausage
- 1 pound of sliced fresh mushrooms
- 1 large onion, chopped
- 3 tablespoons of olive oil
- 6 garlic cloves, minced
- 1 tablespoon of dried oregano
- 1-1/2 cups dry red wine or beef broth, divided
- 2 cans (14-1/2 ounces of each) stewed tomatoes, cut up
- 1 can (15 ounces) tomato sauce
- 1 cup of beef broth
- 4 cups of shredded part-skim mozzarella cheese
- 4 cups of shredded fontina cheese
- Minced fresh parsley, optional

Directions:

- Cook the pasta following the package instructions. In the meantime, on medium heat, cook sausage in a Dutch oven until it is not pink; drain and set the sausage aside.
- Sauté onion and mushrooms in the same Dutch oven with oil until tender. Put it on oregano and garlic; cook for approximately about another minute. Mix in a cup of wine, then boil. Cook until the liquid reduces by 1/2. Mix in the remaining wine, tomatoes, sausage, broth, and tomato sauce, boil. Lower heat: let it simmer while covered for approximately about 15 mins.
- Drain the pasta. In each of two greased 13-in by 9-in baking dishes, slather half a cup of sauce. Split 1/2 of the pasta among the dishes; arrange each in a layer with 2 1/2 cups sauce and a cup each of the cheeses. Repeat the layers.
- Bake for approximately about 25 mins at 350 degrees while covered. Remove the cover, then bake for approximately about another 5 - 10 mins until the cheese is melted and bubbly. If desired, garnish with parsley.

Nutritional Value: Calories 280 | Carbohydrates 24 g | Fat 5 g | Protein 9 g

Recipe 17. Pepper and Egg Curry

This curry recipe is so quick and easy to finish your leftover hard-cooked eggs.

Serving Size: 4

Preparation Time: 20 minutes

Cooking Time: 30 minutes

Total Time: 50 minutes

Ingredients:

- 2 teaspoons of canola oil
- 1 onion, chopped
- 1 green bell pepper, 1-inch dice
- 1 jalapeño pepper, chopped
- 2 teaspoons of finely chopped fresh ginger
- 2 tablespoons of all-purpose flour
- 1 tablespoon of curry powder
- 1 teaspoon of ground cumin
- 2 cups of chicken broth
- ¼ cup of nonfat plain yogurt
- 2 tablespoons of chopped fresh parsley, divided
- 2 teaspoons of lemon juice
- 4 hard-cooked eggs, wedges

Directions:

- Heat the oil in the big saucepan on medium heat. Put in the bell pepper and onion; cook and stir for approximately about roughly 5 minutes or till onions start to color. Put in the ginger and jalapeno; mix for approximately about 60 seconds. Whisk in the cumin, curry powder and flour and cook for approximately about 60 seconds. Slowly stir in the broth; cook while stirring for approximately about roughly 60 seconds or till becoming thick and smooth.
- Take pan out of heat and mix in the lemon juice, 1.5 tablespoon of parsley, and yogurt. Stir the eggs to sauce. Sprinkle on remaining half a tablespoon of the parsley and serve.

Nutritional Value: Calories 300 | Carbohydrates 14 g | Fat 4.5 g | Protein 14 g

Recipe 18. Peppercorn Crusted Filet Mignon

The flavor is quite impressive! This recipe is very colorful and delicious. This dish is loaded with cheesy and savory flavors that you love.

Serving Size: 2

Preparation Time: 5 minutes

Cooking Time: 5 minutes

Total Time: 10 minutes

Ingredients:

- 2 (6 ounces) filet mignon steaks
- 1 tablespoon of coconut oil
- 1 tablespoon of black peppercorns
- 1/2 teaspoon of sea salt
- 1 tablespoon of coconut oil

Directions:

- Heat a medium pan over medium-high heat and add 1 tablespoon coconut oil.
- Place peppercorns in a plastic kitchen bag or parchment pouch and place on cutting board another counter. Crack peppercorns with a heavy rolling pin or pan until broken.
- Add cracked peppercorns to the small mixing bowl with coconut oil and mix to combine.
- Sprinkle steaks with salt, then rub with peppercorn mixture, coating evenly on both sides.
- Place seasoned steaks in a hot oiled pan and cook for approximately about 2 - 4 minutes per side, for rare to medium-rare. Carefully flip halfway through cooking and disturb only this once.
- Transfer seared steaks a cutting board and let rest for approximately about at least 5 minutes.
- Serve warm with your favorite grilled veggies. Or slice with a sharp knife and serve.

Nutritional Value: Calories 170 | Carbohydrates 24 g | Fat 0.5 g | Protein 14 g

Recipe 19. Pesto Veggie Pinwheels

Yummy and tasty. This is a good family recipe, which will also make a nice meal for a group of friends. Enjoy this delicacy.

Serving Size: 4

Preparation Time: 10 minutes

Cooking Time: 40 minutes

Total Time: 50 minutes

Ingredients:

- 3 whole eggs
- 1 egg, beaten for brushing
- 1 cup of grated cheese
- 1 cup of almond flour
- 3 tablespoons of coconut flour
- 4 tablespoons of cream cheese, softened
- 1/4 teaspoon of yogurt
- 1 cup of cold butter
- 1 cup of mushrooms, chopped
- 1 cup of basil pesto
- 2 cups of baby spinach
- Salt to taste

Directions:

- Mix coconut and almond flour, Xanthan gum, and 1/2 teaspoon salt in a bowl. Add cream cheese, yogurt, and butter; mix until it is crumbly. Incorporate three eggs in succession and mix until the dough is formed into an oval. Make the dough flat on a flat, clean surface, wrap it in plastic wrap and chill for an hour.
- Dust a clean, flat area with almond flour. Cut off the dough and then roll out to 15x12 inches. Spread pesto over the top using a spatula, leaving a 2-inch border along one side. A bowl mixes baby mushrooms and spinach, season with salt and black pepper, and spreads the mixture on top of the pesto. Sprinkle with cheese, and wrap as tightly as possible, starting at the lower end. Refrigerate for approximately about 10 minutes. Preheat the oven to 350 F. Take the pastry from the fridge onto a flat surface, and then use the sharp edge of a knife, cut it into 24 small discs. Lay them out in a baking tray, brush with the remaining egg and bake for approximately about 25 minutes until they are golden. Allow cooling.

Nutritional Value: Calories 241 | Carbohydrates 3.4 g | Fat 39 g | Protein 20 g

Recipe 20. Prosciutto Vegetable Egg Cups

I like to make a bigger batch of these delicious breakfast bombs on weekends to store in the refrigerator for those busy weekday mornings. They are super convenient to heat up and even eat on the go! The vegetable combinations of this recipe are limitless—play with your favorite veggie combos and make this recipe uniquely yours.

Serving Size: 2

Preparation Time: 15 minutes

Cooking Time: 20 minutes

Total Time: 35 minutes

Ingredients:

- Extra-virgin olive oil for greasing
- 4 prosciutto slices
- ½ cup of shredded mozzarella cheese
- ¼ cup of heavy (whipping) cream
- ½ Roma (plum) tomato, diced
- 2 large eggs
- ¼ green bell pepper, diced
- 1 tablespoon of chopped scallions, green tops only
- 2 to 3 fresh basil leaves, chopped
- ¼ teaspoon of sea salt
- ½ teaspoon of freshly ground black pepper

Directions:

- Preheat the oven to 375°F. Grease 4 cups of a standard muffin tin with oil. Line each cup with one slice of prosciutto until fully covered, overlapping if necessary. In a medium bowl, whisk together the mozzarella, cream, tomato, eggs, bell pepper, scallion greens, basil, salt, and black pepper. Evenly divide the egg batter among the cups.
- Bake for about 15 to 20 minutes until the eggs are cooked throughout and golden. Cool for 5 minutes in the pan on a wire rack. Set 2 egg cups each on two plates and serve warm.

Nutritional Value: Calories 170 | Carbohydrates 24 g | Fat 0.5 g | Protein 14 g

Recipe 21. Rigatoni and Spicy Sausage Casserole

A baked Rigatoni recipe with mushrooms.

Serving Size: 6

Preparation Time: 20 minutes

Cooking Time: 1 hour

Total Time: 1 hour 20 minutes

Ingredients:

- 4 ounces of hot Italian sausage
- 1 teaspoon of extra-virgin olive oil
- 1 large onion, chopped
- 3 cloves of garlic, very finely chopped
- 8 ounces of mushrooms, sliced
- 1 teaspoon of crumbled dried rosemary
- 2 14-ounces cans of diced tomatoes, or plum tomatoes (chopped)
- ¼ cup of dry red or white wine
- ½ teaspoon of salt, divided
- Freshly ground pepper, to taste
- 12 ounces of whole-wheat rigatoni, mostaccioli or penne
- ½ cup of part-skim ricotta cheese
- ¾ cup of fresh breadcrumbs, preferably whole-wheat
- ¼ cup of freshly grated Parmesan cheese

Directions:

- Set the oven at a heat of 400°F to preheat. Use cooking spray to coat a 3-quart shallow baking dish. Place on a large pot of water to boil.
- Break sausage into a large nonstick skillet into crumbles (remove the casing); over medium heat, cook and stir for approximately about 5 - 7 minutes, or until cooked through and browned. Allow to drain in a paper towel-lined basin.
- Next, wipe out the pan, pour in oil, and heat over medium-high heat. Put in onion and cook for approximately about 5 minutes, occasionally stirring, until softened. Add garlic and cook, stirring, for approximately about around 1 minute more. Place in rosemary and mushrooms; keep cooking and stirring for approximately about 3 minutes longer, or until the mushrooms start to give off the liquid. Stir in the cooked sausage, wine, and tomatoes (and their juices). Bring to a simmer; uncover and cook for approximately about 5 minutes. (The sauce will be thin.) Dust with pepper and 1/4 teaspoon of salt to season.
- Meanwhile, cook pasta for approximately about 8 to 10 minutes or following the package directions, or until just tender. Drain.
- Put the pasta into the sauce and toss to coat. Scatter 1/2 in the coated baking dish. Next, dot with spoonful of ricotta and lay the leftover pasta on top. Use foil to cover and bake for 20 minutes.
- Combine Parmesan and breadcrumbs in a small bowl. Dust with pepper and the leftover 1/4 teaspoon of salt to season. Then sprinkle the pasta with the breadcrumb mixture; uncover and continue to bake for approximately about 10 minutes more, or until the top is golden.

Nutritional Value: Calories 241 | Carbohydrates 1.1 g | Fat 17.7 g | Protein 18.8 g

Recipe 22. Scallop, Bacon, and Pea Pasta

This pasta is a mash-up of comfort food and ocean freshness! Bay scallops are small round scallops and are the most affordable of the scallop varieties. They are the perfect size for a pasta dish and cook up very quickly. This dish is finished with peas, Parmesan, and parsley for a light-tasting, healthy meal.

Serving Size: 6

Preparation Time: 30 minutes

Cooking Time: 25 minutes

Total Time: 55 minutes

Ingredients:

- 8 ounces of whole-grain linguine
- 3 slices of bacon, chopped
- 5 tablespoons of extra-virgin olive oil, divided
- 1 pound of bay scallops, cleaned and dried
- 1 ½ teaspoons of kosher salt or sea salt, divided
- ½ teaspoon of freshly ground black pepper, divided
- 6 to 7 garlic cloves, minced
- 4 tablespoons of all-purpose flour
- 1 ½ cups of unsalted seafood stock
- 1 cup of milk
- 1 cup of frozen spring peas
- 1 teaspoon of dry mustard
- ½ teaspoon of celery salt
- ¼ teaspoon of cayenne pepper
- Zest and juice of ½ medium lemon
- ¼ cup of freshly grated Parmesan cheese
- ¼ cup of fresh flat-leaf Italian parsley leaves, chopped

Directions:

- Bring a large pot of water to a boil. Cook the pasta according to package directions. Reserve ¼ cup pasta water and drain the rest. Set pasta aside.
- Heat a Dutch oven or large skillet over medium heat. Add the chopped bacon and cook for approximately about 8 to 10 minutes, frequently stirring, until the bacon is crispy. Spoon onto a paper towel-lined plate. Discard the bacon fat.
- In the same pot or skillet, heat 3 tablespoons of olive oil. Add the scallops and cook for approximately about 2 – 3 minutes, or until lightly browned on the outside. Remove from pan and serve with bacon.
- Sauté 1 – 2 minutes until aromatic with the remaining 2 tablespoons olive oil and garlic.
- Stir in the flour and simmer for approximately about 1–2 minutes, until the roux is lightly colored. Turn the heat up to medium-high and whisk in the stock. Slowly whisk in the milk and saved pasta liquid, then continue to whisk until the sauce has thickened.
- Stir in the peas, remaining 1 teaspoon salt, remaining ¼ teaspoon black pepper, dry mustard, celery salt, cayenne pepper, lemon zest and juice, and Parmesan cheese. Stir in the scallops, bacon, and parsley.

Nutritional Value: Calories 302 | Carbohydrates 15.7 g | Fat 8.9 g | Protein 18 g

Recipe 23. Scalloped Creamy Oysters

The heavy cream, leeks and dry vermouth add depth and richness to this delicious dish. The crushed saltines give it an added crunch.

Serving Size: 8

Preparation Time: 28 minutes

Cooking Time: 1 hour 10 minutes

Total Time: 1 hour 38 minutes

Ingredients:

- 4 tablespoons of butter, unsalted
- 2 halved, trimmed, thin-sliced leeks
- 1 tablespoon of flour, all-purpose
- 1/2 cup of vermouth, dry
- 1/2 cup of cream, heavy
- 2 x 16-ounces of containers of drained oysters, fresh, with 2 tablespoons of brine reserved
- 20 crushed saltines

Directions:

- Oil and heat the pan. Add the leeks. Stir occasionally while cooking till tender, six to seven minutes. Add the flour. Stir and cook for one minute.
- Add the vermouth. Stir and cook till bubbly and thickened, two to three minutes. Add the cream. Return to simmer. Remove from the heat. Fold in the oysters in brine.
- Transfer the mixture to 11" x 7" casserole dish. Top with saltine crumbles. Bake till bubbly around edges and golden brown, approximately about 40 to 45 minutes. Allow to stand for five minutes and serve.

Nutritional Value: Calories 241 | Carbohydrates 1.1 g | Fat 17.7 g | Protein 18.8 g

Recipe 24. Sea Scallops with Pesto-White Wine Sauce

Scallops, pesto, and white wine—a trio that was meant to be!

Serving Size: 2

Preparation Time: 25 minutes

Cooking Time: 15 minutes

Total Time: 40 minutes

Ingredients:

- ½ cup of low-sodium vegetable stock
- 1 teaspoon of ground black pepper
- 4 garlic cloves, chopped
- ½ teaspoon of sea salt
- ¼ cup of low-carb dry white wine
- 2 tablespoons of pesto
- 2 tablespoons of avocado oil or extra-virgin olive oil
- 3 cups of zoodles (spiralized zucchini)
- ¼ cup of grape tomatoes halved
- 8 ounces of sea scallops
- ¼ cup of thinly sliced fresh basil
- ½ lemon

Directions:

- Season the scallops with salt and pepper. In a pan, Add the scallops and cook on each side for approximately about 2 to 3 minutes, until golden brown.
- Add the vegetable stock and wine and simmer for approximately about 2 minutes, stirring and scraping up any bits from the bottom of the pan. Stir in the pesto. Add the zoodles and tomatoes and mix well. Return the scallops to the pan and cover with a lid for approximately about 30 seconds to a minute to warm them up. Divide evenly between two bowls. Garnish with fresh basil, squeeze the lemon juice over the dish, and serve.

Nutritional Value: Calories 241 | Carbohydrates 1.1 g | Fat 17.7 g | Protein 18.8 g

Recipe 25. Serrano Ham Frittata with Salad

Yummy and tasty. This is a good family recipe, which will also make a nice meal for a group of friends. Enjoy this delicacy.

Serving Size: 2

Preparation Time: 10 minutes

Cooking Time: 25 minutes

Total Time: 35 minutes

Ingredients:

- 2 tablespoons of olive oil
- 3 slices of serrano ham, chopped
- 1 tomato, cut into chunks
- 1 cucumber, sliced
- 1 small red onion cut into slices
- 1 tablespoon of balsamic vinegar
- 4 eggs, beaten
- 1 cup of Swiss Chard Chopped
- Black pepper and salt to taste
- 1 green onion cut into slices

Directions:

- Whisk together vinegar, one tablespoon of olive oil, and pepper into the salad bowl. Add the tomatoes and red onion, and the cucumber, and mix with olive oil to coat. Sprinkle with serrano ham. The remaining olive oil is heated in a skillet over medium-high temperatures. Cook onions and Swiss Chard for three minutes.
- Add salt and pepper, cooking for two minutes. Pour the eggs into the top, lower the heat to a simmer, cover, then simmer for four minutes. Transfer the pan into the oven. Bake until the top is golden within approximately about 5 minutes, at 390 F. Serve the salad sliced and served alongside the salad.

Nutritional Value: Calories 354 | Carbohydrates 7 g | Fat 26 g | Protein 20 g

Recipe 26. Spinach Dumplings

Spinach is without a doubt one of the healthiest green veggies available. To add to its already impressive list of advantages, here's a dish made using steam that is guaranteed to wow you with its tastes. So don't waste any more time and try a healthier version of the traditional dumplings by following the instructions below.

Serving Size: 2

Preparation Time: 28 minutes

Cooking Time: 1 hour 10 minutes

Total Time: 1 hour 38 minutes

Ingredients:

- 8.8 ounces of flour

- ¼ cup of cold water
- 1 tablespoon of tiny prawns (dried)
- Handful rice noodles (vermicelli)
- 2 eggs
- ⅛ cup of chopped parsley
- ¼ cup of boiling water
- 8.8 ounces of rinsed and chopped spinach
- 3 mushrooms (finely diced)
- Salt, to taste
- ½ teaspoon of sugar
- Pepper, to taste
- 2 teaspoons of Sesame oil

Directions:

- Pour warm water into a dish and soak rice noodles and prawns in it until soft.
- Chop both ingredients into tiny bits in a food processor.
- In a separate dish, whisk together all the eggs and cook until dry scrambled.
- Combine prawns, noodles, spinach, eggs, mushrooms, and parsley in a mixing bowl, then season with salt, pepper, sugar, and sesame oil. Set aside the bowl.
- To create the dumpling wrappers, combine flour and boiling water in a mixing bowl, then add cold water while stirring to form a dough.
- Knead the dough until smooth, then cover it with a thin towel and set aside for approximately about 20 minutes.
- Form tiny balls out of the dough. Roll the dough balls into thin discs using a rolling pin.
- Fill the middle of these discs with the spinach filling, then fold the sides to close the dumpling.
- Steam for approximately about 5 minutes in a steamer that has been prepared. The spinach dumplings are ready to eat.

Nutritional Value: Calories 302 | Carbohydrates 15.7 g | Fat 8.9 g | Protein 18 g

Recipe 27. Super Green Salmon Salad

The combination of crisp greens and flaky salmon create the perfect blend of Omega 3 and B vitamins to encourage the best brain function possible. The B vitamins keep memory sharp, and nerves protected, while the Omega 3s allows the brain to stay fat and happy!

Serving Size: 2

Preparation Time: 10 minutes

Cooking Time: 5 minutes

Total Time: 15 minutes

Ingredients:

- 1/4 cup of honey
- 1 tablespoon of whole grain mustard
- 1 tablespoon of Dijon mustard
- 1 tablespoon of extra virgin olive oil
- 1 clove of garlic, minced
- 2 (4ounces) skinless salmon portions
- 1/2 cup of Romaine lettuce, roughly chopped
- 1/2 cup of kale, roughly chopped
- 1/2 cup of spinach
- 1/2 cup of baby arugula
- 1/2 large tomato, cut into wedges
- 1/2 large avocado, pitted and sliced into strips
- 2 tablespoons of corn kernels
- 2 tablespoons, cut into extra thin strips
- 2 strips of nitrate-free turkey bacon, cooked and minced

Directions:

- Whisk together honey, whole grand and Dijon mustard, and garlic together. Pour half into a shallow dish with the salmon portions. Marinate for approximately about two hours. Refrigerate the remaining half to use as a salad dressing.
- Lightly spray a skillet with nonstick spray and heat over medium heat. Sauté salmon until cooked through.
- In a large bowl, toss together kale, romaine, arugula, and spinach with the desired amount of dressing. Separate in the serving bowls. Top with corn, avocado, onion, tomato, bacon, and cooked chicken. Drizzle with additional dressing if desired

Nutritional Value: Calories 434 | Carbohydrates 6 g | Fat 26 g | Protein 42 g

Recipe 28. Veggie and Bacon Hash with Egg Nests

I like to prepare this brunch dish on a late Saturday morning for my husband and me. The combination of bacon, onion, sweet potatoes, and smoked paprika just can't be beaten.

Serving Size: 2

Preparation Time: 21 minutes

Cooking Time: 25 minutes

Total Time: 46 minutes

Ingredients:

- 1 avocado, sliced
- 2 bacon slices, chopped
- ½ teaspoon of smoked paprika
- ½ head of cauliflower, cut into ¼ inch dice
- ½ teaspoon of freshly ground black pepper
- ½ zucchini, cut into ½ inch cubes
- ½ white onion, chopped
- ½ red bell pepper, cut into ½ inch squares
- ⅓ cup of sweet potato, cut into ¼ inch dice
- ½ teaspoon of sea salt
- 4 large eggs

Directions:

- In a medium skillet, cook the bacon until slightly crispy. Remove from the pan and place on a plate lined with paper towels.
- Add the cauliflower, zucchini, onion, bell pepper, sweet potato, smoked paprika, salt, and black pepper. Cook for approximately about 8 to 10 minutes, occasionally stirring until the vegetables become tender and golden. Return the bacon to the pan.
- Make 4 holes in the hash and crack an egg into each hole. Cover and cook for approximately about 5 minutes, or until your desired doneness of the egg is reached.
- Divide evenly between two plates and garnish with avocado slices.

Nutritional Value: Calories 302 | Carbohydrates 15.7 g | Fat 8.9 g | Protein 18 g

Recipe 29. Watercress Salad with Grilled Asparagus

Asparagus contains a lot of potassium and thus stimulates kidney activity, which gently drains the body. The watercress and other herbs bring high-dose minerals and vitamins, especially vitamin C. In addition, secondary plant substances support the body in the fight against free radicals. The low-calorie content makes this dish a natural figure flatterer. Thanks to the blaze of colors of edible flowers, the dish is also a feast for the eyes. Edible flowers are, for example, dandelion, borage or violet flowers, pansies, daisies, and calendula.

Serving Size: 4

Preparation Time: 10 minutes

Cooking Time: 20 minutes

Total Time: 30 minutes

Ingredients:

- 800 grams of asparagus, white or green
- 4 tablespoons of oil
- 2 tablespoons of vinegar
- 2 teaspoon of forest honey
- 1 teaspoon of mustard
- 50 ml of yogurt
- 100 grams of watercress
- 100 grams of mixed fresh herbs, e.g., brown, dandelion leaves, parsley, chives, etc.
- 100 grams of lettuce
- 100 grams of cocktail tomatoes
- 1 carrot
- 1 handful of edible flowers

Directions:

- Peel the asparagus (with green asparagus, it is sufficient to peel only the lower third), cut off the woody ends. Also, cut off the tips and cut the stalks in half lengthways. Cut into bite-sized pieces.
- Mix the asparagus pieces with 2 tablespoons of oil and place them on a baking sheet lined with baking paper. Add the asparagus tips—grill under the grill of the oven for 5 minutes. If necessary, turn carefully in between.
- In the meantime, whisk together vinegar, honey, yogurt, 2 tablespoons of oil, salt, and pepper to make a salad dressing.
- Wash the herbs and lettuce and spin dry. Roughly pick up. Quarter the tomatoes and grate the carrot. Mix everything with the salad dressing. Arrange on plates, add the grilled asparagus, and decorate with edible flowers.

Nutritional Value: Calories 241 | Carbohydrates 1.1 g | Fat 17.7 g | Protein 18.8 g

Recipe 30. White Lasagna with Mushrooms

It is a meatless dish. It is the family's favorite dish. White lasagna comes from Italy. Lasagnas originated in Italy during the middle centuries. It is traditionally identified as the city of Naples. Mushrooms make the white lasagna more delicious. It is ready in 2 hours. White lasagna is a light meal. It is also a traditional dish. You can cook this recipe for lunch or dinner.

Serving Size: 4

Preparation Time: 30 minutes

Cooking Time: 2 hours

Total Time: 2 hours 30 minutes

Nutritional Value: Calories 434 | Carbohydrates 6 g | Fat 26 g | Protein 42 g

Ingredients:

- 1/4 cup of white wine
- salt and pepper, for taste
- 1 tablespoon of freshly chopped rosemary
- 1 tablespoon of newly cut oregano
- 1 tablespoon of freshly chopped thyme
- 2 tablespoons of olive oil
- 2 spicy Italian sausages, casings removed
- 2 cups of mushrooms, thinly sliced
- 4 tablespoons of butter
- 2 cups of whole milk
- pinch of cayenne pepper
- pinch of nutmeg
- ½ pound of lasagna noodles, cooked
- 1 onion, finely chopped
- 3 cloves of garlic, finely chopped
- 1/4 cup of flour
- 1/2 cup of thinly sliced mozzarella cheese
- ½ of grated Parmesan cheese

Directions:

- Take a large skillet and heat the olive oil over medium heat. Then add sausage and fry until done by crushing it into small pieces with a spatula.
- Then add mushrooms and cook until tender for four to five minutes. Cook until the liquid has entirely evaporated after deglazing the pan with wine. — season with salt, pepper, and herbs and reserve the mixture.
- Take a middle pan and thaw the butter over medium heat. Then garlic and sauté for another minute until fragrant.
- Stir in the flour and cook for approximately about a few more minutes. Slowly whisk in the milk, then whisk continuously until there are no more lumps.
- Heat béchamel until thick enough to cover the back of the spoon. Season with pepper, nutmeg, salt, and cayenne pepper. Exterminate the fire and stay aside.
- Start by layering the noodles in a separate loaf pan or small frying pan. Next, spread a layer of béchamel over the noodles and cover it with the layer of the sausage mushroom mixture.
- Do it again until the fillings and noodles are used and finish with the layer of béchamel on the top part.
- Top with shredded cheese. Bake lasagna until cheese is golden and sausage is bubbly for approximately about 20 to 30 minutes.

CONCLUSION WITH DISCLAIMER

This diet plan is, without a doubt, effective and works well in reducing weight. However, consult your physician before beginning the diet plan and ask for a calorie reduction to achieve a more well-rounded diet, as well as the addition of any dietary supplement that contains nutrients essential for the body.

A diet with 1,200 calories per day is considered a low-calorie diet plan since it provides fewer calories than your body requires daily.

Helping someone lose weight by reducing the number of calories they consume daily is one way to do it. However, people don't need to get healthier only by reducing their body weight. In other cases, having a lower weight might even make a person less healthy, mainly if they consume food that isn't good for them or doesn't get enough essential nutrients in their diet.

Also, sticking to a very low-calorie diet may be challenging, especially for those who already have trouble meeting their daily food requirements. Finally, a person needs to choose a diet and exercise routine that they will be able to maintain for the rest of their life, regardless of the weight reduction method they pick.

A dietitian or nutritionist may assist with the creation of a customized diet and nutrition plan that includes the appropriate amount of indulgent and nutrient-dense foods.

INDEX

ABOUT THE AUTHOR 5

BOOK 1 | THE 7 SECRETS OF DR. NOWZARADAN DIET PLAN ... 6

INTRODUCTION 7

CHAPTER 1. HOW TO GET STARTED 9

CHAPTER 2. THE SECRET PRINCIPLES 11

CHAPTER 3. THE 7 SECRETS OF DR NOWZARADAN'S DIET PLAN - 12

CHAPTER 4: THE DISEASES THAT ONLY THE NOWZARADAN DIET CAN CURE 14

CHAPTER 5: THE TRICKS AND TIPS TO STAY ON THE NOWZARADAN DIET PLAN 15

BOOK 2 | THE NEW DR. NOWZARADAN DIET PLAN AND COOKBOOK ENCYCLOPEDIA ON A BUDGET ... 17

INTRODUCTION 18

CHAPTER 1. ALL ABOUT THE NOWZARADAN DIET PLAN 19

CHAPTER 2. BREAKFAST RECIPES 20

RECIPE 1. BACON AND CHEESE CLOUD EGGS 20
RECIPE 2. BACON AND MUSHROOM "TACOS" 20
RECIPE 3. BROCCOLI WAFFLES 20
RECIPE 4. CANADIAN BACON EGGS BENEDICT 21
RECIPE 5. CAULIFLOWER-BASED WAFFLES 21
RECIPE 6. CHEESE WAFFLES 21
RECIPE 7. CHORIZO FRITTATA 22
RECIPE 8. CHILI OMELET WITH AVOCADO 22
RECIPE 9. COCONUT CREPES WITH VANILLA CREAM .. 22
RECIPE 10. CRABMEAT FRITTATA WITH ONION 23
RECIPE 11. CREAMY OATMEAL 23
RECIPE 12. CRESPELLE AL MASCARPONE 23
RECIPE 13. GOAT CHEESE FRITTATA WITH ASPARAGUS .. 24
RECIPE 14. HAM AND EGG CASSEROLE 24
RECIPE 15. JACKFRUIT VEGETABLE FRY 24
RECIPE 16. MEXICAN EGGS 25
RECIPE 17. MORNING HERBED EGGS 25
RECIPE 18. MUSHROOM AND CHEESE CAULIFLOWER RISOTTO .. 25
RECIPE 19. POACHED EGGS 25
RECIPE 20. ROLLED SMOKED SALMON WITH AVOCADO .. 26
RECIPE 21. SCRAMBLED EGGS WITH MUSHROOMS AND SPINACH .. 26
RECIPE 22. SERRANO HAM FRITTATA WITH SALAD 26
RECIPE 23. SESAME AND POPPY SEED BAGELS 27
RECIPE 24. SNAZZY BAKED EGGS 27
RECIPE 25. SOFT BANANA BREAD 27
RECIPE 26. SPINACH NESTS WITH EGGS AND CHEESE .. 28
RECIPE 27. SWEET CHIA BOWLS 28
RECIPE 28. TUNA AND EGG SALAD WITH CHILI MAYO .. 28
RECIPE 29. TURKEY BACON AND SPINACH CREPES 29
RECIPE 30. WESTERN OMELET QUICHE 29
RECIPE 31. ZUCCHINI AND PEPPER CAPRESE GRATIN .. 29
RECIPE 32. ALMOND AND MAPLE QUICK GRITS 30
RECIPE 33. BACON STUFFED MUSHROOMS 30
RECIPE 34. BACON-WRAPPED CHICKEN WINGS 30
RECIPE 35. BAKED ASPARAGUS WITH CHEESY SAUCE .. 31
RECIPE 36. BAKED BEANS 31
RECIPE 37. BAKED CHICKEN THIGHS 31
RECIPE 38. BARLEY PORRIDGE 32
RECIPE 39. BITE-SIZED BAKED CHICKEN 32
RECIPE 40. BREAKFAST QUINOA 32
RECIPE 41. BREAKFAST SAUSAGE PINEAPPLE SKEWERS .. 33
RECIPE 42. BUTTERED CARROT-ZUCCHINI WITH MAYO .. 33
RECIPE 43. CAULIFLOWER FRIED RICE WITH BACON .. 33
RECIPE 44. CHEESY SICILLIAN TORTELLINI 34
RECIPE 45. CHEESE WRAPS 34
RECIPE 46. ALFREDO 34
RECIPE 47. CHICKPEA FRITTERS 34
RECIPE 48. GLAZED CARROTS 35
RECIPE 49. CORN MEAL MUSH WITH POLISH SAUSAGE .. 35
RECIPE 50. CHICKPEAS BOWLS 35
RECIPE 51. FRIED CODFISH 36
RECIPE 52. GARLIC AND TOMATO BRUSCHETTA 36
RECIPE 53. GARLIC STEAMERS 36
RECIPE 54. GARLIC MASHED POTATOES 37
RECIPE 55. GAZPACHO WITH MELON AND HAM 37
RECIPE 56. GNOCCHI IN CREAM SAUCE 37
RECIPE 57. GROUPER WITH WINE SAUCE 38
RECIPE 58. HAM AND SUN-DRIED TOMATO ALFREDO .. 38
RECIPE 59. HONEY ALMOND RICOTTA SPREAD WITH PEACHES .. 38
RECIPE 60. LEMON PARSLEY SWORDFISH 38
RECIPE 61. MUSSELS WITH HERBED VINAIGRETTE 39
RECIPE 62. PEPPY CASSEROLE 39
RECIPE 63. PESTO FISH FILLET 39
RECIPE 64. PITA WITH GREENS, FRIED ONIONS, AND BACON .. 40
RECIPE 65. PORK ONIONS 40
RECIPE 66. ROSEMARY BAKED CHICKEN DRUMSTICKS .. 40
RECIPE 67. SHREDDED BEEF 41
RECIPE 68. SMOKEY SPANISH GARLIC SHRIMP 41
RECIPE 69. STEAMED BALSAMIC ARTICHOKES 41
RECIPE 70. STEWED MUSSELS AND CLAMS W/ TOMATOES & OLIVES .. 42
RECIPE 71. TAHINI PINE NUTS TOAST 42
RECIPE 72. TOASTED BAGUETTE WITH TOMATOES AND ANCHOVIES .. 42
RECIPE 73. TOMATO-BASIL POACHED COD 43
RECIPE 74. TORTELLINI IN CHICKEN BROTH 43
RECIPE 75. TUNA WITH LEMON BUTTER SAUCE 43
RECIPE 76. VANILLA-CREAM MORNING OATMEAL 44
RECIPE 77. FRUIT AND NUTS 44
RECIPE 78. PUMPKIN AND CINNAMON CREAM 44
RECIPE 79. TOMATO AND PROSCIUTTO SANDWICHES .. 45
RECIPE 80. VEGETARIAN SPANISH TOAST WITH ESCALIVADA .. 45

CHAPTER 3. LUNCH RECIPES 46

RECIPE 81. ASPARAGUS AND BEEF SHIRATAKI 46
RECIPE 82. BAKED CHICKEN 46
RECIPE 83. BAKED CHICKEN NUGGETS 46
RECIPE 84. BARBECUED PORK CHOPS 47
RECIPE 85. BBQ BEEF SLIDERS 47
RECIPE 86. BBQ PULLED CHICKEN 47

Recipe	Page
RECIPE 87. BEEF AND CHEESE AVOCADO BOATS	48
RECIPE 88. BEEF, BELL PEPPER AND MUSHROOM KEBABS	48
RECIPE 89. BEEF BURGERS WITH LETTUCE AND AVOCADO	48
RECIPE 90. BEEF CHEESE AND EGG CASSEROLE	49
RECIPE 91. BEEF PATTIES TOPPED WITH BROCCOLI MASH	49
RECIPE 92. BEEF SAUSAGE AND OKRA CASSEROLE	50
RECIPE 93. BRAISED CHICKEN WITH TOMATO AND GARLIC	50
RECIPE 94. BROCCOLI AND CARROT TURKEY BAKE	50
RECIPE 95. BUFFALO CHICKEN SALAD WRAP	51
RECIPE 96. BURGUNDY BEEF WITH MUSHROOMS	51
RECIPE 97. CABBAGE AND BROCCOLI CHICKEN CASSEROLE	51
RECIPE 98. CAULIFLOWER AND BEEF CASSEROLE	52
RECIPE 99. CHICKEN AND BRUSSELS SPROUT BAKE	52
RECIPE 100. CHICKEN CURRY	53
RECIPE 101. CHICKEN WITH NOODLES	53
RECIPE 102. CILANTRO BEEF BALLS STUFFED WITH MASCARPONE	53
RECIPE 103. COCONUT-OLIVE BEEF WITH MUSHROOMS	54
RECIPE 104. COUNTRY SPARE RIBS WITH WHITE BEANS	54
RECIPE 105. CREAMY CHICKEN WITH CARAMELIZED LEEKS	55
RECIPE 106. EGGPLANT BEEF LASAGNA	55
RECIPE 107. FETA AND KALE CHICKEN BAKE	55
RECIPE 108. GREEN BEAN AND BROCCOLI CHICKEN STIR FRY	56
RECIPE 109. GRILLED BEEF STEAKS AND VEGETABLE MEDLEY	56
RECIPE 110. GROUND PORK STUFFED MUSHROOMS	57
RECIPE 111. HAM AND CHEESE STUFFED CHICKEN	57
RECIPE 112. HERBY VEGGIES AND CHICKEN CASSEROLE	57
RECIPE 113. HONEY SPICED CAJUN CHICKEN	58
RECIPE 114. JUICY BEEF MEATBALLS	58
RECIPE 115. JUICY CHICKEN WITH BROCCOLI AND PINE NUTS	58
RECIPE 116. LEMONGRASS PRAWNS	59
RECIPE 117. MARINATED FRIED CHICKEN	59
RECIPE 118. OAXACAN CHICKEN	60
RECIPE 119. OLIVE CAPERS CHICKEN	60
RECIPE 120. OREGANO CHICKEN THIGHS	60
RECIPE 121. PAN-FRIED CHICKEN WITH ANCHOVY TAPENADE	61
RECIPE 122. PANCETTA AND CHEESE STUFFED CHICKEN	61
RECIPE 123. PARMESAN CHICKEN MEATBALLS	61
RECIPE 124. PEANUT-CRUSTED CHICKEN	62
RECIPE 125. PESTO CHICKEN CACCIATORE	62
RECIPE 126. PIMIENTO CHEESE PORK MEATBALLS	62
RECIPE 127. PORK CHOPS WITH NUTMEG	63
RECIPE 128. PORK WITH APPLE SAUCE	63
RECIPE 129. PORK WITH SCALLIONS AND PEANUTS	63
RECIPE 130. PROSCIUTTO BROCCOLI CHICKEN STEW	64
RECIPE 131. RISOTTO W/ GREEN BEANS, SWEET POTATOES, & PEAS	64
RECIPE 132. ROASTED PORK STUFFED WITH HAM AND CHEESE	64
RECIPE 133. ROSEMARY BUTTERED PORK CHOPS	65
RECIPE 134. SAFFRON SHRIMP	65
RECIPE 135. SALMON CASSEROLE	65
RECIPE 136. SALMON MEATBALLS WITH GARLIC	66
RECIPE 137. SALMON WITH MUSHROOM	66
RECIPE 138. SALSA CHICKEN	66
RECIPE 139. SEARED SCALLOPS WITH APRICOT ORZO SALAD	67
RECIPE 140. SHRIMP AND ORZO	67
RECIPE 141. SHRIMP QUESADILLAS	67
RECIPE 142. SPINACH CHICKEN	68
RECIPE 143. STEWED PORK WITH CAULIFLOWER AND BROCCOLI	68
RECIPE 144. STIR FRY GROUND PORK	68
RECIPE 145. TACO CASSEROLE	69
RECIPE 146. TAMARI CHICKEN THIGHS AND CAPERS	69
RECIPE 147. TERIYAKI CHICKEN WINGS	70
RECIPE 148. THYME CHICKEN WITH MUSHROOMS AND TURNIP	70
RECIPE 149. TILAPIA BROCCOLI PLATTER	70
RECIPE 150. TURKEY AND VEGETABLE CASSEROLE	71
RECIPE 151. TURKEY BACON-WRAPPED BEEF TENDERLOIN	71
RECIPE 152. TURNIP AND PORK PACKETS WITH GRILLED HALLOUMI	71
RECIPE 153. ZUCCHINI AND BELL PEPPER CHICKEN GRATIN	72
RECIPE 154. ZUCCHINI BEEF LASAGNA	72
RECIPE 155. CABBAGE ROLL CASSEROLE WITH VEAL	73
RECIPE 156. CHICKEN STIR-FRY	73
RECIPE 157. CHICKEN WITH ZUCCHINI NOODLES	73
RECIPE 158. FALAFEL SALAD WITH LEMON-TAHINI DRESSING	74
RECIPE 159. GLAZED RIBS	74
RECIPE 160. KALE AND GROUND BEEF CASSEROLE	74
RECIPE 161. LEMON GARLIC THIGHS WITH ASPARAGUS	75
RECIPE 162. PORK AND PEPPERS CHILI	75
RECIPE 163. PORK CHOPS AND TOMATO SAUCE	76
RECIPE 164. ROSEMARY BAKED CHICKEN DRUMSTICKS	76
RECIPE 165. SHRIMP LUNCH ROLLS	76

CHAPTER 4. DINNER RECIPES — 77

Recipe	Page
RECIPE 166. ALMOND-CRUSTED ZUCCHINI CHICKEN STACKS	77
RECIPE 167. ARTICHOKE AND SPINACH CHICKEN	77
RECIPE 168. ASPARAGUS AND LEMON SALMON	77
RECIPE 169. BACON AND PARSNIP CHICKEN BAKE	78
RECIPE 170. BACON TOPPED TURKEY MEATLOAF	78
RECIPE 171. BAKED CHEESY CHICKEN TENDERS	78
RECIPE 172. BAKED CHICKEN LEGS WITH TOMATO SAUCE	79
RECIPE 173. BAKED CHICKEN WRAPPED IN SMOKED SALMON	79
RECIPE 174. BAKED ZUCCHINI WITH CHEESE AND CHICKEN	79
RECIPE 175. BALSAMIC CHILI ROAST	80
RECIPE 176. BEEF AND BELL PEPPER FRITTATA	80
RECIPE 177. BEEF AND MUSHROOM MEATLOAF	81
RECIPE 178. BROWN BASMATI RICE PILAF	81
RECIPE 179. CABBAGE AND BEEF STEAKS	81
RECIPE 180. CHICKEN AND CHEESE STUFFED PEPPERS	82
RECIPE 181. CHICKEN AND CHORIZO TRAYBAKE	82
RECIPE 182. CHICKEN AND SAUSAGE GUMBO	83
RECIPE 183. CHICKEN CACCIATORE	83
RECIPE 184. CHICKEN RELLENO CASSEROLE	83
RECIPE 185. CHICKEN TIKKA	84
RECIPE 186. CHICKEN, TOMATO AND GREEN BEANS	84
RECIPE 187. CHICKEN WITH GARLIC AND FENNEL	84
RECIPE 188. CHICKEN WITH POTATOES OLIVES AND SPROUTS	85
RECIPE 189. CITRUS PORK	85
RECIPE 190. COCONUT CHICKEN AND MUSHROOMS	85
RECIPE 191. COCONUT FRIED SHRIMP WITH CILANTRO SAUCE	86
RECIPE 192. COD SALAD WITH MUSTARD	86
RECIPE 193. CREAMY CHICKEN FRIED RICE	87
RECIPE 194. CUMIN PORK AND BEANS	87
RECIPE 195. FETA AND MOZARELLA CHICKEN	87
RECIPE 196. GINGERED GRILLED CHICKEN	88
RECIPE 197. GRILLED BEEF ON SKEWERS WITH FRESH SALAD	88
RECIPE 198. GRILLED CHICKEN	88

RECIPE 199. GRILLED PORK SKEWERS WITH CHILI DIPPING SAUCE 89
RECIPE 200. GRILLED STEAK WITH GREEN BEANS 89
RECIPE 201. GRILLED SWORDFISH WITH LEMON, CAPERS, & OLIVES 89
RECIPE 202. HAWAIIAN CHICKEN 90
RECIPE 203. KABOBS WITH PEANUT CURRY SAUCE 90
RECIPE 204. LEMON AND GARLIC SCALLOPS 90
RECIPE 205. LEMON-PARSLEY CHICKEN BREAST 91
RECIPE 206. MACKEREL AND ORANGE MEDLEY 91
RECIPE 207. MEATBALLS AND SAUCE 91
RECIPE 208. MUSHROOM AND BEEF STIR-FRY 92
RECIPE 209. MUSSELS CURRY WITH LIME 92
RECIPE 210. MUSTARD CHICKEN WITH ROSEMARY 93
RECIPE 211. NUTMEG SALMON AND MUSHROOMS 93
RECIPE 212. OKRA AND SAUSAGE HOT POT 93
RECIPE 213. OVEN-BAKED SALAMI AND CHEDDAR CHICKEN 94
RECIPE 214. PAELLA WITH CHICKEN, LEEKS, AND TARRAGON 94
RECIPE 215. PAN-SEARED SQUIDS AND SAUSAGE 94
RECIPE 216. PANCETTA, BEEF AND BROCCOLI BAKE 95
RECIPE 217. PAPRIKA PORK AND SCALLIONS 95
RECIPE 218. PARMESAN BEEF STUFFED MUSHROOMS 95
RECIPE 219. PEACH-MUSTARD PORK SHOULDER 96
RECIPE 220. PESTO CHICKEN BREASTS WITH SUMMER SQUASH 96
RECIPE 221. PINEAPPLE GLAZED CHICKEN 96
RECIPE 222. PIZZAIOLA STEAKS 97
RECIPE 223. PORK AND SALSA 97
RECIPE 224. PORK AND ZUCCHINI STEW 98
RECIPE 225. PORK CHOPS WITH GREEN BEANS AND AVOCADO 98
RECIPE 226. PORK MEATBALLS 98
RECIPE 227. PORK ROAST WITH CRANBERRY 99
RECIPE 228. PORK SAUSAGE SAUERKRAUT 99
RECIPE 229. PORK STEW WITH SHALLOTS 99
RECIPE 230. PORK WITH DATES SAUCE 100
RECIPE 231. PORK WITH MUSHROOMS BOWLS 100
RECIPE 232. PUMPKIN AND BLACK BEANS CHICKEN 100
RECIPE 233. RED WINE BEEF ROAST AND VEGETABLES 101
RECIPE 234. ROASTED CHICKEN 101
RECIPE 235. ROASTED CHICKEN THIGHS 101
RECIPE 236. ROASTED LEMON SWORDFISH 102
RECIPE 237. ROSEMARY CHICKEN WITH AVOCADO SAUCE 102
RECIPE 238. ROSEMARY PORK MEDALLIONS 103
RECIPE 239. SALMON AND BRUSSELS SPROUTS 103
RECIPE 240. SAUCY CHICKEN LEGS WITH VEGETABLES 103
RECIPE 241. SCALLION AND EGG BEEF BOWLS 104
RECIPE 242. SCALLOPS AND ROSEMARY POTATOES 104
RECIPE 243. SESAME PORK BITES 105
RECIPE 244. SHRIMP WITH CILANTRO SAUCE 105
RECIPE 245. SMOKED SAUSAGE CASSEROLE 105
RECIPE 246. SPICED WINTER PORK ROAST 106
RECIPE 247. SRIRACHA TUNA KABOBS 106
RECIPE 248. STUFFED CHICKEN BREASTS 106
RECIPE 249. SWEET PORK CHOPS WITH SPAGHETTI SQUASH 107
RECIPE 250. TANDOORI CHICKEN 107
RECIPE 251. THYME BEEF AND BACON CASSEROLE 108
RECIPE 252. TURMERIC CHICKEN WINGS WITH GINGER SAUCE 108
RECIPE 253. TURNIP GREENS AND ARTICHOKE CHICKEN 108
RECIPE 254. VEGETABLE BAKE AND SAUSAGE 109
RECIPE 255. WINTER CHICKEN AND VEGETABLES 109

CHAPTER 5. SIDES & SOUPS RECIPES ----------------------------------- 110
RECIPE 256. BABY SPINACH SALAD 110
RECIPE 257. BACON AND GORGONZOLA SALAD 110
RECIPE 258. BAKED POTATO WITH THYME 110
RECIPE 259. BEAN AND BARLEY SOUP 111
RECIPE 260. BEAN SOUP 111
RECIPE 261. BELL PEPPERS CAKES 111
RECIPE 262. BLACK BEAN SOUP 112
RECIPE 263. BUTTERNUT SQUASH SOUP 112
RECIPE 264. CAPRESE SALAD STACKS ANCHOVIES 112
RECIPE 265. CAULIFLOWER BUTTERNUT SOUP 113
RECIPE 266. CAULIFLOWER CHEESE SOUP 113
RECIPE 267. CAULIFLOWER SOUP WITH CRISPY BACON 113
RECIPE 268. CAULIFLOWER-WATERCRESS SALAD 114
RECIPE 269. CHEDDAR AND TURKEY MEATBALL SALAD 114
RECIPE 270. CHEESY BEEF SALAD 115
RECIPE 271. CHEESY CHICKEN SOUP WITH SPINACH 115
RECIPE 272. CHICKEN, AVOCADO AND EGG BOWLS 115
RECIPE 273. CHICKEN SALAD WITH PARMESAN 116
RECIPE 274. CHICKPEA AND KALE SOUP 116
RECIPE 275. CHORIZO AND TOMATO SALAD WITH OLIVES 116
RECIPE 276. CLAM CHOWDER 117
RECIPE 277. CORIANDER SEEDS CABBAGE 117
RECIPE 278. CREAM SOUP WITH AVOCADO AND ZUCCHINI 117
RECIPE 279. CREAMY WHITE CHICKEN CHILI 118
RECIPE 280. CRISPY GARLIC BAKED POTATO WEDGES 118
RECIPE 281. CUMIN BLACK BEANS AND PEPPERS 118
RECIPE 282. CURRY EGGPLANT 119
RECIPE 283. FIERY SHRIMP COCKTAIL SALAD 119
RECIPE 284. GREEN LENTIL AND OLIVE SALAD 119
RECIPE 285. GREEN SALAD WITH FETA AND BLUEBERRIES 120
RECIPE 286. GRILLED AVOCADO CAPRESE CROSTINI 120
RECIPE 287. KALE-POPPY SEED SALAD 120
RECIPE 288. LETTUCE, BEET AND TOFU SALAD 121
RECIPE 289. MINESTRONE SOUP 121
RECIPE 290. MOROCCAN SWEET POTATO SOUP 121
RECIPE 291. MUSHROOM CREAM SOUP WITH HERBS 122
RECIPE 292. MUSHROOM SAUSAGES 122
RECIPE 293. PARMESAN ARTICHOKES 123
RECIPE 294. PARSLEY RED POTATOES 123
RECIPE 295. PEACH AND CARROTS 123
RECIPE 296. PLANTAIN AND CORN SOUP 123
RECIPE 297. POTATO SOUP 124
RECIPE 298. QUINOA AND SCALLOPS SALAD 124
RECIPE 299. REFRIED BEANS W/ BAKED TORTILLA OR PITA CHIPS 125
RECIPE 300. ROASTED CORN SALAD 125
RECIPE 301. ROASTED GARLIC SOUP 125
RECIPE 302. ROASTED VEGETABLES 126
RECIPE 303. ROSEMARY CARROTS 126
RECIPE 304. SAUSAGE AND PESTO SALAD WITH CHEESE 126
RECIPE 305. SMOKED MACKEREL LETTUCE CUPS 127
RECIPE 306. SMOKED SALMON, BACON AND EGG SALAD 127
RECIPE 307. SPICY BRUSSELS SPROUTS 127
RECIPE 308. SPINACH AND BRUSSELS SPROUT SALAD 128
RECIPE 309. SPINACH AND LENTIL SOUP 128
RECIPE 310. SPINACH SALAD WITH GOAT CHEESE AND NUTS 129
RECIPE 311. SPINACH SALAD WITH PANCETTA AND MUSTARD 129

RECIPE 312. SPLIT PEA CREAM SOUP 129
RECIPE 313. SWEET BUTTERNUT 130
RECIPE 314. SWEET CORN SOUP 130
RECIPE 315. TAHINI BEANS 130
RECIPE 316. THYME SWEET POTATOES 131
RECIPE 317. TOASTED ORZO PASTA 131
RECIPE 318. TUNA BITES 131
RECIPE 319. TURKEY BACON AND TURNIP SALAD 132
RECIPE 320. TURKEY GINGER SOUP 132
RECIPE 321. VEGETABLE BEEF STEW 132
RECIPE 322. VEGETARIAN CHILI MAC 133
RECIPE 323. VEGGIE FRITTERS 133
RECIPE 324. WONTON SOUP 133
RECIPE 325. ZUCCHINI AND LEEK TURKEY SOUP 134

CHAPTER 6. SNACKS RECIPES ------------------------------- 135

RECIPE 326. APPLE CRISP 135
RECIPE 327. AVOCADO TUNA BITES 135
RECIPE 328. BAKED EGGPLANT CHIPS WITH SALAD AND AIOLI 135
RECIPE 329. BAKED SCOTCH EGGS 136
RECIPE 330. CASHEW AND CARROT MUFFINS 136
RECIPE 331. CHEESE AND NUT ZUCCHINI BOATS 136
RECIPE 332. CHEESE CHIPS 137
RECIPE 333. CHEESY MASHED SWEET POTATO CAKES 137
RECIPE 334. CHERRY CLAFOUTI 138
RECIPE 335. CINNAMON PEACH COBBLER 138
RECIPE 336. FAT-FREE FRIES 138
RECIPE 337. GINGER AND PUMPKIN PIE 139
RECIPE 338. GINGER SNAPS 139
RECIPE 339. GOAT CHEESE AND RUTABAGA PUFFS 139
RECIPE 340. GRILLED FRUIT 140
RECIPE 341. HALLOUMI AND CHEDDAR STICKS 140
RECIPE 342. HOISIN MEATBALLS 140
RECIPE 343. HONEY GRANOLA 141
RECIPE 344. HOT MARINATED SHRIMP 141
RECIPE 345. JALAPENO VEGETABLE FRITTATA CUPS 141
RECIPE 346. LEAFY GREENS AND CHEDDAR QUESADILLAS .. 142
RECIPE 347. LEMON ZEST PUDDING 142
RECIPE 348. LENTIL SWEET BARS 142
RECIPE 349. MINI TERIYAKI TURKEY SANDWICHES 143
RECIPE 350. PESTO VEGGIE PINWHEELS 143
RECIPE 351. PLUM CAKE 143
RECIPE 352. PORK BEEF BEAN NACHOS 144
RECIPE 353. PUMPKIN PIE 144
RECIPE 354. RASPBERRY AND GOAT CHEESE FOCACCIA BITES 145
RECIPE 355. ROSEMARY FETA CHEESE BOMBS 145
RECIPE 356. SALMON APPLE SALAD SANDWICH 145
RECIPE 357. SALMON SPINACH AND COTTAGE CHEESE SANDWICH 146
RECIPE 358. SHRIMPS CEVICHE 146
RECIPE 359. SPINACH CHIPS WITH AVOCADO HUMMUS 147
RECIPE 360. VEGAN RICE PUDDING 147
RECIPE 361. AVOCADO CAPRESE WRAP 147
RECIPE 362. BRUSSELS SPROUTS WITH PISTACHIOS 148
RECIPE 363. CARAMELIZED ONIONS 148
RECIPE 364. CREAMY PANINI 148
RECIPE 365. ZINGY ZUCCHINI BITES 148

CHAPTER 7. 93+1 MEAL PLANS -------------------------------- 150

CONCLUSION -- 159

BOOK 3 | THE NEW DR. NOWZARADAN DIET PLAN AND COOKBOOK FOR BEGINNERS 160

INTRODUCTION --- 161

CHAPTER 1. THE 1200-CALORIE DIET -------------------------- 162

CHAPTER 2. FOLLOWING THE 1200-CALORIE DIET ---------- 163

CHAPTER 3. CAN IT HELP YOU LOSE WEIGHT? --------------- 165

CHAPTER 4. BREAKFAST RECIPES ---------------------------- 166

RECIPE 1. BAKED BEANS 166
RECIPE 2. BEEF AND SPINACH STROGANOFF 166
RECIPE 3. BAKED MAC AND CHEESE 166
RECIPE 4. EGGPLANT LASAGNA 167
RECIPE 5. GROUND PORK WONTON RAVIOLI 167
RECIPE 6. HERB-ROASTED EGGPLANT 168
RECIPE 7. POTATO PANCAKES 168
RECIPE 8. SEARED TUNA WITH WHITE BEAN SALAD 169
RECIPE 9. STEWED MUSSELS AND CLAMS W/ TOMATOES & OLIVES 169
RECIPE 10. TOMATO-BASIL POACHED COD 169

CHAPTER 5. LUNCH RECIPES -------------------------------- 171

RECIPE 11. ASIAN FLANK STEAK WITH EDAMAME AND SOBA 171
RECIPE 12. BAKED VEGETABLES 171
RECIPE 13. BUFFALO WINGS 171
RECIPE 14. CURRIED CHICKEN MEATBALLS WITH RICE 172
RECIPE 15. GREEN BEAN CASSEROLE 172
RECIPE 16. NUT-CRUSTED CHICKEN BREASTS 172
RECIPE 17. ROAST PORK LOIN WITH ROSEMARY AND GARLIC 173
RECIPE 18. ROSEMARY BRAISED CHICKEN W/ MUSHROOM SAUCE 173
RECIPE 19. STEAK FAJITAS 174
RECIPE 20. TUNA NOODLE CASSEROLE 174

CHAPTER 6. DINNER RECIPES ------------------------------- 176

RECIPE 21. AFRICAN CHICKEN AND RICE 176
RECIPE 22. CHICKEN AND VEGGIE UNFRIED RICE 176
RECIPE 23. PASTA WITH ALFREDO SAUCE 176
RECIPE 24. PORK SHOULDER ROAST 177
RECIPE 25. PORK TENDERLOIN WITH CHERRY SAUCE 177

CHAPTER 7. SOUP RECIPES --------------------------------- 178

RECIPE 26. CHEESY CAULIFLOWER SOUP 178
RECIPE 27. CHICKEN AND BEAN SOUP 178
RECIPE 28. CHICKEN BARLEY SOUP 178
RECIPE 29. CHICKEN NOODLE SOUP 179
RECIPE 30. CREAM OF BROCCOLI SOUP 179
RECIPE 31. CREAM OF POTATO SOUP 180
RECIPE 32. CREAMY CHICKEN VEGETABLE SOUP 180
RECIPE 33. FRENCH ONION SOUP 180
RECIPE 34. HAM AND BEAN SOUP 181

CHAPTER 8. SNACKS RECIPES ------------------------------ 182

RECIPE 35. CREAMED PEAS 182
RECIPE 36. CREAMED SPINACH 182
RECIPE 37. EGG SALAD SANDWICH 182

RECIPE 38. GELATIN WITH PEACHES AND COTTAGE CHEESE 183
RECIPE 39. HAM SALAD SANDWICH 183
RECIPE 40. HOT SHREDDED CHICKEN SANDWICH 183
RECIPE 41. MARINATED TOMATO SLICES 184
RECIPE 42. POTATO SALAD 184
RECIPE 43. SOFT CAULIFLOWER SALAD 184
RECIPE 44. TURKEY BACON BRUSSELS SPROUTS 185

CHAPTER 9. MEAL PLANS 186

CONCLUSION 187

BOOK 4 | HIGH PROTEIN LOW CARB DR. NOW RECIPES   188

CHAPTER 1. RECIPES 189

RECIPE 1. ASPARAGUS CASSEROLE 189
RECIPE 2. BACON AND PARSNIP CHICKEN BAKE 189
RECIPE 3. BAKED MAC AND CHEESE 189
RECIPE 4. BERRIES AND GRILLED CALAMARI 190
RECIPE 5. BROWN RICE PILAF WITH BUTTERNUT SQUASH 190
RECIPE 6. CABBAGE AND BEEF STEAKS 191
RECIPE 7. CHEESY BAKED BEANS 191
RECIPE 8. CHICKEN MOMOS 191
RECIPE 9. CILANTRO-LIME SHRIMP AND PEPPERS 192
RECIPE 10. COCONUT AND LEMONGRASS TURKEY SOUP 192
RECIPE 11. CREAMED PEAS 193
RECIPE 12. CRISPY POLLOCK AND GAZPACHO 193
RECIPE 13. GINGER SESAME PORK SOUP 194
RECIPE 14. GINGERED HONEY SALMON 194
RECIPE 15. GLAZED MISO COD WITH BABY BOK CHOY 194
RECIPE 16. HAM AND BEAN SOUP 195
RECIPE 17. HERBED CHICKEN PAPRIKASH 195
RECIPE 18. JACKFRUIT VEGETABLE FRY 196
RECIPE 19. LAMB CHOPS WITH LEMON AND MINT ASPARAGUS 196
RECIPE 20. LOADED SHRIMP PASTA 197
RECIPE 21. LOBSTER CASSEROLE 197
RECIPE 22. MUSTARD MAPLE CHICKEN WITH POTATO WEDGES 197
RECIPE 23. PAN-SEARED BUTTER SCALLOPS 198
RECIPE 24. PISTACHIO-CRUSTED SCALLOPS 198
RECIPE 25. ROSEMARY BRAISED CHICKEN W/ MUSHROOM SAUCE 199
RECIPE 26. ROSEMARY PORK ROAST 199
RECIPE 27. SALMON-KALE SUMMER ROLLS 199
RECIPE 28. SEAFOOD PAELLA 200
RECIPE 29. SPANISH RICE CASSEROLE WITH CHEESY BEEF 201
RECIPE 30. SPICY CARROT AND LIME SOUP 201
RECIPE 31. SPINACH AND BRUSSELS SPROUT SALAD 201
RECIPE 32. STOUT-STEAMED SHELLFISH WITH CHARRED ONIONS 202
RECIPE 33. STRIP STEAK WITH CREAMY PEPPERCORN SAUCE 202
RECIPE 34. TURKEY AND QUINOA STUFFED PEPPERS 203
RECIPE 35. VIOGNIER STEAMED CLAMS WITH PARSNIPS & BACON 203
RECIPE 36. WHITE CABBAGE AND LENTILS WITH RELISH 204
RECIPE 37. ZUCCHINI AND PEPPER CAPRESE GRATIN 204

CONCLUSION 206

BOOK 5 | AND A HUGE BONUS FOR YOU... LOW-CALORIE KETO DIET COOKBOOK   207

CHAPTER 1. ALL ABOUT KETO EXPLAINED 208

CHAPTER 2: FUNDAMENTALS OF THE KETOGENIC DIET 210

CHAPTER 3: RECIPES 213

RECIPE 1. ALMOND HALIBUT AND VEGETABLE CURRY 213
RECIPE 2. BEEF AND BELL PEPPER FRITTATA 213
RECIPE 3. BELL PEPPER CREAM PAN WITH PUMPKIN 214
RECIPE 4. BUTTERNUT SQUASH SOUP 214
RECIPE 5. CARROT CAKE QUINOA 215
RECIPE 6. CHEESE SOUP WITH MUSHROOMS 215
RECIPE 7. CHEESY MASHED SWEET POTATO CAKES 216
RECIPE 8. CHICKEN CASSEROLE 216
RECIPE 9. CHICKEN SOUVLAKI 217
RECIPE 10. CREAM OF MUSHROOM SOUP 217
RECIPE 11. EGGPLANT LASAGNA 217
RECIPE 12. EIGHT LAYER CASSEROLE 218
RECIPE 13. GRILLED CHICKEN WINGS 218
RECIPE 14. KETO PIZZA CASSEROLE 219
RECIPE 15. MIXED SEAFOOD LASAGNA 219
RECIPE 16. PENNE AND SAUSAGE CASSEROLES 220
RECIPE 17. PEPPER AND EGG CURRY 220
RECIPE 18. PEPPERCORN CRUSTED FILET MIGNON 221
RECIPE 19. PESTO VEGGIE PINWHEELS 221
RECIPE 20. PROSCIUTTO VEGETABLE EGG CUPS 221
RECIPE 21. RIGATONI AND SPICY SAUSAGE CASSEROLE 222
RECIPE 22. SCALLOP, BACON, AND PEA PASTA 223
RECIPE 23. SCALLOPED CREAMY OYSTERS 223
RECIPE 24. SEA SCALLOPS WITH PESTO-WHITE WINE SAUCE 224
RECIPE 25. SERRANO HAM FRITTATA WITH SALAD 224
RECIPE 26. SPINACH DUMPLINGS 224
RECIPE 27. SUPER GREEN SALMON SALAD 225
RECIPE 28. VEGGIE AND BACON HASH WITH EGG NESTS 225
RECIPE 29. WATERCRESS SALAD WITH GRILLED ASPARAGUS 226
RECIPE 30. WHITE LASAGNA WITH MUSHROOMS 226

CONCLUSION WITH DISCLAIMER 228

Made in United States
North Haven, CT
16 March 2023